Icelandic Herbs and
Their Medicinal Uses

Icelandic Herbs

and Their Medicinal Uses

ANNA RÓSA RÓBERTSDÓTTIR

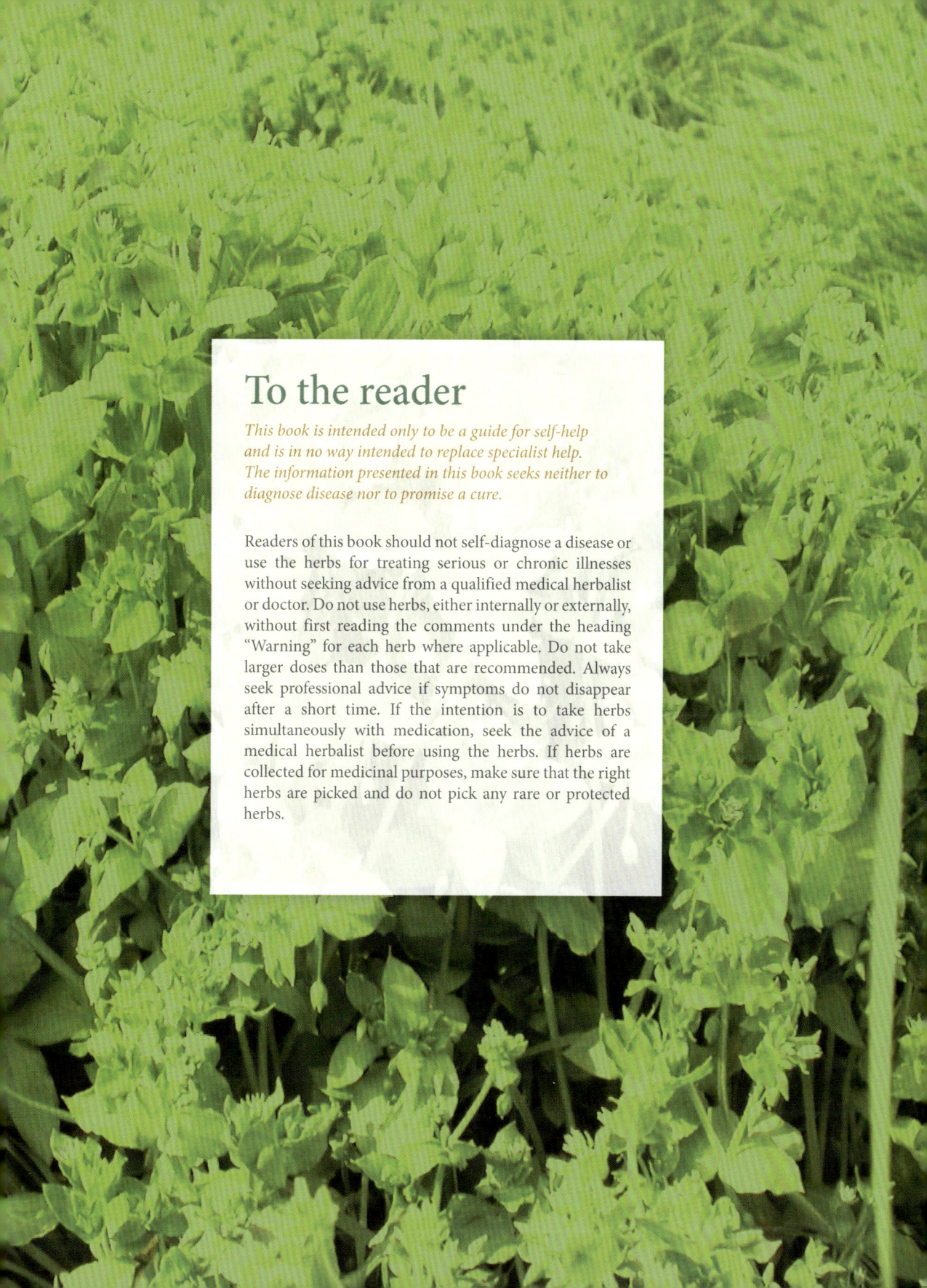

To the reader

This book is intended only to be a guide for self-help and is in no way intended to replace specialist help. The information presented in this book seeks neither to diagnose disease nor to promise a cure.

Readers of this book should not self-diagnose a disease or use the herbs for treating serious or chronic illnesses without seeking advice from a qualified medical herbalist or doctor. Do not use herbs, either internally or externally, without first reading the comments under the heading "Warning" for each herb where applicable. Do not take larger doses than those that are recommended. Always seek professional advice if symptoms do not disappear after a short time. If the intention is to take herbs simultaneously with medication, seek the advice of a medical herbalist before using the herbs. If herbs are collected for medicinal purposes, make sure that the right herbs are picked and do not pick any rare or protected herbs.

Translated from the Icelandic by Shelagh Smith

All photos © Erling Ólafsson, except page 37 © Hrafn Óskarsson, pages 133, 134, and 135 © Hörður Kristinsson, pages 3 and 163 © Shutterstock.

Published by
North Atlantic Books
Berkeley, California

Cover photo by Erling Ólafsson
Cover design by Jasmine Hromjak
Book design by Harri

Printed in the United States of America

Icelandic Herbs and Their Medicinal Uses is sponsored and published by the Society for the Study of Native Arts and Sciences (dba North Atlantic Books), an educational nonprofit based in Berkeley, California, that collaborates with partners to develop cross-cultural perspectives, nurture holistic views of art, science, the humanities, and healing, and seed personal and global transformation by publishing work on the relationship of body, spirit, and nature.

North Atlantic Books' publications are available through most bookstores. For further information, visit our website at www.northatlanticbooks.com or call 800-733-3000.

Library of Congress Cataloging-in-Publication Data

Anna Rósa Róbertsdóttir, author.
  [Anna Rósa grasalæknir og íslenskar lækningajurtir. English]
  Icelandic herbs and their medicinal uses / Anna Rósa Róbertsdóttir.
      p. ; cm.
  Translation of Anna Rósa grasalæknir og íslenskar lækningajurtir: notkun þeirra, tínsla og rannsóknir. Reykjavík : Anna Rósa grasalæknir ehf, 2011.
  Includes bibliographical references and index.
  Summary: "A comprehensive guide on Icelandic medicinal herbs, including uses, preparations—such as infusions, decoctions, tinctures, and syrups—harvesting, and drying."—Provided by publisher.
  ISBN 978-1-62317-022-6 (paperback) — ISBN 978-1-62317-023-3 (ebook)
  I. Title.
  [DNLM: 1. Plants, Medicinal—Iceland. 2. Phytotherapy—Iceland. QV 770 GI3]
  RS177.I2
  615.3'21094912—dc23
                    2015030994

1 2 3 4 5 6 7 8 9 UNITED 21 20 19 18 17 16

Contents

Foreword ix
Acknowledgments x
Introduction 1

Harvesting 3
Uses of Herbs 6
Alpine Bistort 12
Angelica 14
Arctic Poppy 18
Bearberry 20
Bilberry 24
Biting Stonecrop 28
Bladderwrack 30
Bogbean 32
Butterwort 36
Caraway 38
Chickweed 42
Cold-weather Eyebright 44
Coltsfoot 48
Common Sea-thrift 50
Couch Grass 52
Cow Parsley 54
Creeping Thyme 56
Crowberry 60
Cuckooflower 64
Daisy 66
Dandelion 68
Devil's Bit Scabious 72
Downy Birch 74
Dulse 78
Field Gentian 82
Fir Clubmoss 84
Grass of Parnassus 86
Greater Burnet 88
Greater Plantain 92
Groundsel 96
Hawkweed 98
Heartsease 100
Heather 102
Hemp-nettle 104
Horsetail 106
Iceland Moss 110
Irish Moss 114
Juniper 116
Kidney Vetch 120
Knotgrass 122
Lady's Bedstraw 126
Lady's Mantle 128
Large-flowered Wintergreen 132

Male Fern 136
Mare's-tail 138
Marsh Marigold 140
Meadow Buttercup 144
Meadowsweet 146
Mountain Avens 150
Nootka Lupine 152
Northern Dock 154
Pineappleweed 158
Polypody 160
Purging Flax 162
Purple Marshlocks 164
Red Clover 166
Ribwort Plantain 170
Rose Bay Willow Herb 174
Roseroot 176
Rowan 180
Scurvy Grass 184
Sea Mayweed 186
Self-heal 188
Sheep's Sorrel 192
Shepherd's Purse 194
Silverweed 198
Sorrel 202
Speedwell 204
Spotted Orchid 206
Stinging Nettle 208
Stone Bramble 212
Sundew 214
Sweet Cicely 216
Sweet Grass 218
Sweet Vernal Grass 220
Valerian 222
Water Avens 226
Water Forget-me-not 228
Water Speedwell 230
White Dead-nettle 232
Wild Strawberry 234
Willow 236
Wood Cranesbill 240
Yarrow 242
Yellow Rattle 246

Glossary 248
Bibliography 252
Research Bibliography 254
Index 280
About the Author 290

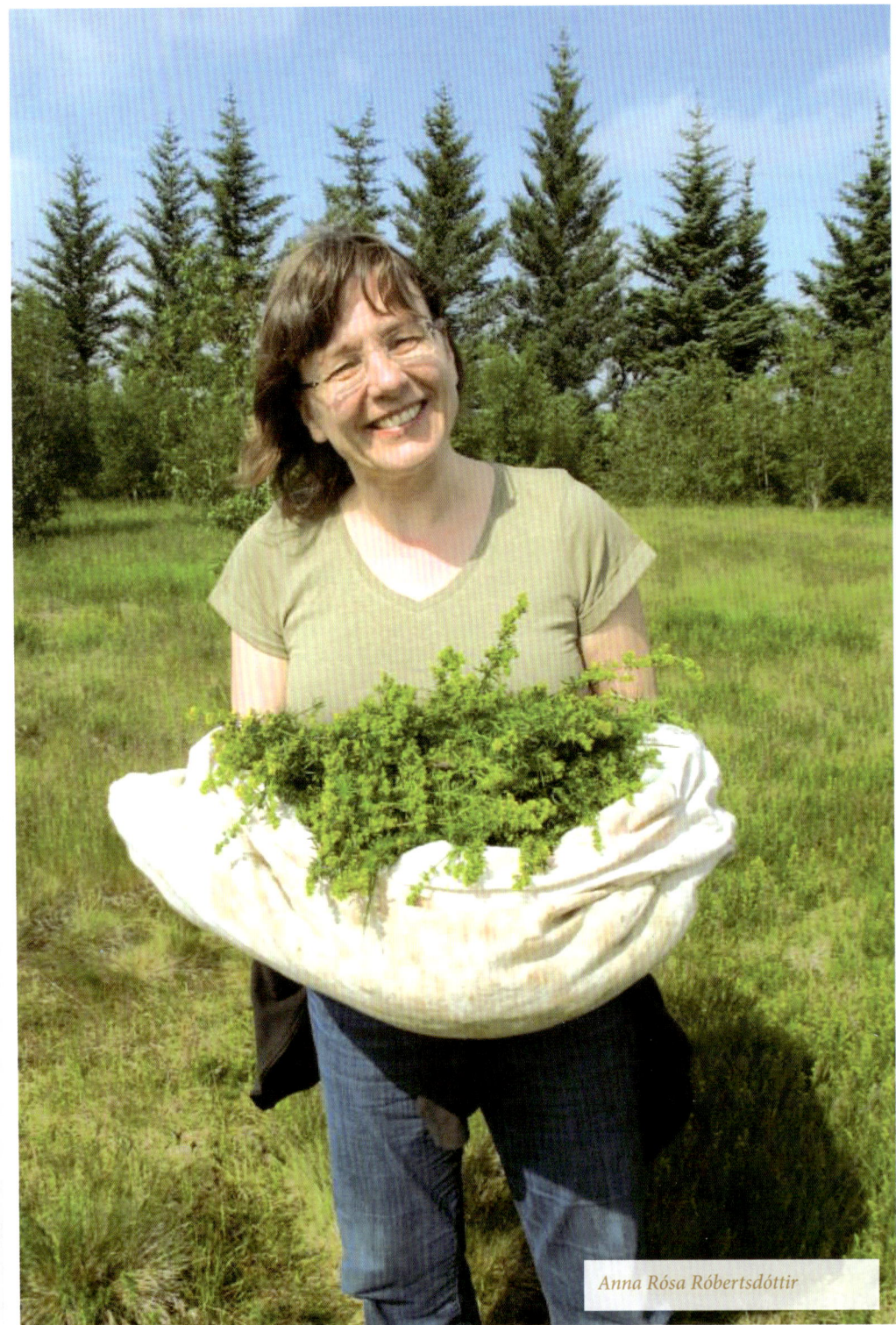

Anna Rósa Róbertsdóttir

Foreword

The North Country presents a fascinating biological region. In the southern hemisphere continents are widely spread and plant populations have long been isolated. In the north, on the other hand, the continents are close together. This has created a unique biome where plants from Scandinavia to the tip of eastern Siberia, and on to Alaska, Canada, Greenland, and Iceland, are closely related, nearly identical, actually identical, or can only be separated through genetic profiles. This region also includes the northern British Isles, the European Alps, the Rocky Mountains, and Appalachia. What this means is that the same herbs or very similar cognates are used throughout this enormous region. It also means that an herbal written about the flora of an isolated island in the north Atlantic is pertinent to herbalists almost everywhere in this bioregion.

Another aspect of Northern herbal flora is that *there is not so much of it.* Unlike the rainforests, where there are thousands of different plant species per acre, in the North Country the sparse amount of flora, the contiguous biological region (supporting cross-pollination), and the short growing season (not supporting as much genetic mutation) have left the plant population smaller (though widespread).

The confluence of these factors means that the herbal folk traditions of these regions depend upon pretty much the same herbs. A Viking in Iceland, a Scottish Highlander, an Aleut medicine man, a Native American medicine woman, a Tyrolean healer, even an occasional Chinese herbalist, and many a Western herbalist, are all going to be using an overlapping selection of medicinal plants.

This is why two herbalists from Minnesota and Alberta find themselves excitedly reading *Icelandic Herbs* and providing a foreword for the American edition: we use many of the same plants. We have used these plants in the clinic and have compared notes with other herbalists. We are, therefore, excited to know what the herbal medicine of Iceland can teach us: either by supporting established uses, introducing similar but new ideas, or completely new approaches. We thank the authoress for making her tradition available to us in an enjoyable, readable, informative manner.

We have both enjoyed visiting with Anna in person. On a visit to Iceland last summer, Robert had the opportunity to walk with Anna among the wild Angelica, Rhodiola, and Creeping Thyme in the pristine countryside. Sharing traditional plant medicine knowledge with another northern herbalist is truly a blessing and gift.

One final word: there is a big difference between an herbal written by a practicing herbalist and one penned by a "journalist." Authenticity rings out in the lines penned by someone who has used the herbs they are discussing. This is the case in *Icelandic Herbs.*

—Matthew Wood, MS (Herbal Medicine), RH (AHG) and Robert Dale Rogers, BSc, RH (AHG)

Acknowledgments

Special thanks go to Erling Ólafsson for his uniquely beautiful photographs and immeasurable assistance.

Ingrid Markan and Harri have, each in their own way, played a major part in this book and get my best thanks for all their help. Many others were involved in one way or another with the proofreading, and my gratitude goes to all of them for the useful comments and suggestions that I received. Thanks go to Albert Eiríksson, Ásdís Ragna Einarsdóttir, Ásdís Káradóttir, Dagný E. Einarsdóttir, Eva G. Þorvaldsdóttir, Eyjólfur Friðgeirsson, Gerður Sigtryggsdóttir, Guðrún Ingólfsdóttir, Jan Triebel, Jónína Yngvadóttir, María Björg Ágústsdóttir, Shelagh Smith, Steinunn Harðardóttir, Steinþór Sigurðsson, Sveinn Kjartansson, and Þórunn Steinsdóttir.

Special thanks for the English version go to Shelagh Smith and Lowana Veal, both of whom did an excellent job in translating and proofreading.

Introduction

Iceland is a small country with a population of about 330,000 people and a relatively short history of herbal medicine. The flora of Iceland consists of about five hundred plants, of which eighty-five are medicinal herbs that are discussed in this book. Most of the medicinal plants are not unique to Iceland; they also grow in Europe, North America, and elsewhere in the world. However few of the herbs are not commonly used elsewhere. There are numerous references to medicinal uses of plants in the old sagas of Iceland, but the old texts that are the most accessible nowadays and quoted in this book were published in 1783 and 1830. In these works, the authors often refer to books from Europe, commonly Germany and Norway.

When discussing herbal medicine with the older generation of Iceland today there is a collective memory for one herb in particular that people remember their grandmother using, namely Yarrow and mainly in ointments. Other herbs that often get mentioned are those that are also used as food, e.g., Iceland Moss, Dulse, Bilberry, and Crowberry. For decades the only herbalists working in Iceland all belonged to one family, which used the same recipes for well over 100 years. These recipes consisted of various herbs made into a few types of decoctions that were prescribed for all ailments. Some descendants of this family are still practicing in this way today and the ingredients in the decoction are a well-kept family secret. It was not until 1990 with the arrival of an Icelandic herbalist educated in the UK that herbalism started to be recognized again in Iceland. Today there are four herbalists working in Iceland, all educated in the U.K. and none of them with any family history of herbalism. Herbalism was illegal by law until 15 years ago in Iceland. However, herbalists were left to their own devices without any action being taken, before it became legal to practice. Many medicinal herbs that are legal to use both in Europe and the U.S. are illegal in Iceland and use is controlled by the Icelandic Medicines Agency. As a consequence of the above restrictions, I have often had to be quite creative in the use of the few herbs that are easy to collect in Iceland. I have commonly used a number of species that are closely related to well-known medicinal herbs elsewhere that I have found to work in a similar way. Here is an example of a few of them: Creeping Thyme, Sea Mayweed, Downy Birch, Lady's Bedstraw, Northern Dock, and Woolly Willow.

Of the medicinal plants in Iceland only about 15–20 are common enough to wildcraft in any quantanties without over-harvesting. It is easy to wildcraft common herbs in Iceland as there is a lot of wilderness within easy access and very little pollution. However it is not common to find forests in Iceland; it is a country composed of heaths, mountains, and marshland with the types of herbs that grow in these conditions. The season to harvest in Iceland is very short, spring comes late and autumn early. Since the growing period is so short in Iceland there has been some speculation that the medicinal herbs are more potent here than elsewhere.

This book is written primarily with the general public in mind because knowledge of medicinal herbs belongs to everyone and not to the chosen few. In my work as a medical herbalist for the past two decades, I have held many courses and have clearly found that there is a growing interest in Icelandic medicinal herbs. I have always felt it important to inform people about Icelandic herbs because it is easy to collect common medicinal herbs in Iceland, which are more often than not categorized as weeds. Medicinal herbs can be used as daily preventives and refreshments, and because individuals should take responsibility for their own health, medicinal herbs can become part of one's daily food intake.

Herbal medicine is the oldest form of medicine and is above all built on experience passed on from person to person, although in recent decades scientists have started to research medicinal herbs more thoroughly. In this book I have chosen to take quotes from ancient Icelandic works to give the reader an insight into how medicinal herbs were used in Iceland centuries ago. More often than not, there are similarities between how herbs were used 200 years ago and how they are used nowadays, though this statement does not hold true for every herb.

First, I present information on the harvesting, drying, and storage of medicinal herbs, together with instructions on how to make use of herbs. I sought a way of explaining in simple terms the use of medicinal herbs at home. In the Glossary at the back of this book, explanations are given for the most common constituents and terminology used in medicinal herbalism.

Erling Ólafsson, an entomologist at the Icelandic Institute of Natural History, took most of the photographs in the book. Through much dedication and passion he strove to take exceptionally clear and distinctive photographs so that the public would easily be able to identify and distinguish the herbs. The importance of good photographs for a book such as this is indisputable, so I was very fortunate to find Erling for the project and I can never thank him enough for his wonderful contribution.

This book contains a summary of the research that has been done on medicinal herbs found in Iceland, but the summary is by no means exhaustive. Most of the research was not done in Iceland, since most species of medicinal herbs similar to those in Iceland are found in other countries as well. I have not evaluated the quality or results of the research—that would provide material for many more books.

The purpose of summarizing the research that has been done on Icelandic medicinal herbs is to give the reader a chance to find out more about the research that awakens their special interest. Each herb has a detailed bibliography, but most research was found in open databases on the internet and is easy to access. Of special interest is the NCBI (National Center for Biotechnology Information) database, which keeps information on thousands of research papers on medicinal herbs. The website is http://www.ncbi.nlm.nih.gov /guide/.

Much of the research was done on isolated constituents of the medicinal herbs in question and not on individual plant parts. If the research was done on a blend of some herbs, this is stated.

The first phase of research on herbs generally consists of *in vitro* tests in test tubes, and if circumstances call for it further research is done on animals (*in vivo* testing). The last phase of research is clinical trials on humans. In this book it is stated whether or not the research is a clinical trial; if the type of research is not specified, this means that it is either *in vitro* or *in vivo* testing.

It should be remembered that the results of *in vitro* or *in vivo* research cannot generally be transferred to humans. However, they do give a good indication of the effects of herbs, which could later lead to further research on people.

Scientific research studies vary greatly in quality, so the results should always be viewed with caution. In clinical trials, for example, the size of the experimental groups matters a great deal, and the same applies to whether or not a placebo has been used. The quality of the herbs themselves is also important as this can differ greatly as well.

It is my deepest hope that this book will awaken interest in the treasures that Icelandic nature holds, while also increasing the knowledge and use of medicinal herbs by individuals so they can improve their general health.

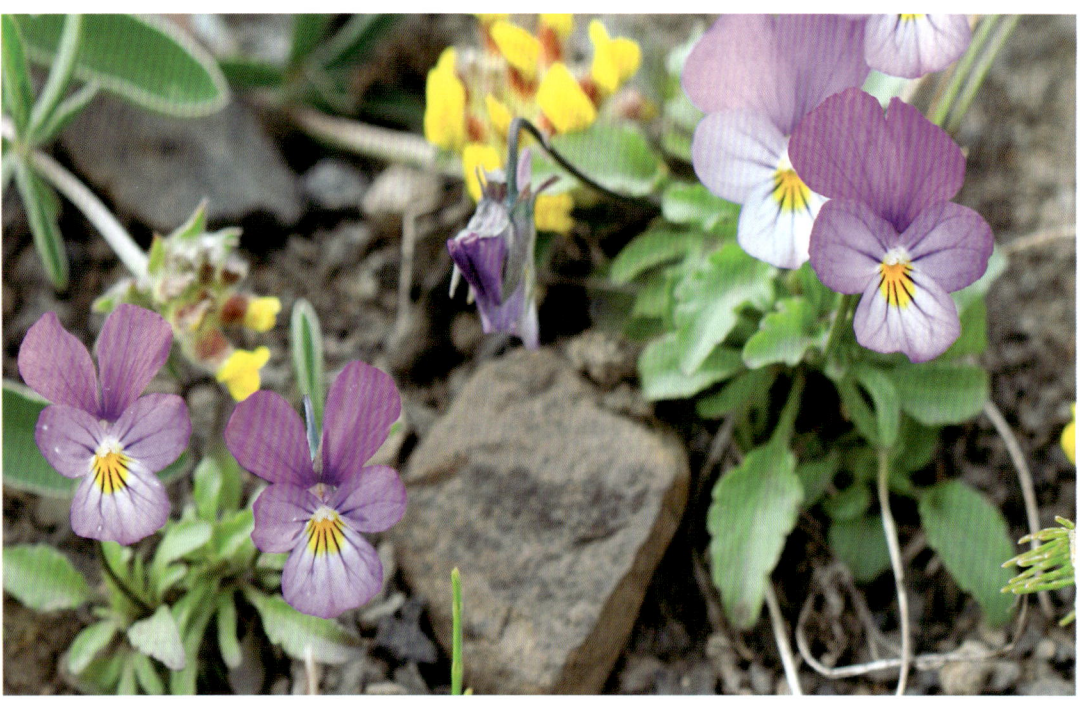

Harvesting

When harvesting, it is important to be completely familiar with the herb that is being harvested, as many herbs look similar and it is easy to confuse them. A good plant handbook with good photos and descriptions of the herbs will make identification easier when harvesting. Damage might result if the wrong herb is collected and then used, so no one should pick herbs without knowing exactly what they are doing.

Icelandic nature is sensitive and many herbs grow only in specific places or are very rare; therefore, everyone should be careful and harvest in moderation. Be aware that some herbs are protected and may not be picked at all. (See the list of protected herbs on the next page.)

Some herbs are not actually rare but are, however, very small and grow sparsely and not in broad swaths. A good example of this is

Butterwort, which is endangered in many countries though it is common in Iceland. It is not recommended to collect Large-flowered Wintergreen, Sundew, Kidney Vetch, or Greater Burnet because of their rarity. It should also be kept in mind that some herbs take a long time to grow (e.g., Roseroot and Iceland Moss), and this should be taken into consideration when picking them.

When harvesting herbs that are prolific and grow in broad swaths, the general rule is to never harvest more than one-third of the herb in each place. Another point to keep in mind when harvesting, is to get permission from the landowner if the herbs are not on public property.

When harvesting medicinal herbs, special care must be taken not to pick herbs from polluted areas. Do not pick where insecticides or chemical fertilizers have been used, alongside roads or other areas where there is traffic, or

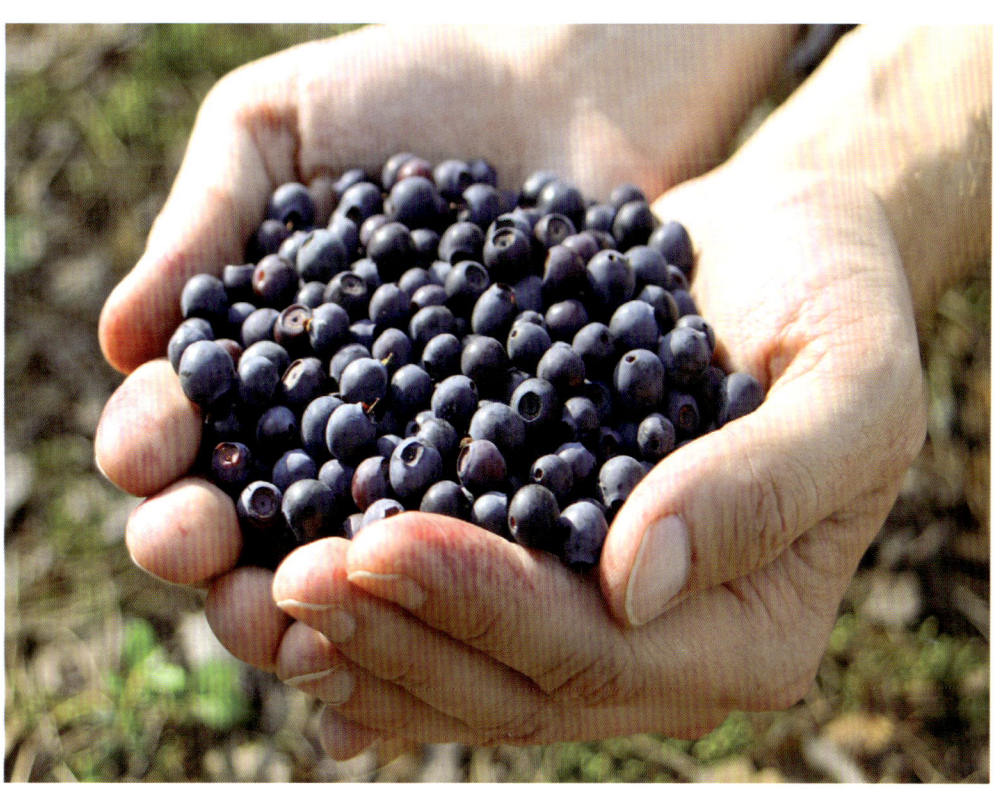

Protected Plants

Icelandic law declares that 31 plant species are protected, which means that it is forbidden to break off the buds, flowers, or roots of plants, to trample on them, dig them up, or damage them in any other way.

Pyramidal Bugle	*Ajuga pyramidalis*	Common Twayblade	*Listera ovata*
Field Garlic	*Allium oleraceum*	Stag's-horn Clubmoss	*Lycopodium clavatum*
Forked Spleenwort	*Asplenium septentrionale*	Wood Sorrel	*Oxalis acetosella*
Maidenhair Spleenwort	*Asplenium trichomanes*	Arctic Poppy	*Papaver radicatum* ssp. *stefanssonii*
Green Spleenwort	*Asplenium viride*	Herb Paris	*Paris quadrifolia*
Hard Fern	*Blechnum spicant* var. *fallax*	Amphibious Bistort	*Persicaria amphibia*
Glossy Moonwort	*Botrychium simplex*	Tormentil	*Potentilla erecta*
Pedunculate Water-starwort	*Callitriche brutia*	Greenland Primrose	*Primula egaliksensis*
Large Yellow-sedge	*Carex flava*	Glaucous Dog Rose	*Rosa dumalis*
Hudson Bay Sedge	*Carex heleonastes*	Burnet Rose	*Rosa pimpinellifolia*
Parsley Fern	*Cryptogramma crispa*	Saxifrage Foliolose	*Saxifraga foliolosa*
Common Heath Grass	*Danthonia decumbens*	Lesser Spurrey	*Spergularia salina*
Eyebright	*Euphrasia calida*	Boreal Starwort	*Stellaria borealis*
Common Marsh-Bedstraw	*Galium palustre*	Water Pygmyweed	*Tillaea aquatica*
Wilson's Filmy-fern	*Hymenophyllum wilsonii*	Common Dog Violet	*Viola riviniana*
Saltmarsh Rush	*Juncus gerardii*		

close to factories and other industrial areas. The same applies to harvesting from beaches. Iceland Moss, for example, is extremely sensitive to all pollution. If herbs are contaminated by heavy metals, they can cause toxicity with internal use.

When harvesting, it is important to use either a pair of scissors or a knife and to avoid pulling or breaking the herb. Some herbs (e.g., Creeping Thyme), break up readily with the roots if they are pulled, so it is extremely important to cut the herb carefully and not break it off. Herbs are best collected in a basket, paper bag, or canvas bag; bags sewn from old sheets are ideal. Do not use nylon or plastic bags for harvesting.

When harvesting medicinal herbs, make sure that the herb is free of any diseases, for instance a fungal disease. This is not uncommon in some herbs, such as Lady's Mantle and Shepherd's Purse.

Herbs should always be picked in dry weather; the only exception is Iceland Moss, which is better to collect when it is wet. The general rule with harvesting is that leaves of herbs are usually collected in early summer before the herb has bloomed and new flower buds are picked at first bloom, while berries and seeds are gathered when they are mature, which is usually in August. Roots are generally harvested in autumn and, in some cases, in spring. It is also very important to know what part of the herb should be collected, as in some cases different medicinal properties apply to different parts of the same herb. A good example of this is Dandelion, the actions of which depend on whether the leaves or the roots are used.

After harvesting, it is essential to process the herbs on the same day, whether for drying or for making fresh tinctures. This applies especially to leaves and flowers, which are more sensitive than roots.

Drying

There are many ways to store herbs, but drying is one of the commonest ways to do so. The herbs must be kept in a dry, heated place. Most Icelandic medicinal herbs can be dried at room temperature.

Leaves, Flowers, and Seeds

The leaves or flowers can be spread out either on paper or on some sort of material. Newspaper should not be used because the ink can seep into the herbs. An ideal solution consists of laying an old sheet on a table and putting the herbs on top of it, but make sure that direct sunlight does not shine on the herbs while they are drying. The herbs should be turned once a day; most herbs dry within a week at room temperature.

Another method is to make a drying rack, which can easily be done with a wooden frame and garden netting. If the herbs are laid on fine netting, the air circulates better around them, which makes drying easier. To see if the herbs are ready for use, rub a bit between your fingers: if they are brittle and break up easily, they are ready.

Tall plants with good stalks, like Meadowsweet, can also be tied together in bunches and hung upside down to dry. It is a good idea to hang these herbal bunches upside down on a clothes-line to dry.

Berries

Berries are full of juice so they do not dry at room temperature like other parts of plants. However, they can be spread out on a baking tray and dried in an oven. Set the oven on the lowest heat and put the berries in the oven with the door half open. Allow the berries to remain at this heat for 1–2 hours with the door half open, then switch off the oven but keep the berries in the warmth for another 2 hours. After that, the berries can be transferred to a drawer lined with paper and allowed to dry at room temperature. To hasten drying, repeat the above process the next day.

Roots

Roots are usually harvested in autumn, when the visible parts of the plant are withering and before the ground freezes. If a garden fork is used instead of a shovel, there is less chance that the roots will be damaged.

Roots have to be thoroughly cleaned in warm water so that all soil and dirt is removed; a nailbrush is good for this as it gets the dents and ridges clean of soil and dirt. The root is then wiped carefully and cut into slices or little pieces. These are then laid on material or paper and dried at room temperature in the same way as the visible parts of the plant. Roots often take longer to dry than leaves and flowers, but this also depends on how thickly they have been cut.

Storage

Medicinal herbs are best stored in air-tight containers. It is good to store dried herbs in glass jars with a good lid, but ensure that the jars are kept out of direct sunlight. Another common method is to keep herbs in paper bags—if the herbs are to be stored for a long time, the bags can be placed in a cake pan to get rid of the air completely. It is not desirable to store herbs in aluminum pans or plastic for a long time.

Most dried herbs keep well for 1–2 years, but after that they begin to lose their quality and medicinal power. However, roots often have a longer shelf life than leaves, flowers, and seeds.

Uses of Herbs

There are many ways of using herbs. The most common methods that are practical for home use are discussed below.

Infusions

When an infusion is made, boiling water is poured over the soft parts of the plant (e.g., leaves, flowers, and seeds). These parts do not have to be boiled as the active constituents are easily released. Normally, 1–2 teaspoons of the dry herb are used for each cup and the daily dose is often 3–4 cups per day. Boiling water is poured over the herbs and the infusion is allowed to stand for 10–15 minutes. Then the herbs are sieved before the infusion is drunk. Many herbs contain volatile oils, so it is important to put a lid over the cup while the herbs are steeping so that the volatile oils do not evaporate. Herbs that contain volatile oils include Angelica, Creeping Thyme, and Pineappleweed.

It is also very convenient to put 2–3 tablespoons of herbs in a vacuum flask (750 ml), pour boiling water over them, and put the lid on. Allow to steep for about 15 minutes before using and drink from the flask throughout the day. The herbs are sieved each time the tea is poured into the cup, but it is best to return them to the flask afterward as this is the best way to get the most out of them. If the tea becomes too strong or bitter later in the day, boiling water can be added.

Some people do not like to drink hot tea, so then the best solution is to make the infusion in the traditional way, cool it down, and keep it in the refrigerator. Herbal infusions can be sweetened with a little honey if necessary, and some spices (e.g., fresh ginger, are ideal for giving the infusion extra flavor). If fresh herbs are used instead of dried ones for infusions, the general rule is to use double the amount of fresh herbs to the dried. It should also be kept in mind that although it is stated above that 1–2 teaspoons of herbs are normally used per cup, this is only a general suggestion and is not always appropriate, thus it is always necessary to know the correct dosage for each herb.

In some instances, cold infusions are also made. This is done to release certain substances that cannot tolerate heat; Greater Plantain and Couch Grass are examples of herbs that are suitable for use in this way. To make cold infusions, pour cold water over the herbs and allow to steep for 8–12 hours. This is often done at night so that the infusion is ready to drink the next day.

Children always need smaller doses; see "Children and Dosage," page 21.

. . . .

Hot Infusion

‣ Use 1–2 teaspoons of finely cut dried herbs or 2–4 teaspoons of fresh herbs.

‣ Place the herbs in a cup (150 ml), add boiling water, and cover with a lid.

‣ Allow the infusion to stand for 10–15 minutes.

‣ Strain the herbs through a sieve.

‣ Drink 3–4 cups a day.

. . . .

Cold Infusion

‣ Put 3–6 teaspoons of dried herbs in a 500 ml container, add cold water, and cover with a lid.

‣ Allow to stand for 8–12 hours.

‣ Strain the herbs with a sieve.

‣ Drink 3–4 cups a day.

Decoctions

A differentiation is made between infusions and decoctions in herbal medicine. Decoctions must be made from the hard parts of plants, such as roots and bark; otherwise, the active constituents are not released from them. To make decoctions, the general dosage is 2–3 tablespoons of roots or bark to a pot of 750 ml cold water (do not use aluminum pots). Bring to a boil, then allow the decoction to simmer on low heat for 30–40 minutes. About one-third of the water will evaporate, so about 500 ml of the decoction is left. The decoction is then strained and the normal dosage of 1–3 cups is used. Decoctions keep well for 3 days in the refrigerator. In China, where it is still traditional to drink decoctions, as opposed to the Western world where decoctions are not as common as they once were, it is customary to use roots and bark much more. The same parts are boiled three times (i.e., after the decoction has been strained the first time, the herbal residue is boiled in fresh water using the same method a second time). This is then repeated a third time; all three decoctions are then mixed together and the blend is used when necessary.

Children always need smaller doses; see "Children and Dosage," page 21.

. . . .

Decoction

- ‣ Use 2–3 tablespoons of roots or bark.
- ‣ Add 750 ml cold water.
- ‣ Place in a pot and boil, uncovered, on low heat for 30–40 minutes.
- ‣ Strain the herbs through a sieve.
- ‣ Drink 1–3 cups a day.

Tinctures

Ancient methods used by herbalists to extract active substances from medicinal herbs involve steeping them in alcohol. The resulting liquid is called a tincture.

Tinctures can be made at different strengths, but with dried herbs a 1:5 ratio is generally used (e.g., 100 g dried herbs to 500 ml alcohol). The strength of the alcohol differs according to which herb is being used, but normally the percentage of alcohol ranges between 25% and 60%. Information on the ratio and strength can be found in the dosage for tinctures for each individual herb in this book where applicable. The usual alcohol strength is 45%, but in this book 40% is most often given instead of 45% because it is assumed that pure vodka or spirits are used in homemade tinctures. When 25% strength is used to make tinctures, the vodka or spirits are diluted with sufficient water to make a 25% solution.

The herbs are placed in a container with a tight-fitting lid (e.g., a glass jar), and covered with alcohol. The lid is then screwed tightly closed, the jar is shaken and left to stand for at least 2 weeks, though it often takes 4–6 weeks for the tincture to be ready. The jar should not be exposed to sunlight, so it is best to keep it in a cupboard. The jar should be shaken every other day. When the tincture is ready, the herbs are strained through a sieve and a muslin cloth (a cloth diaper is ideal for this). Wring the cloth thoroughly to extract as much of the liquid out as possible. The tincture is then put into a glass bottle with a tight cap, labeled with the name and date, and stored away from the light. Tinctures keep well because the alcohol preserves the active constituents as soon as they are released. The usual shelf life is 3–4 years.

Tinctures can also be made with apple cider vinegar or glycerol instead of alcohol.

If tinctures are made with fresh herbs, the ratio is 1:2 (i.e., 100 g of herbs to 200 ml of alcohol). The easiest way is to fill the jar with fresh herbs, compact them slightly, and then add the alcohol to cover the herbs completely. The method described for dried herbs is then used.

It is not recommended to blend many different herbs in one jar when making tinctures. A much better practice is to make tinctures from single herbs and then mix the ready-made tinctures together, because then it is possible to alter the herbal ratio of the tincture when necessary.

The common dosage for tinctures that are made with dried herbs is 1 teaspoon three times a day, but if tinctures are made with fresh herbs, the dose is often 1–2 teaspoons three times a day. In this book, the dosage for the use of tinctures is given according to each individual herb. Keep in mind that herbalists rarely work with one herb at a time when prescribing tinctures, but instead often blend 4–6 types of herbs. See "Herbal Blends," page 20.

Children always need smaller doses; see "Children and Dosage," page 21.

Tinctures from Dried Herbs

- Fill the jar with fresh herbs and compress lightly.
- Cover well with alcohol (see different strengths for each herb).
- Close the lid well and label the jar with the name of the herb and date.
- Store at room temperature for 4–6 weeks; shake every other day.
- Strain the herbs through a sieve and muslin cloth, wringing well.
- Pour the tincture into a glass bottle, labeled with the name and date. Keep away from the light.

Tinctures from Fresh Herbs

- Fill the jar with fresh herbs and compress lightly.
- Cover well with alcohol (see different strengths for each herb).
- Close the lid well and label the jar with the name of the herb and date.
- Store at room temperature for 4–6 weeks; shake every other day.
- Strain the herbs through a sieve and muslin cloth, wringing well.
- Pour the tincture into a glass bottle, labeled with the name and date. Keep away from the light.

Powders

Medicinal herbs ground into powders in a mortar or coffee grinder can be mixed with cold or hot water or sprinkled over food. The powder can also be put into capsules and taken like any other medication. Externally, the powder can also be mixed with an ointment or sprinkled directly over wounds or rashes, which was the common method for skin disorders in the past. Another old method that was often practiced consisted of sniffing powders for nosebleeds. Knotgrass was one of the herbs used this way.

Herbal Syrups

Sugar and honey are preservatives and have been used in herbal syrups for centuries. They also have soothing properties, so are normally used in herbal syrups for coughs and throat infections. The base for herbal syrups is either a strong infusion or decoction, preferably double strength, but a tincture can be added to increase the effect and preserve it even more. Usually an equal amount of infusion/decoction and sugar/honey is used. Icelandic herbs that are suitable as cough syrups include Creeping Thyme, Angelica, Heather, and Yarrow. The normal dosage of herbal syrup is 1–2 teaspoons three times a day.

Herbal Syrup

- 500 ml strong infusion or decoction (double strength).
- 500 g sugar, raw sugar, or honey.
- 10 ml tincture.
- Boil the sugar/honey in the tea on low heat and stir until the sugar/honey has dissolved.
- Add the tincture last. Remove from the heat and allow to cool.
- Pour into disinfected bottles, labeled with the name and date. Keep away from the light.
- Keeps for 6–12 months.

Infused Oils

The herb is usually heated in a base oil in a double boiler on low heat for 2–4 hours. Base oils include olive oil, sunflower oil, almond oil, and many other types of oils. Another method of making infused oils is to put fresh herbs in a clear glass jar, fill it with base oil to cover the herbs completely, and place it in the sun. Often the jar is kept exposed to the sun for up to 2 weeks until the oil is ready. This method is more suitable for sunnier countries than Iceland.

Infused oils keep for 6–12 months. Many Icelandic medicinal herbs are suitable for use in this form (e.g., Yarrow, Downy Birch, Chickweed, and Meadowsweet).

Volatile or Essential Oils

Essential oils are distilled from herbs—mostly from the flowers or seeds of the plant—using distillation equipment. A large quantity of herbs is needed to get a few milliliters of essential oil, so this kind of oil is rarely homemade. These oils are very concentrated and often need to be blended into a base oil before being used externally. Base oils include olive oil, sunflower oil, almond oil, and many other types of oils. Essential oils are not recommended for internal use unless under professional supervision.

Ointments and Creams

In the old days, ointments were usually made by boiling medicinal herbs in sheep fat or unsalted butter. Nowadays, however, it is far more common to use infused oils in ointments and thicken these with various types of wax (e.g., beeswax). Ointments keep for up to 1 year without preservatives. White cream is often made by blending water or an herbal infusion with oil and binding agents that bind the water and the oil. If no preservatives are used, white creams do not keep well. However, many medicinal herbs and essential oils can help to extend their shelf life.

Poultices

Herbal poultices are made with fresh or dried herbs as well as powders. They are usually used for nerve, joint, or muscle pain, but also for injuries such as strains and broken bones and to draw out pus from infected wounds or abscesses.

Poultices are made by boiling the herbs for about 2 minutes in a little water, so that the water just covers the herbs. The water is then drained away, a little oil is applied to the skin so the herbs do not stick to it, and the poultice is then laid directly onto the skin. It is then covered with a muslin cloth. A heat wrap can also be put over the poultice to keep it warm. Poultices are often kept on for 2–3 hours and renewed if necessary.

Compresses

Sometimes it can be useful to lay a compress or muslin cloth moistened with an infusion, decoction, or tincture on inflammations and bruises, or to relieve headaches and lower fevers. Hot compresses are especially good when dealing with sports injuries, bruises, or inflammations, while cold compresses are generally used to lower fevers and for headaches.

A normal infusion or decoction can be used, but it is also possible to double the strength. Tinctures are diluted with water; the recommended use is 25 ml tincture to 500 ml water. A muslin cloth or handkerchief is moistened with the infusion, decoction, or diluted tincture and squeezed well. A little oil is applied to the skin to prevent the cloth from sticking to it and then the compress is applied. Cling wrap is used to cover the compress, which is kept on the injury or sore spot for 1–2 hours. Repeat if necessary.

Eyebaths

Inflammation or itching in the eyes can be reduced if the eyes are rinsed with herbal infusions or diluted tinctures. The herbal infusion should not be strong as this could irritate the eyes.

. . . .

Eyebath

‣ Place 1 teaspoon of herbs in a cup, add hot water, and allow to steep for 10 minutes. Strain through a coffee filter so that no herbal residue remains in the infusion.

‣ When the infusion is cold, pour it into an eyebath (available in pharmacies). Hold this against the eye, tilt the head back, and blink a few times. Rinse both eyes.

‣ Repeat two to three times a day.

It is also possible to fill the eyebath with boiling water and add 2–3 drops of tincture to it. Allow to cool and then use as above. Eyebright has long been used traditionally in eyebaths, but Heather and other herbs can also be used.

Gargles and Mouthwashes

Many astringent medicinal herbs make good rinses for gingivitis, mouth ulcers, wounds, and throat infections as they strengthen the mucous membranes of the mouth and throat. The mouth can be rinsed with a conventional infusion that has steeped for at least 20 minutes before straining, but double strength infusions are frequently used. Decoctions and diluted tinctures can also be used as gargles and mouthwashes.

For mouthwashes, 5 ml tincture to 1 dl hot water is recommended. The infusion, decoction, or diluted tincture is usually swallowed after gargling, the recommended dose being 1 cup three times a day. Many Icelandic medicinal herbs are suitable for gargles and mouthwashes (e.g., Lady's Mantle, Eyebright, Silverweed, Water Avens, Strawberry leaves, and Creeping Thyme).

Vaginal Douches

Vaginal douches are used for infections, itching, and soreness in the vagina (e.g., fungal infections). Conventional infusions, decoctions, or diluted tinctures can be used for douching, preferably using the infusion or decoction at double strength.

The easiest way of rinsing the vagina is to use a vaginal douche bag, using 1 dl twice to three times a day. If a diluted tincture is used, 5 ml tincture to 1 dl warm water is recommended. Common medicinal herbs for douching include Lady's Mantle, Yarrow, and White Dead-nettle.

Herbal Baths

Herbal baths can relieve joint pain and inflammation and soothe rashes and wounds, as well as being useful for hemorrhoids. A conventional infusion or decoction can be made, of which ½–1 liter is put in the bath water, but infusions or decoctions at double strength can also be used. It is also possible to put the herbs in a muslin cloth and allow boiling water to run through it. Cold water can then be run through the bag until the bath water reaches a suitable temperature.

This method is only possible to use with leaves, flowers, or seeds, not with roots or bark, which need boiling water to release their active constituents. The muslin cloth should contain 100–200 g herbs.

Juices and Shakes

Medicinal herbs may be pressed in a juicer or blended with water in a food processor and used fresh for medicinal purposes, both internally and externally. Another good idea is to add fresh herbs to any shake using vegetables, fruit, seeds, etc. Fresh juice can also be poured into ice-cube bags and frozen for later use.

Herbal Blends

Herbalists seldom work with one herb at a time, but instead blend a few herbs together. In Western herbal medicine, 4–6 different herbs are generally combined for internal use, but in Eastern herbal medicine, the general practice is to combine far more herbs. One reason for blending herbs is that one herb could enhance the action of another, as research has shown.

There are often many theories on how to blend herbs, but it would take too long to describe them for the purposes of this book.

Dosage

All doses in this book apply to dried herbs, unless otherwise stated. They also apply to adults and not to children. When 1 teaspoon of herbs is mentioned, this means 1 teaspoon of finely chopped dried herbs.

The dosage applies to individuals of average weight; those who are petite or very thin need a lower dose than the average person. Similarly, older people need a lower dose than is commonly recommended.

Children and Dosage

In this book, the doses that are given for each herb are always intended for adults, as children need much smaller doses. If infants are breastfed, the mother should take the adult dose of the herb as the effects will enter the breast milk and the infant will benefit as a result.

. . . .

The following doses usually apply for children:

- ‣ 0–6 months: $\frac{1}{20}$ of adult dosage.
- ‣ 6 months to 2 years: $\frac{1}{10}$ of adult dosage.
- ‣ 2–5 years: $\frac{1}{5}$ of adult dosage.
- ‣ 5–12 years: $\frac{1}{4}$–$\frac{1}{2}$ of adult dosage.

After 12 years of age, adult dosage applies for children. Keep in mind that children of the same age can be of different heights and sizes, so the dosage must be adjusted according to their weight. Tinctures are best given to children in fruit juice or tasty drinks as they rarely taste nice. Also, children generally are less keen on hot infusions compared to adults, so it is better to cool down a traditional infusion and give it to them as a cold drink. Another method is to make a conventional infusion, pour it into lollipop molds and freeze.

. . . .

Measurements

- ‣ 1 ml = 20 drops
- ‣ 5 ml = 1 teaspoon
- ‣ 20 ml = 1 tablespoon
- ‣ 150 ml = 1 cup

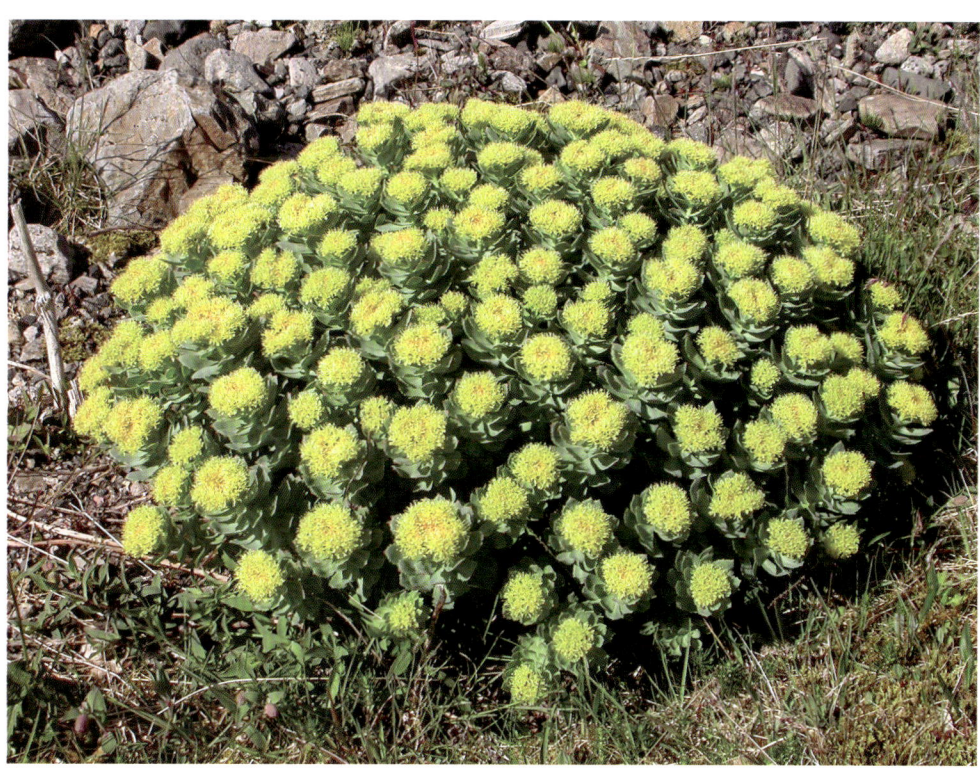

Alpine Bistort

Bistorta vivipara
Polygonaceae—Kornsúra

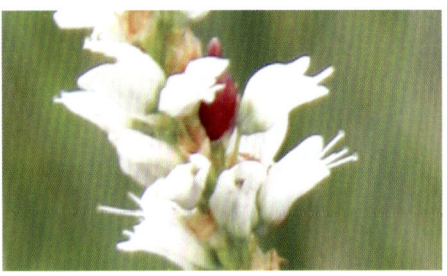

Action

Astringent, hemostatic, and vulnerary.

Uses

Alpine Bistort is not used much in Western herbal medicine nowadays. It is thought to be good as a rinse for sore throats and gingivitis and to ease diarrhea. It is also used to stop bleeding and heal wounds and abscesses. In China, Alpine Bistort is used in a similar way to stop bleeding and diarrhea and to lower fevers, as well as being used as an anti-inflammatory and externally for wounds, hemorrhoids, rashes, and snake bites.

Research

In China, Alpine Bistort is used with another Chinese herb, *Pedicularis muscicola*, for snake bites. Research shows that this blend is effective.[1]

Dosage

Tincture: 1–3 ml three times a day (1:5, 25%).

Infusion: 1 teaspoon in a cup three times a day.

Decoction: 1 teaspoon in a cup three times a day.

Infusions, decoctions, tinctures, compresses, and ointments for external use.

Habitat

Alpine Bistort is common all over Iceland and grows in all soil types.

Parts Used

The entire plant is used, including the root.

Harvesting

Alpine Bistort is collected in early summer and the roots harvested in autumn.

Constituents

Polyphenols, tannins, and flavonoids.

History

In the past, Alpine Bistort was used as food. The entire plant was eaten and the seeds, which were called field corn, were mulled and were thought to be good for baking or with milk. A foreign relative, *Polygonum bistorta*, is a well-known medicinal herb and sources report that it has similar properties.

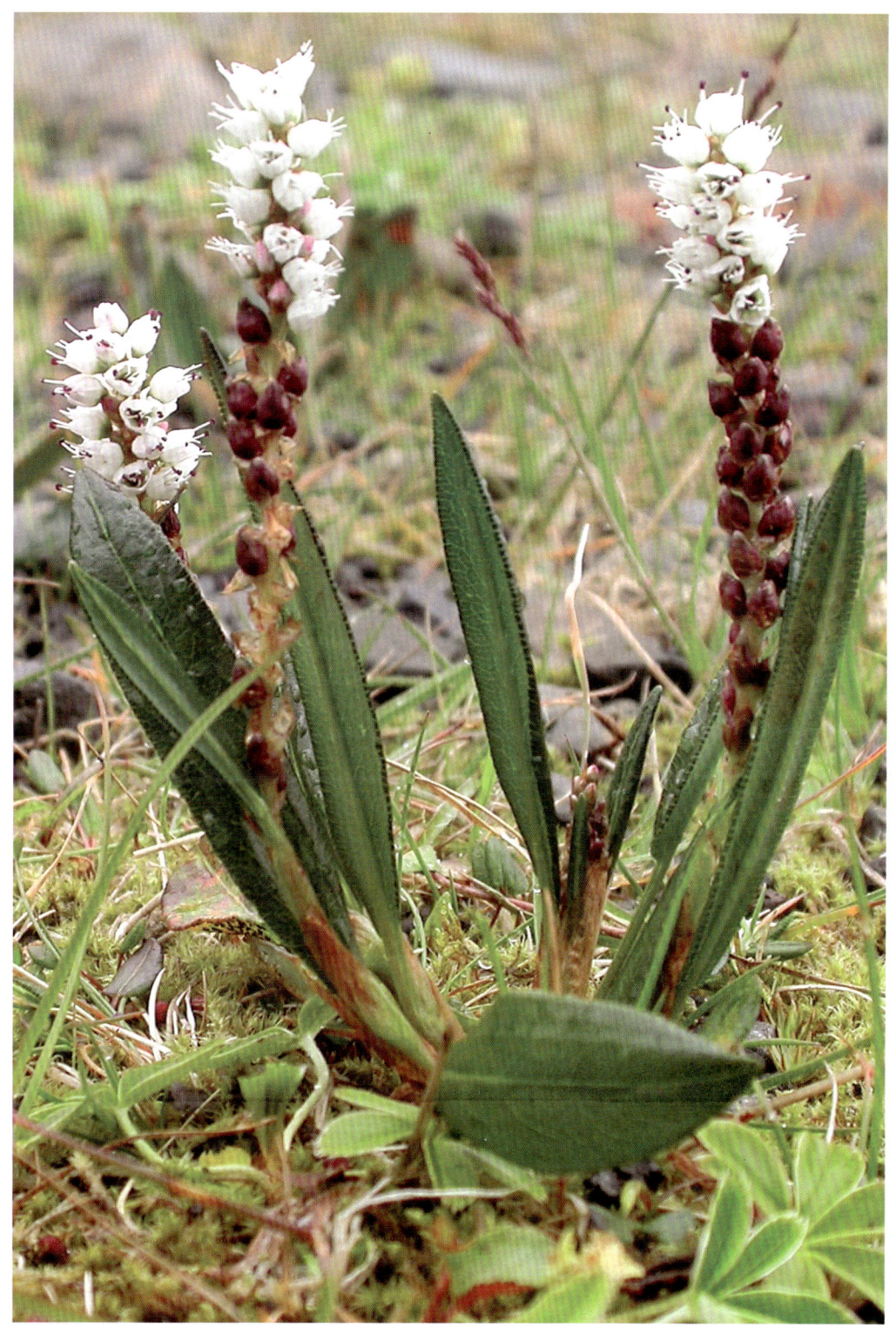

Angelica

Angelica archangelica
Apiaceae—Ætihvönn

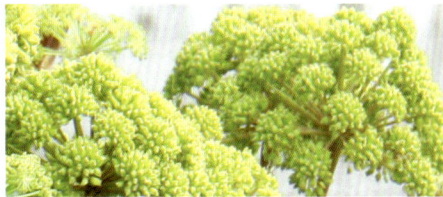

Habitat

Angelica grows all over Iceland and is mainly found alongside streams and on river banks.

Parts Used

Roots, leaves, and seeds.

Harvesting

The leaves are collected before bloom in early summer, the seeds are collected in August, and the roots are harvested in the autumn.

Constituents

Essential oils, sesquiterpenes, resins, phytosterols, phenolic acids, fatty acids, coumarin, and tannins.

History

Angelica has an ancient history as a medicinal herb and is considered extremely versatile. Worldwide, over 60 different species of Angelica are found and most of them are used for medicinal purposes, especially in Asia where Dong Quai (*A. sinensis*) is extremely popular. The Latin name *archangelica* is associated with the archangels and one folk tale speaks of Angelica appearing before an angel in a dream as a cure for the Black Death. Angelica was said to provide good protection against evil spirits and

Wine, in which this herb has been soaked, or the juice thereof, thins blood, opens veins, stimulates sweating and menstrual bleeding, promotes birth and placental birth, heals palpitations. The root may steep in vinegar, then let it dry again and smell it or have a piece of it under the tongue. It is said to be good against unclean and bad air, if this vinegar is drunk. The root strengthens the stomach, eliminates wind, kills worms in the intestines, and is good for stitches and old coughs, chest pains and toothache when it is chewed often. Angelica seeds, taken with honey or alcohol in which they have soaked for a long time, heal jaundice. They also eliminate flatulence from the intestines. The herb is called the best remedy for plagues and poison; it moves stagnant blood, heals internal injuries and eliminates all bad fluids.

Björn Halldórsson, Uses of Herbs, *1783*

witchcraft, and it was held in such high esteem that it was also called "The Root of the Holy Spirit." In the past, Angelica was frequently grown in gardens in Iceland, as it was used both in cooking and for medicinal purposes. Angelica stems were peeled and eaten, both raw and boiled, and it was considered healthy to chew the root when virulent plagues swept over. Angelica roots were often consumed in Iceland in the past; they were kept in soil during the winter and eaten new, when necessary, with dried fish and butter. Angelica was also exported centuries ago; it was used as currency and fines were imposed for stealing it.

The Native Americans used many species of Angelica as remedies and food, and usually the root was used. The herb was considered beneficial for headaches, both internally and externally. It was also extensively used for digestive disturbances and was, for instance, given to children to eliminate worms. It was also reputed to be good for colds, fevers, and back pain, but was not recommended for use by

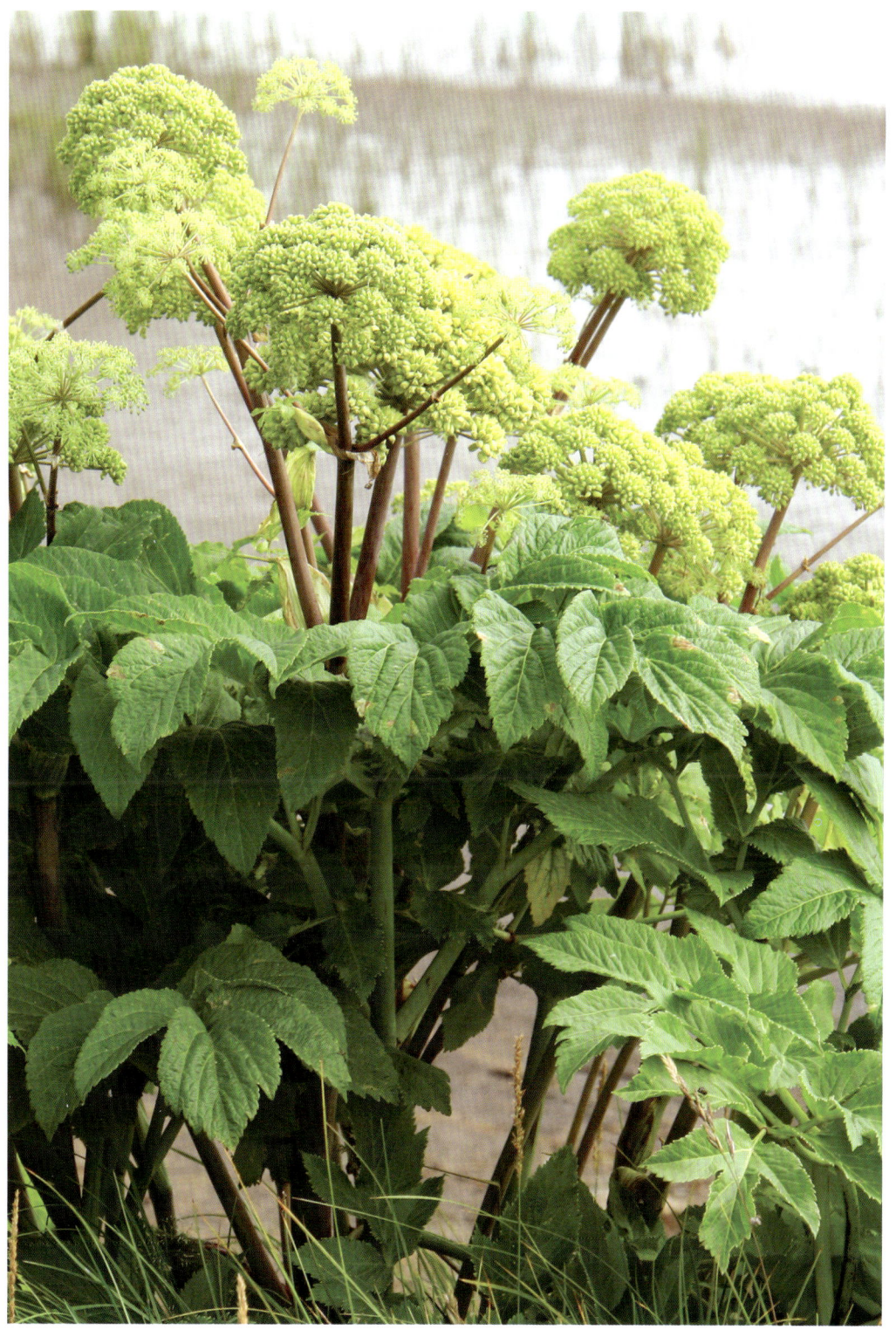

pregnant women. Angelica root was reported to protect against nightmares if a compress was placed on the head and ears, and it was thought to bring good luck for fishing and betting.

Angelica root is used to flavor alcohol, namely liqueurs such as Chartreuse and Bénédictine, Vermouth, Dubonnet, and Icelandic Brennivín. Essential oil is extracted from the root. In Britain and mainland Europe, an age-old custom consisted of boiling Angelica stalks in sugar and eating them as candy or using them as cake decorations. Both *A. sylvestris* and *Ligusticum scoticum* have been used for medicinal purposes in a similar way to Angelica, but they are said to be less effective and there are fewer references to them.

Action

Carminative, antispasmodic, expectorant, diaphoretic, diuretic, antibacterial, antifungal, emmenagogue, cholagogue, and stimulates blood circulation.

. . . .

Uses

Angelica has been a popular medicinal herb for centuries for respiratory diseases such as colds, coughs, sore throats, influenza, bronchitis, and asthma, especially for the fevers that accompany these illnesses. It is also considered very good for bloating, sluggish digestion, loss of appetite, flatulence, and colon spasms. Angelica stimulates blood circulation to the outer limbs and is said to work well against both atherosclerosis and Buerger's Disease, the symptoms of which are constriction of the veins in the hands and feet. It is also considered effective for benign enlargement of the prostate gland, frequent urination, and cystitis. Angelica has been used for arthritis, both internally and externally, and has been given to those who are recuperating after a chronic illness, especially to stimulate blood circulation. It is also thought to be diuretic and good for headaches.

Research

In vitro testing on the essential oil of Angelica root has shown that it has antiseizure properties.[1]

When the effects of two isolated constituents, one from the seed of Angelica and the other from the root of *Peucedanum ostruthium*, were compared to known seizure medication, their anticonvulsant properties were found to be similar to that of the medication.[2,3] Icelandic research with *in vitro* tests has revealed that a blend of Angelica and Wood Cranesbill has inhibiting effects on the breakdown of the enzyme acetylcholinesterase, which indicates that Angelica might have a positive effect on memory.[4] Further Icelandic *in vitro* research studies on the essential oil, a tincture of Angelica seeds, and an extract from the leaves have shown inhibiting effects on the growth of cancer cells.[5-7] Research on isolated constituents of Angelica root has revealed positive effects on liver and skin cells and inhibiting effects on *Helicobacter pylori,* which causes gastritis and stomach ulcers.[8] *In vitro* and *in vivo* tests show that Angelica has a positive effect on liver damage caused by alcohol use[9] and it also heals stomach ulcers,[10] as well as being antifungal, antibacterial, antispasmodic, sedative, anti-inflammatory, and analgesic. These tests also show that Angelica stimulates uterine contractions[11] and dilates veins.[12]

Dosage

Tincture: 2–5 ml (leaves), 0.5–2 ml (root), 1–3 ml (seeds) three times a day (1:5, 40%).

Infusion: 1–2 teaspoons in a cup three times a day.

Decoction: 1 teaspoon in a cup, boiled for 2 minutes and allowed to stand for about 15 minutes. 1 cup three times a day.

Warning

It is not recommended to use *A. archangelica* or other Angelica species during pregnancy. Angelica can cause photosensitivity, so sun tanning and tanning lamps are not recommended while using the herb. There is a possibility that Angelica could affect blood-thinning medication. The use of Angelica should be stopped 1 week before planned surgery.

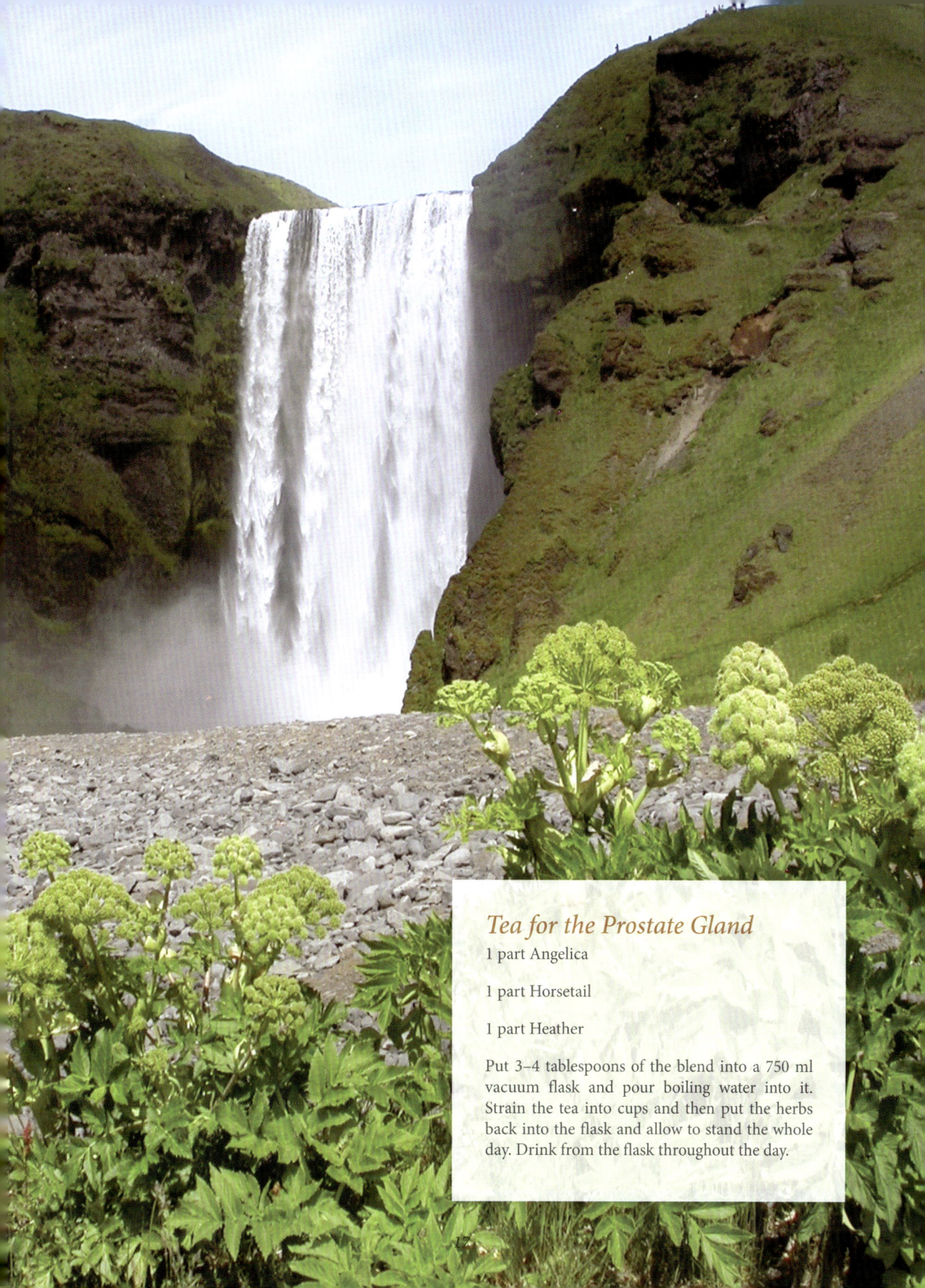

Tea for the Prostate Gland

1 part Angelica

1 part Horsetail

1 part Heather

Put 3–4 tablespoons of the blend into a 750 ml vacuum flask and pour boiling water into it. Strain the tea into cups and then put the herbs back into the flask and allow to stand the whole day. Drink from the flask throughout the day.

Arctic Poppy

Papaver radicatum
Papaveraceae—Melasól

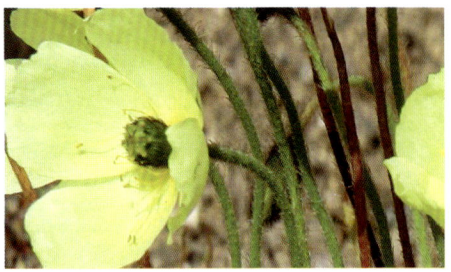

Habitat

Arctic Poppy grows mainly in the West Fjords and East Iceland and is rare elsewhere in the country. It is usually yellow, but can also have white or pink flowers although these are very rare so are protected.

Parts Used

Flower.

Harvesting

Arctic Poppy is collected in bloom in June.

Constituents

Not known.

History

The most well known species of the Papaveraceae family is the Opium Poppy (*P. somniferum*), which was popular in tincture form in Europe in the 16th century for its sedative effects. It is also narcotic and addictive and was therefore quickly abused. Morphine, codeine, and heroin are all processed from the Opium Poppy. Mature Poppy seeds do not have any narcotic effects and are used mainly in baking. In Iceland these seeds are called Birch seeds, despite there being no relation to Birch at all.

The Old Icelandic name for Arctic Poppy is "sleep grass." There are very few references to its use as a medicinal herb, either in Iceland or in other countries. Iceland Poppy (*P. croceum*) is an imported species that grows sparsely around farmhouses, but there is little reference to its medicinal use. Iceland Poppy is thought to be analgesic and good for scurvy as the leaves contain vitamin C. The flowers and leaves are also thought to be mild diaphoretics. Iceland Poppy is slightly toxic compared to Opium Poppy. However, there is reason to be cautious when using both it and Arctic Poppy.

Action

Sedative and analgesic.

Uses

It is not known if Arctic Poppy is used in Western herbal medicine nowadays. In the past, it was considered useful for insomnia and as a painkiller.

Dosage

Tincture: 1–2 ml three times a day (1:5, 40%).

Infusion: ½ teaspoon in a cup three times a day.

Warning

Large doses of Arctic Poppy are not recommended and it should not be given to children or taken during pregnancy.

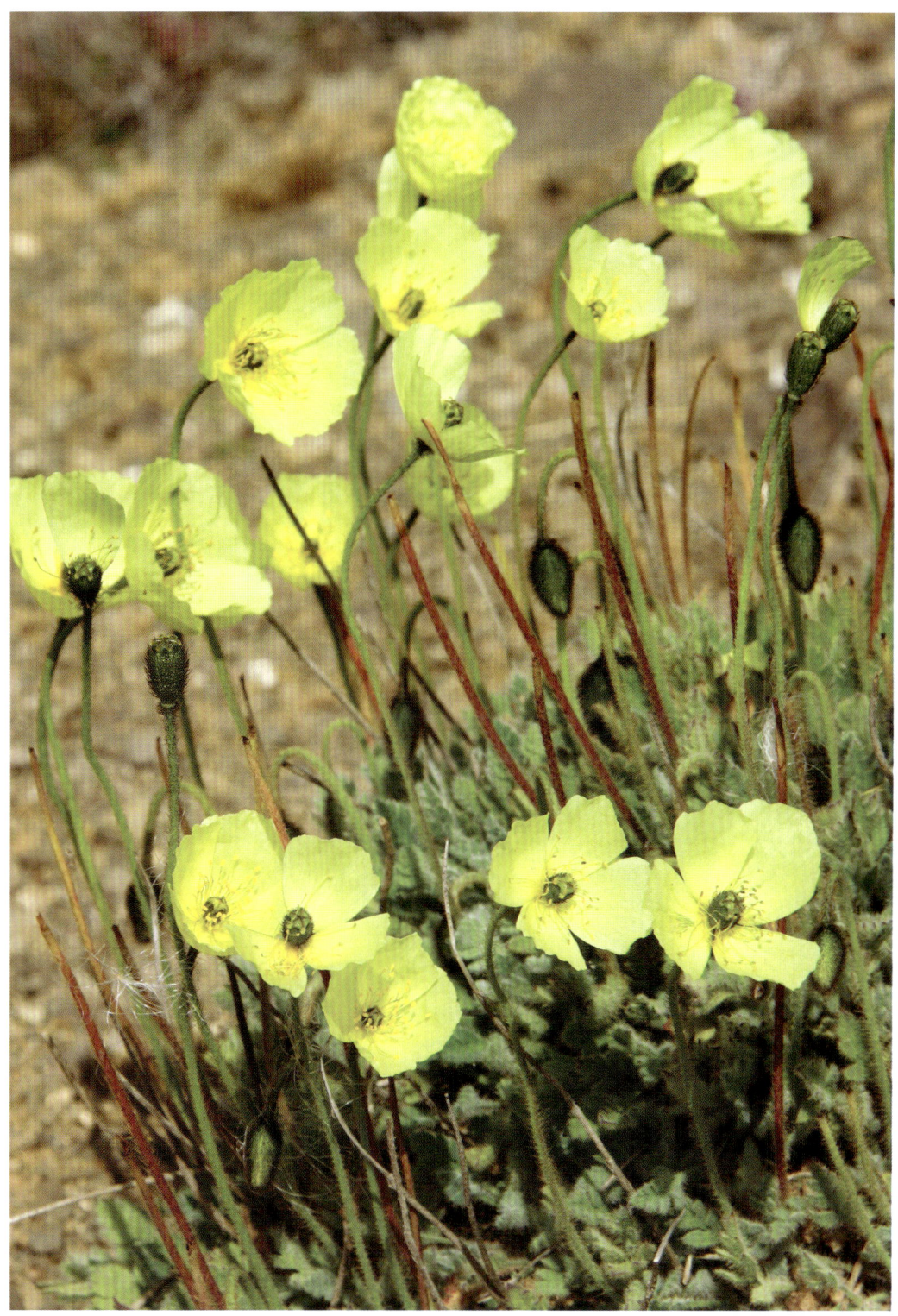

Bearberry

Arctostaphylos uva-ursi
Ericaceae—Sortulyng

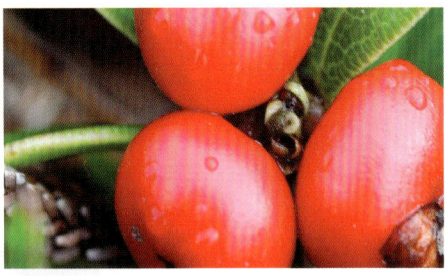

Habitat

Bearberry is common all over Iceland and grows mainly on heaths and woodlands.

Parts Used

Leaves.

Harvesting

Bearberry is collected in early summer.

Constituents

Hydroquinones (arbutin), iridoids, flavonoids (quercitrin), polyphenolic acids, triterpenes, tannins, and essential oils.

History

The berries of Bearberry are called "lice crumbs" in Icelandic, as it was believed that one would become infested with lice if they were eaten. The English name and the Latin *uva-ursi* both mean "bear's berry," which refers to bears' love for the berries.

References to Bearberry can be found dating back to the 13th century and it has been a popular medicinal herb ever since. In the past it was used to make ink, tan leather, and dye yarn. An extract was made from the berries and used as a sauce with meals as it was thought to stimulate blood and increase appetite. The berries were also preserved in sugar, vinegar, and wine. Old Icelandic folklore states that it is good to carry Bearberry on the body as this would protect against evil spirits and ghosts.

Native Americans have a long tradition of using Bearberry for healing. For instance, they used it for urinary tract infections and to strengthen the kidneys and bladder. Bearberry was thought to be diuretic and it was also used both to stimulate and to reduce menstrual bleeding and to prevent miscarriage. It was also considered to be good for colds, coughs, blood spitting, backache, and diarrhea, while the fresh berries were thought to be laxative. The Native Americans also used Bearberry externally (e.g., for rashes, wounds, itching, abscesses, burns, acne, dandruff, disorders of the scalp, and for promoting hair growth). They used it as a rinse for gingivitis, mouth ulcers, and conjunctivitis, and an infusion of Bearberry was used to bathe those who were afflicted with broken bones and arthritis.

Bearberry was mixed with tobacco and smoked at holy ceremonies; it was used as a hallucinatory drug, for headaches, and for good luck. Smoke from the leaves was also thought to be good for earache. In addition, the leaves were burned to drive away evil spirits, and were placed in a shoe when a spouse died to protect against evil. The Native Americans ate the berries in many different ways (e.g., fresh, sugared, fried, in

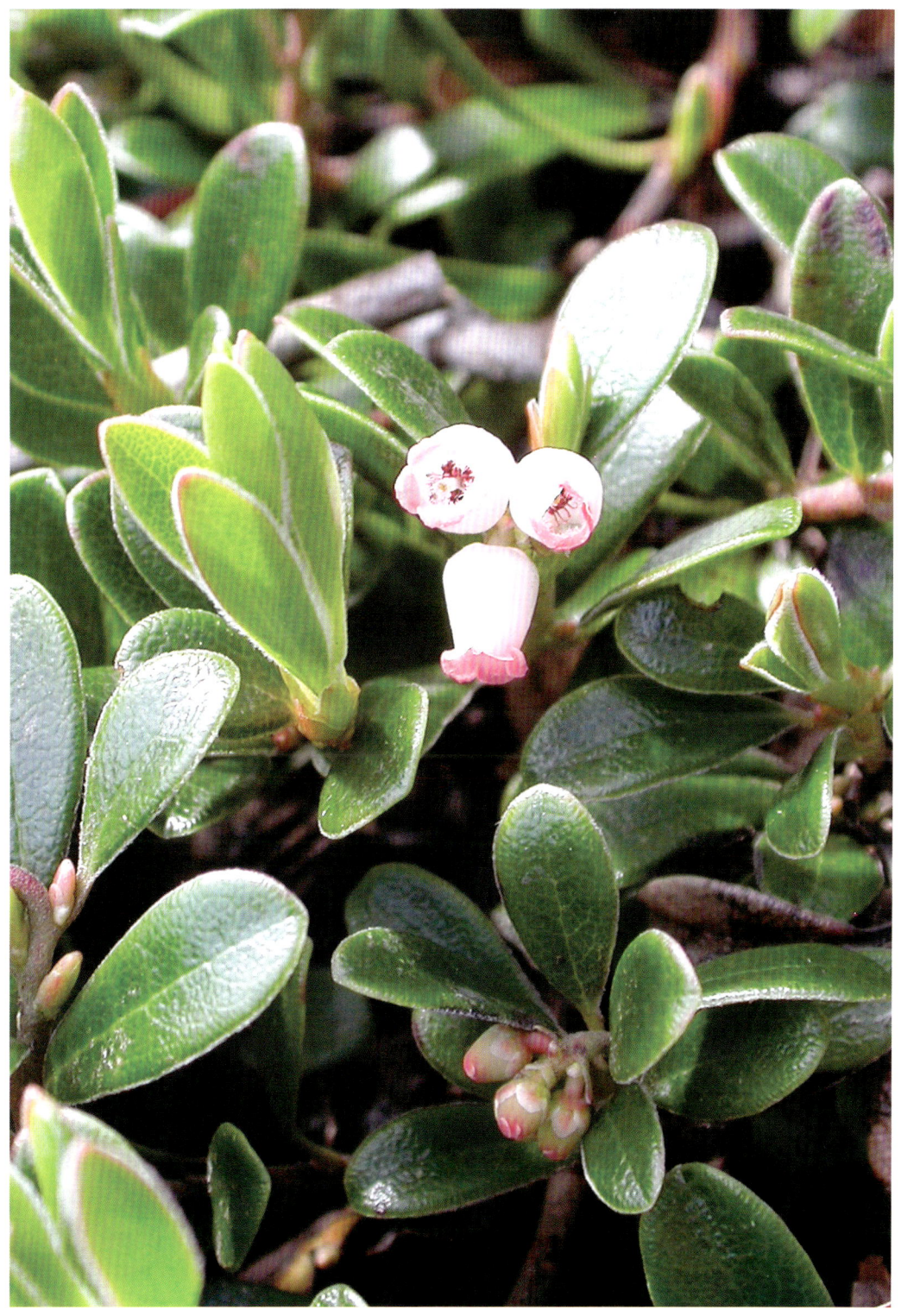

soups and oil, with salmon roe, ice cream, meat, and fish).

Action

Diuretic, astringent, antibacterial, and vulnerary. Good for urinary infections.

. . . .

Uses

Bearberry is first and foremost an effective medicinal herb for the urinary system. It has a tonic effect on the mucous membrane of the ureter and is used extensively for both chronic and acute cystitis and other infections and inflammation in the urinary system. However, Bearberry is not recommended if there is an existing kidney infection. Bearberry is also traditionally used for bladder and kidney stones and for sores in the kidneys or bladder. Bearberry is also thought to be good for children who wet the bed. It can be used for heavy menstrual bleeding and menstrual cramps and as a douche for vaginal infections. Bearberry has also been used for diarrhea and dysentery because of its astringent properties. There are references to the use of Bearberry for diabetes, arthritis, and sexually transmitted diseases, and for strengthening eyesight. Bearberry is thought to be good for healing wounds and skin disorders.

People are advised to drink plenty of liquid when taking Bearberry and to avoid acid-forming food (i.e., food that lowers the pH-balance of the body), such as fruit juice and acid-forming fruit.

Research

Clinical research has revealed the strong antibacterial properties of Bearberry, but only when the urine is alkaline (pH 8); when the urine was more acidic (pH 6) there was no effect.[1] *In vitro* tests on Bearberry have shown that it has antibacterial function[2-4] and an antiviral effect on the herpes simplex virus 2, the influenza virus A2, and the vaccinia virus,[4] as well as antioxidant[5] and anti-inflammatory effects.[4,6,7] Research has also shown that Bearberry has diuretic action[8] but has no effect on kidney stones.[9] Other research on Bearberry has revealed its antitussive[4] effects and its

lightening effect on the skin.[10] One of Bearberry's active constituents is hydroquinone, which lightens the skin,[4,10] and so it is used in cosmetics for this reason. In the USA, England, and Nigeria it is forbidden to use more than 2% of hydroquinone in cosmetics, as it has come to light that a higher percentage could cause skin diseases. Cases are also known in which a percentage lower than 2% has caused skin diseases and allergic reactions.[4]

Dosage

Tincture: 2–4 ml three times a day (1:5, 25%).

Cold infusion: 1–2 teaspoons in a cup of cold water, allowed to steep overnight. 1 cup three times a day.

A pinch of bicarbonate of soda is added to the infusion as this is said to increase the efficacy of it.

Infusions, tinctures, compresses, and ointments for external use.

Warning

Pregnant and lactating women should not use Bearberry; the same applies to those with kidney disease. Neither large doses nor continuous use for more than 2 weeks at a time are recommended. Large doses of Bearberry can cause vomiting.

Tea for Cystitis

2 parts Bearberry

1 part Heather

1 part Lady's Bedstraw

Put 3–4 tablespoons of the blend into a 750 ml vacuum flask and pour boiling water into it. Sieve the tea into cups and then put the herbs back into the flask and allow to stand the whole day. Drink from the flask throughout the day.

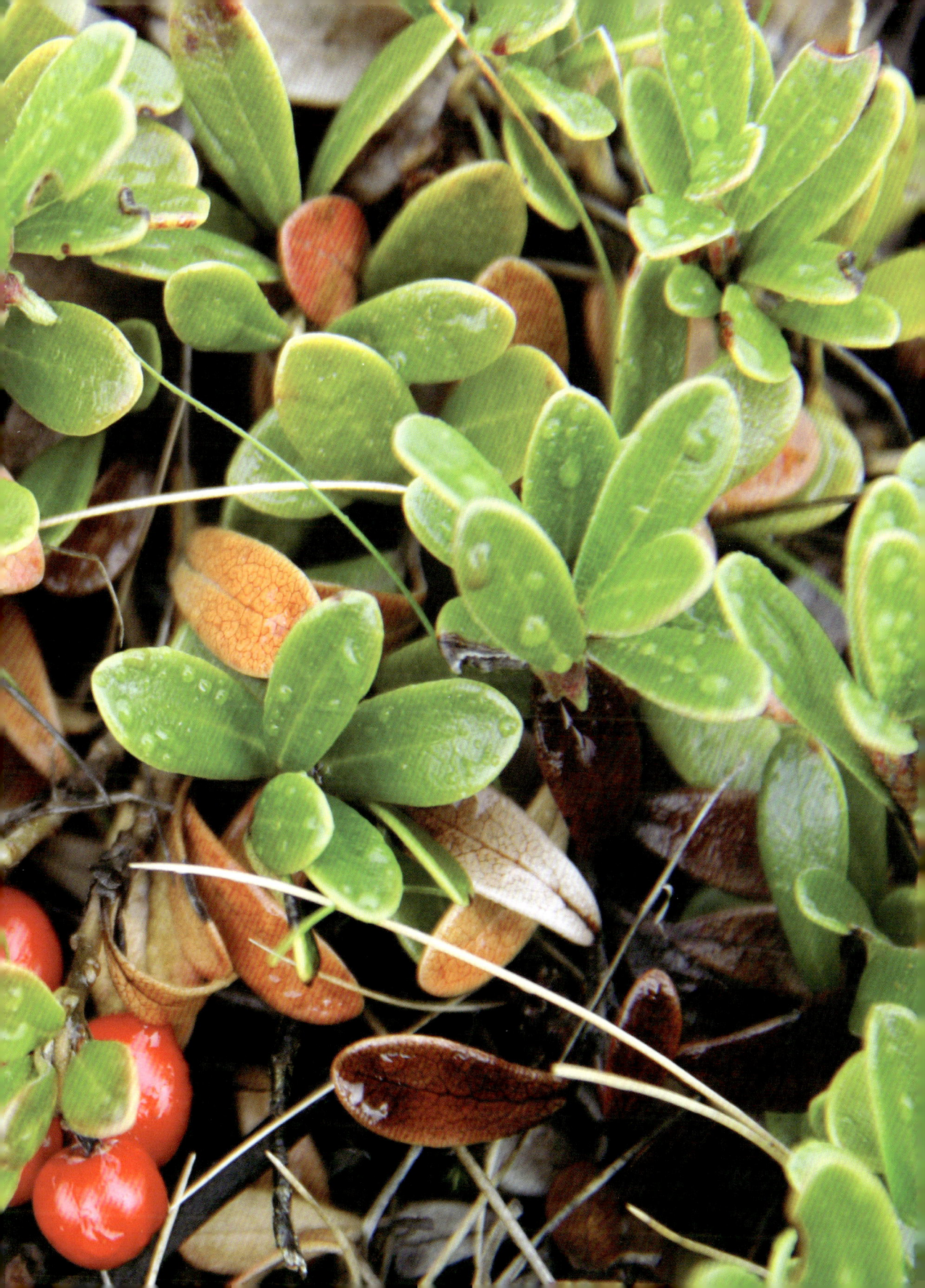

Bilberry

Vaccinium myrtillus
Ericaceae—*Aðalbláber*

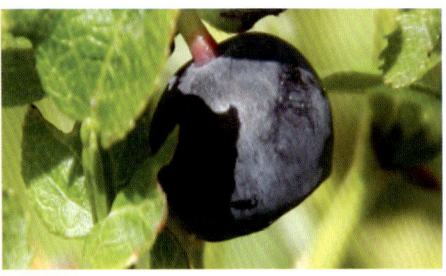

Habitat

Found all over Iceland except for the South.

Parts Used

Berries and leaves.

Harvesting

Leaves are collected in early summer, while berries are picked in late autumn.

Constituents

Berries: Anthocyanosides, vitamins A, B, and C, tannins, pectin, and organic acids. Leaves: Tannins, flavonoids (quercetin), caffeic acid, and organic acids.

History

Bilberry has been used in healing for at least one thousand years, but reference to its use as a medicine in Germany dates back to the 12th century. Bilberry was first researched in Britain during World War II when it was given to pilots in the form of Bilberry jam, with the belief that it improved vision, particularly for night flights. Ever since then, the effects of Bilberry on vision and eye diseases have been researched. Before insulin was discovered, Bilberry leaves were used to lower blood sugar.

Bilberry is rich in nutrients and has a long use as a culinary herb, particularly to make juices, jams, and desserts. In Iceland, a popular dish is made with Bilberries, Icelandic skyr, and cream. The berries have also been used to dye yarn. Dried Bilberries, often as a standardized extract in capsule form, have been used as a popular food supplement in North America and Europe for the past few decades. In comparison, Blueberries (*Vaccinium uliginosum*) have been less used for medicinal purposes and have not been researched as much as the Bilberry. This does not mean, however, that the Blueberry is not an effective healing herb.

Action

Astringent, anti-inflammatory, diuretic, antibacterial, antioxidant, hypoglycemic, and nourishing. Strengthens the eyes and venous system.

Uses

Traditionally, the berries were used, dried and boiled, for diarrhea, especially in children. They are antibacterial and are effective against *Helicobacter pylori*, which causes gastritis and stomach ulcers. They are also known to help colitis. Fresh Bilberry contains fructose, which stimulates digestion and has laxative properties. The berries and leaves are reported to be good for gingivitis and sore throats, externally for healing wounds, and as a douche for vaginal discharges. Both the berries and leaves are

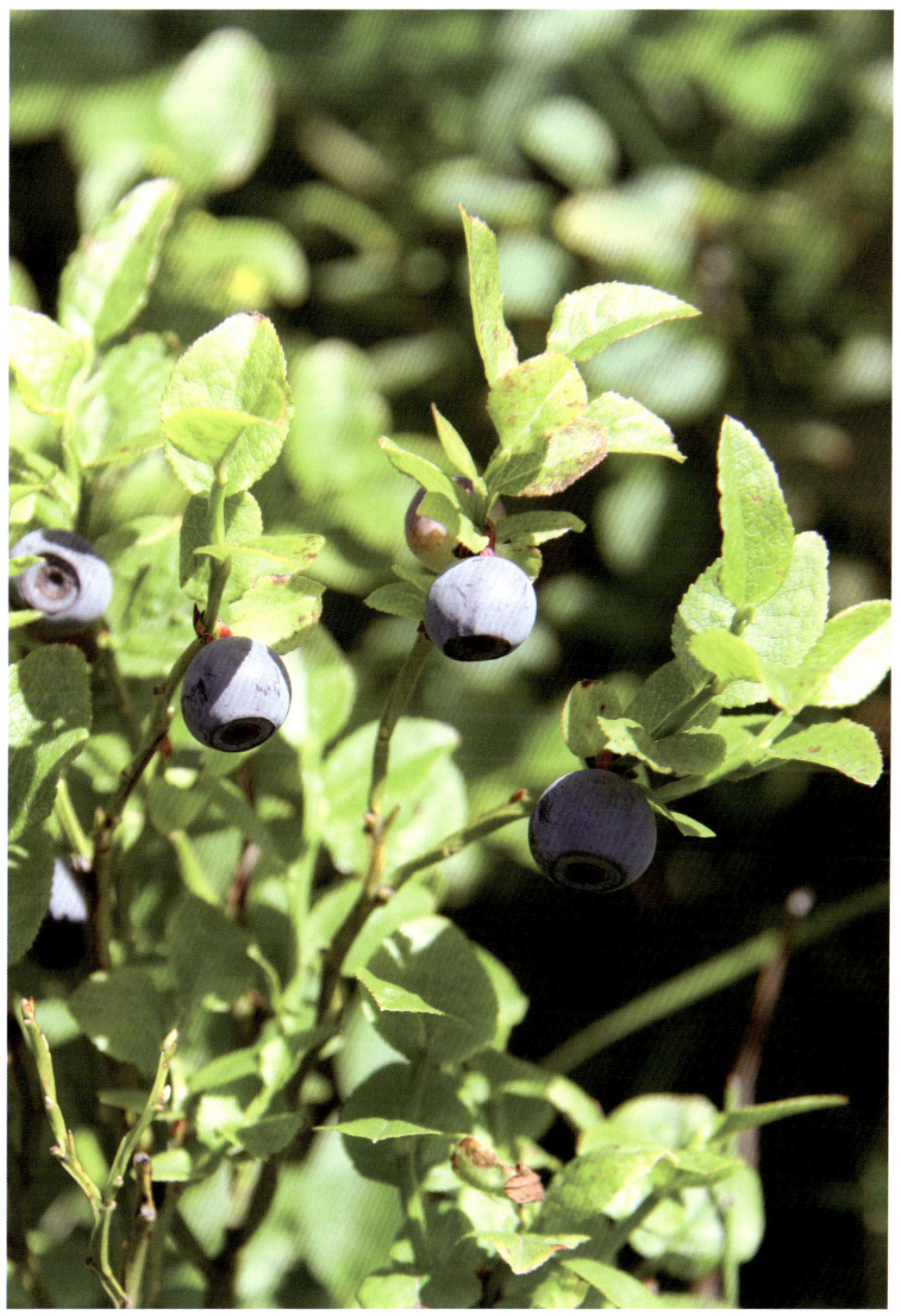

diuretic and good for cystitis and are traditionally used to lower blood sugar. They are good for relieving period pains.

Bilberries have a high antioxidant content, which is thought to boost the immune system, lessen the danger of cardiovascular disease, and reduce wrinkles. They are reputed to be effective against varicose veins, vasculitis, atherosclerosis, Raynaud's Disease, hemorrhoids, and nose-bleeds. They also strengthen capillary veins. Bilberries have long been popular for a variety of eye diseases and for retinal diseases related to high blood pressure and diabetes. They are thought to strengthen eyesight and are considered effective against glaucoma, cataracts, and night blindness. Bilberries are rich in vitamins and have also been used against anemia and scurvy.

Research

In much of the following research, Bilberry extract in capsule form was used in which the active compound, anthocyanoside, had been standardized.

Various human clinical studies have been done to find out the effectiveness of Bilberry on eyesight, the oldest trials being from the 1970s. Recent double-blind trials using a placebo are better than the older trials, and in most cases confirm older research. These clinical trials indicate the positive effects of Bilberry on retinal diseases and eye diseases related to high blood pressure as well as those related to diabetes, night blindness, glaucoma, nearsightedness, and cataracts,[1-6] though recent studies have debunked older research, to some extent, on night blindness.[7,8] Additionally, in vitro and in vivo tests show positive effects of Bilberry in the treatment of eye disease.[9-15]

There has been some clinical research on the effectiveness of Bilberry in the treatment of vascular disease, with positive results (e.g., Raynaud's Disease, varicose veins, hemorrhoids and vasculitis). Bilberry is also thought to reduce edema, pain, cramps, and itching due to dysfunction in the vascular system.[16-21] Two clinical trials show that Bilberry reduces bleeding between periods caused by IUDs[22] and also surgical bleeding.[23] Several in vitro and in vivo tests indicate that Bilberry strengthens the cardiovascular system and protects against atherosclerosis.[24-30]

In vitro testing shows that Bilberry has a high concentration of antioxidants[31-43] and the berries also have anti-inflammatory properties.[1] Both in vitro and in vivo testing show that Bilberry inhibits the growth of cancer cells, particularly in the colon and breast, as well as in leukemia.[44-53] In one such test, it became apparent that out of the 10 different berry types that were researched, Bilberry was the most effective.[54]

In vitro tests on both leaves and berries show antibacterial properties.[55] Bilberry leaves are effective against tuberculosis bacteria[56] and the berries are considered to be active against Streptococcus pneumonia, the cause of pneumonia, meningitis, and otitis.[57] It has also been shown that Bilberry is effective against Helicobacter pylori, which causes gastritis and stomach ulcers,[58,59] and on the parasite Giardia duodenalis, a common cause of diarrhea.[60] Both leaves and berries of Bilberry have been used traditionally to lower blood sugar; some research confirms this efficacy,[61,62] and some does not.[63] Some research has also indicated that the external application of Bilberry can protect the skin from the damaging effects of the sun.[64,65] In addition, one clinical trial showed that Bilberry could be effective for period pains and premenstrual tension.[66]

Although Blueberry (Vaccinium uliginosum) has not been researched as much as Bilberry, some recent research has been done on it. In vitro testing on Blueberry shows its inhibitory effect on cancer cells,[67,68] its lowering effect on blood sugar,[69] and its antioxidant properties.[70,71] In addition, in vitro tests show that Blueberry reduces necrosis and the damaging effect of light on the retina, increasing the possibility of retinal repair after damage caused by light.[72]

Dosage

Tincture: 1–5 ml three times a day (1:5, 40%).

Infusion: 1–2 teaspoons in a cup three times a day.

Decoction: 1–2 teaspoons in a cup three times a day.

Fresh berries: 1–2 tablespoons three times a day.

Infusions, decoctions, tinctures, compresses, and ointments for external use.

Warning

When taken for an extended period of time, large doses of standardized capsules of Bilberry extract can have an effect on blood-thinning medication. Diabetes patients who take insulin should not consume Bilberry leaves without consulting a specialist. It is not advisable to use Bilberry leaf for longer than 3 weeks at a time.

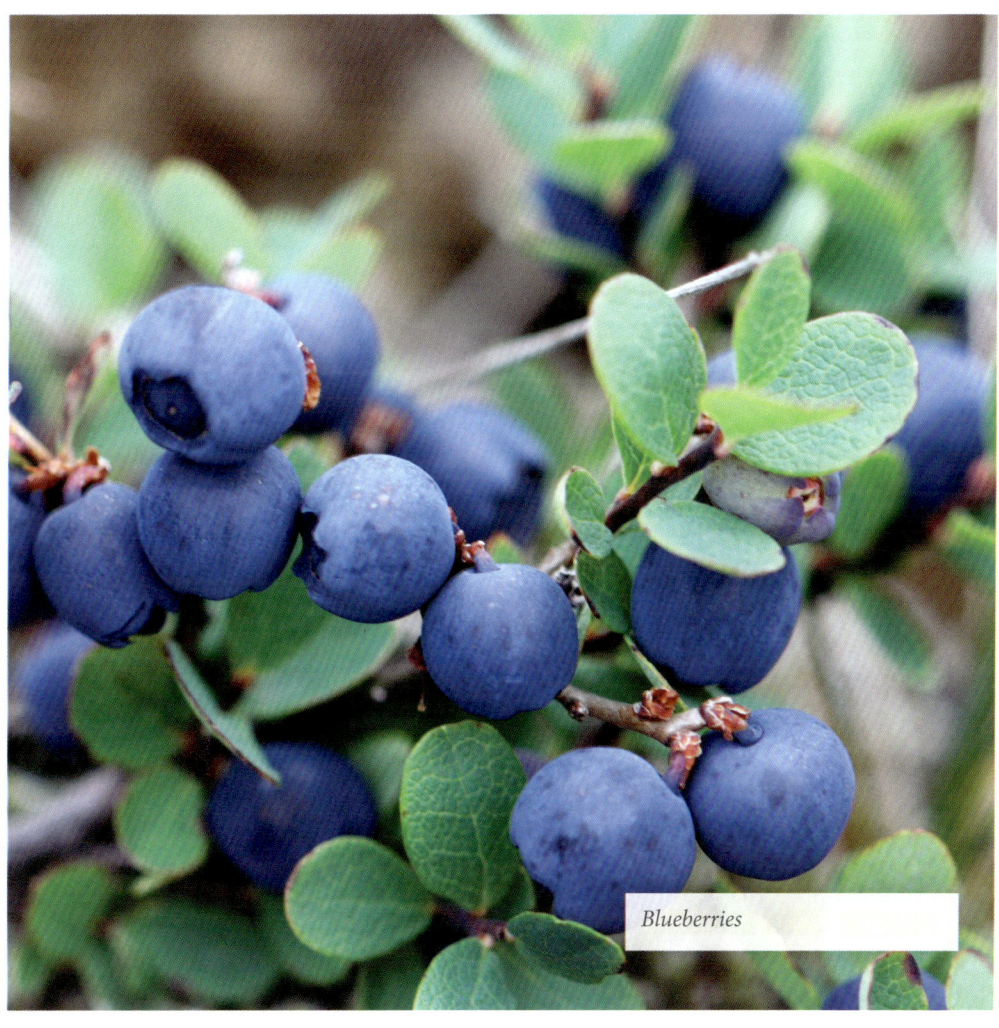

Blueberries

Biting Stonecrop

Sedum acre

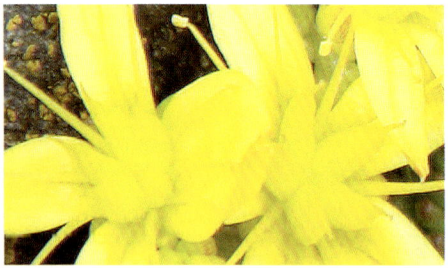

Crassulaceae—Helluhnoðri

Habitat

Biting Stonecrop is found all over Iceland and grows mainly in gravel, cliffs, and scree.

Parts Used

The entire plant is used, except for the root.

Harvesting

Biting Stonecrop is collected all summer.

Constituents

Flavonoids (rutin), alkaloids, mucilage, and tannins.

History

The Latin name *acre* indicates that the leaves have a strong taste. Other English names (e.g., Wall pepper and Wall ginger, also refer to the taste). In older times, Biting Stonecrop was part of a well-known British recipe for eliminating worms from the bowels. Another old Latin name is *vermicularis*, which indicates that Biting Stonecrop was thought to be auspicious for

> This herb is blood cleansing, fluid thinning, dissolving, and prevents infection. It causes vomiting and diarrhea. It is therefore good against scurvy, kidney stones, colds, coughs, constipation and impurities in the stomach.
>
> *Oddur Jónsson Hjaltalín,*
> Icelandic Botany, *1830*

killing worms; the appearance of the plant indeed resembles worms.

In old sources, there are conflicting opinions about whether Biting Stonecrop was good as a medicine; some found it useful for various things, others were against it on the grounds that, due to its strength and toxicity, it was not thought safe to use, especially internally. It has been used for scurvy, both as a mouthwash for gingivitis and in an infusion to wash wounds characteristic of scurvy. Biting Stonecrop has also been used for edema, fever, cancer, and epilepsy as well as for lowering blood pressure. The herbalist Pliny, who lived around AD 60, recommended Biting Stonecrop for insomnia but not for internal use: "Wrap the herb in a black cloth and place it under the pillow of the patient, without his knowledge, otherwise it will have no effect." In China, many species related to Biting Stonecrop are used topically to heal wounds.

Action

Astringent, rubefacient, causes blisters, removes warts, vulnerary.

Uses

Biting Stonecrop is not used much in Western herbal medicine today. The fresh juice from the leaves is used on warts and corns. Be careful that the juice does not get onto the skin as it can cause blisters. It is also possible to use the juice to heal

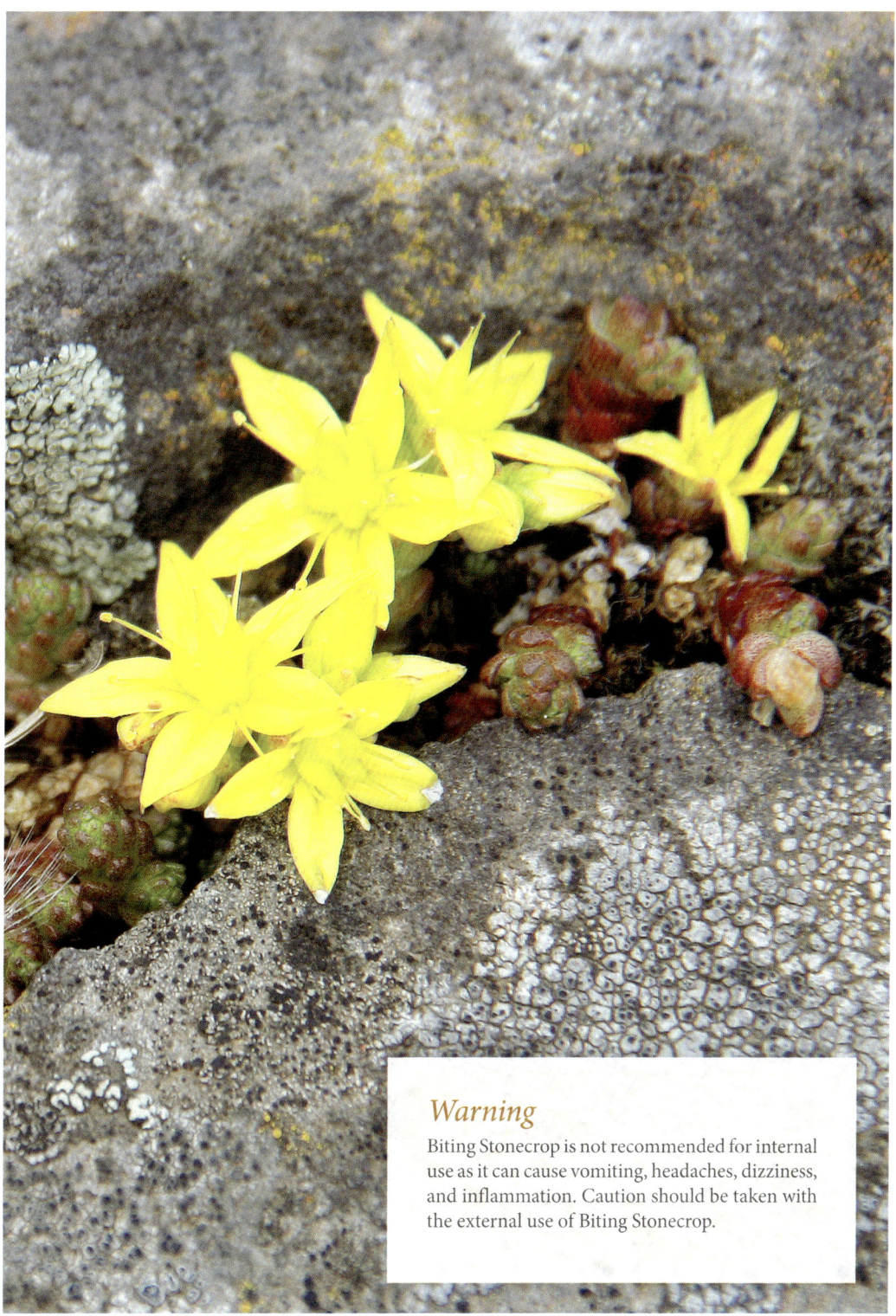

Warning

Biting Stonecrop is not recommended for internal use as it can cause vomiting, headaches, dizziness, and inflammation. Caution should be taken with the external use of Biting Stonecrop.

Bladderwrack

Fucus vesiculosus
Fucaceae—Bóluþang

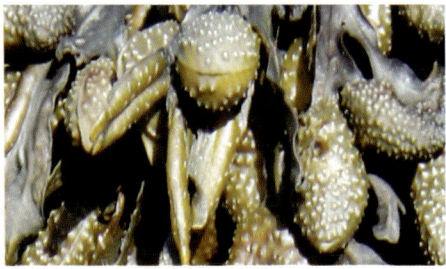

Habitat

Bladderwrack is common on stony beaches all over Iceland.

Parts Used

The entire seaweed.

Harvesting

Early summer.

Constituents

Phenols, polysaccharides (fucoidan), iodine, vitamins, and minerals.

History

It was traditionally used as a fertilizer for potatoes and vegetables in Iceland and Britain. Bladderwrack is rich in minerals and is ideal for cooking (e.g., in soups); the newly formed fronds are best for eating. Iodine used to be extracted from Bladderwrack.

Action

Stimulates the thyroid gland, stimulates metabolism, and is nourishing.

Uses

Bladderwrack is thought to stimulate the production of thyroid hormones and is traditionally used for hypothyroidism. When weight gain is caused by an underactive thyroid, Bladderwrack can help the person lose weight. It is also considered to be effective for arthritis, used both internally and externally.

Research

Most of the following research is based on the isolated polysaccharide fucoidan that is found in Bladderwrack. Both *in vitro* and *in vivo* tests indicate the blood-thinning properties of fucoidan. In one such test it was shown that fucoidan had a much stronger effect than the blood-thinning drug heparin.[1-5] Bladderwrack is also an antioxidant[6-11] and anti-inflammatory.[3,4] It lowers cholesterol[12] and blood sugar,[13] heals wounds,[14] protects the skin against aging[15] and prolongs the menstrual cycle.[12] Research shows that Bladderwrack stimulates the immune system,[16-18] protects white blood cells against radiation,[19] and has an inhibiting effect on HIV[20] as well as cancer cells.[4,21] Research also shows that it reduces oxalates in urine, a high content of which indicates the presence of kidney stones.[22]

Dosage

Tincture: 4–8 ml three times a day (1:5, 25%).

Infusion: 1–2 teaspoons in a cup three times a day.

Infusions, tinctures, compresses, and ointments used externally.

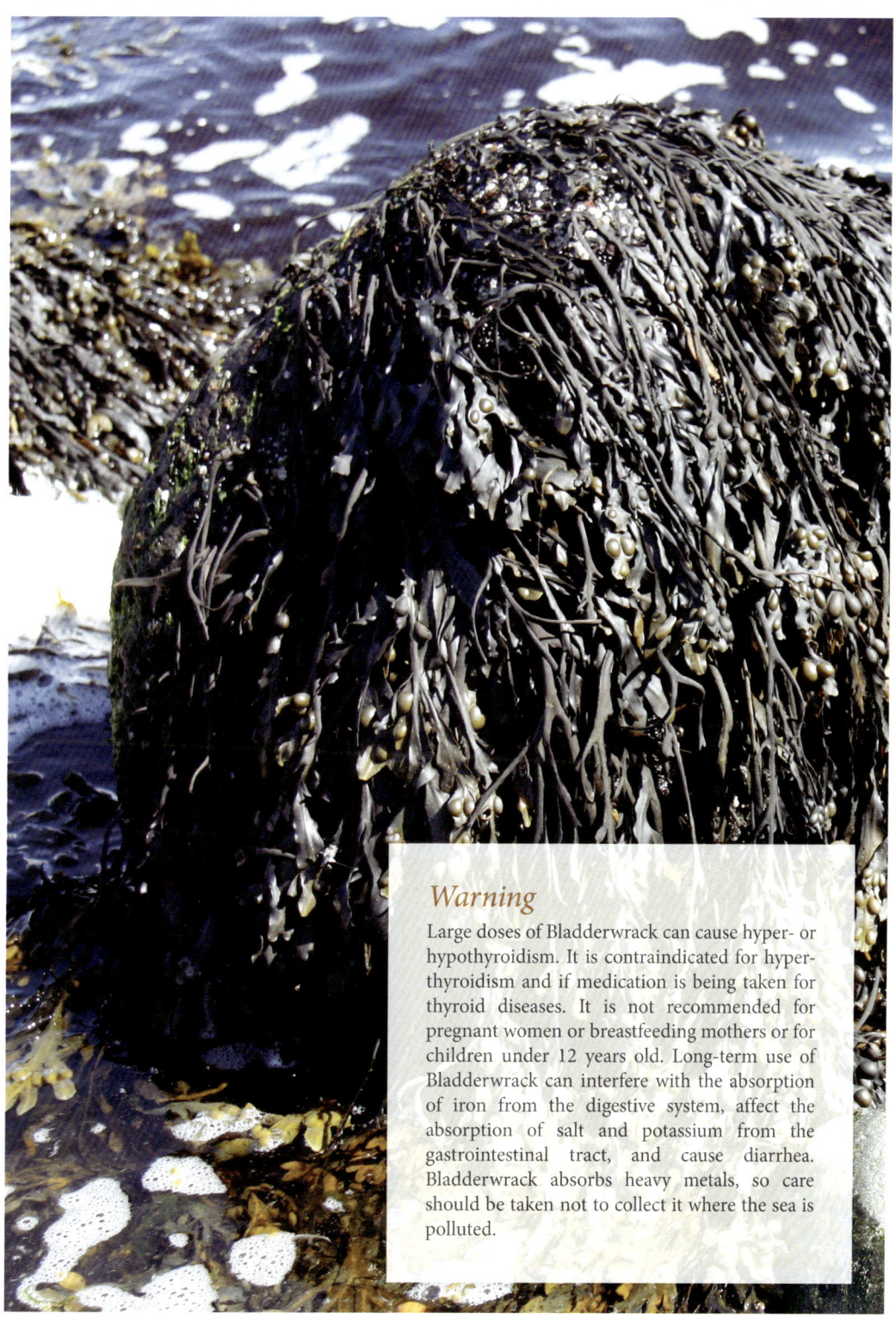

Warning

Large doses of Bladderwrack can cause hyper- or hypothyroidism. It is contraindicated for hyperthyroidism and if medication is being taken for thyroid diseases. It is not recommended for pregnant women or breastfeeding mothers or for children under 12 years old. Long-term use of Bladderwrack can interfere with the absorption of iron from the digestive system, affect the absorption of salt and potassium from the gastrointestinal tract, and cause diarrhea. Bladderwrack absorbs heavy metals, so care should be taken not to collect it where the sea is polluted.

Bogbean

Menyanthes trifoliata
Menyanthaceae—*Horblaðka*

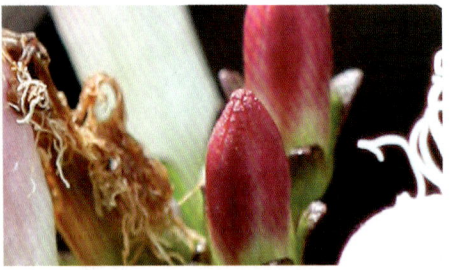

Habitat

Bogbean is common all over Iceland and grows in wetlands and small lakes.

Parts Used

Leaves.

Harvesting

Bogbean is collected after blooming in June.

Constituents

Iridoids, alkaloids, lactones, flavonoids (rutin), triterpenes and phenolic acids.

History

The Icelandic name "Horblaðka" (emaciation leaf) arose because the plant is so bitter that livestock would starve to death rather than eat it. Another name for Bogbean is Riding Grass, as rhizomes of the plant, which are both tough and firm, were believed to make good back protection for packhorses. The names "kveisugras" (colic herb) and "ólúagras" (not tired herb) were also used for Bogbean and refer to its healing powers.

This herb is considered to be particularly good against scurvy and leprosy, edema and joint pain, also for foot pain, and with the last-mentioned it works best in unboiled milk. It is very good for paralysis, also for colds, colic, stomach and colon pain, and eye diseases. It works against fatigue and kills worms in people, drunk both as a juice, pressed from the herb, and also as a decoction. The herb can be steeped in ale and then it becomes a blood cleanser and is healthy for depressed people. Poor folk in Sweden brew the herb instead of hops, which makes a healthy but not tasty ale. Bitter, it is said to be, and so is the bread made in hard times from the root of this herb. For this, the roots are collected, ground and cooked together with flour of rye and other grains.

Björn Halldórsson, Uses of Herbs, *1783*

Of all the Icelandic medicinal herbs, Bogbean is by far the most bitter. The Native Americans have been using Bogbean as a medicinal herb for a very long time. Unlike European herbalists, they have also used the root, not just the leaves. Bogbean is thought to be good against colds and flu, flatulence, constipation, and arthritis. It was also used for stomach cramps and blood spitting, and for recuperating after illness. Topically, Bogbean compresses were used for inflammation and snake bites. When life was tough, the roots were also dried and ground down for cooking, even though they were not considered to be tasty. Bogbean has been used to brew beer.

Action

Hepatic, cholagogue, carminative, diuretic, febrifuge, and laxative.

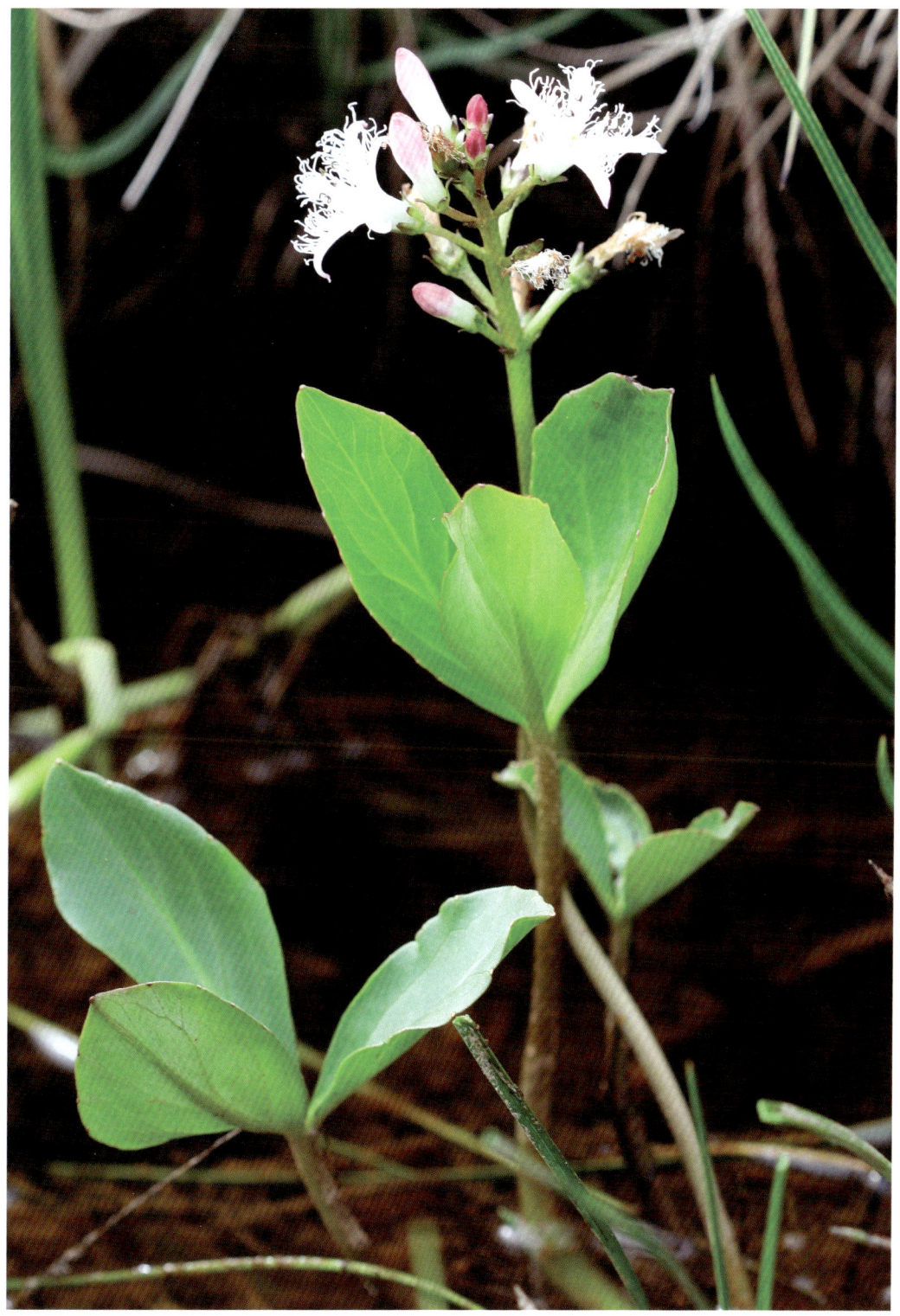

Uses

Bogbean is extremely bitter; bitter herbs characteristically stimulate all digestive juices, which helps in the absorption of nutrients from the digestive tract. It is considered good for liver and gallbladder diseases, as well as being a laxative and relieving colic and flatulence. Bogbean is also used internally for skin diseases, to increase appetite, and to stimulate slow digestion. There is a long tradition of using Bogbean for arthritic diseases such as rheumatism, osteoarthritis, fibromyalgia, and gout, especially when accompanied by little appetite, weight loss, and weakness. Bogbean, like many other bitter herbs, is seldom given alone, but is instead blended with other herbs. In Chinese herbal medicine, Bogbean is thought to be good as an analgesic and hypnotic as well as being a febrifuge.

Research

In vitro tests done at the University of Iceland on Bogbean indicated that it contains active constituents that could possibly help with mitigating autoimmune diseases.[1] *In vitro* research done on 100 herbs showed that Bogbean was one of seven herbs that showed the greatest potential in suppressing the growth of cancer cells.[2] Bogbean has also shown efficacy in balancing the immune system and as an anti-inflammatory.[3] It is also thought that Bogbean could have anticoagulant properties and so have an effect on blood-thinning medication.[4]

Dosage

Tincture: 1–3 ml three times a day (1:5, 25%).

Infusion: 1 teaspoon in a cup three times a day.

Warning

Large doses of Bogbean can cause irritation in the digestive tract, diarrhea, stomach cramps, nausea, vomiting, and headaches. Those suffering from colitis, dysentery, or diarrhea should not take Bogbean. It is not recommended to use Bogbean with blood-thinning medication or during pregnancy.

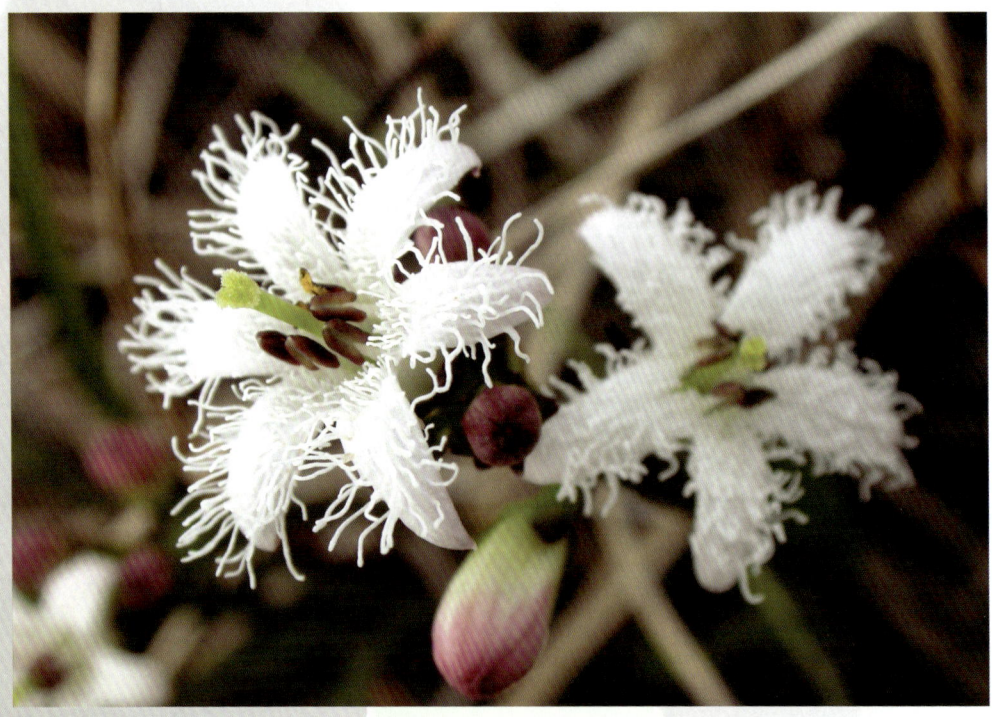

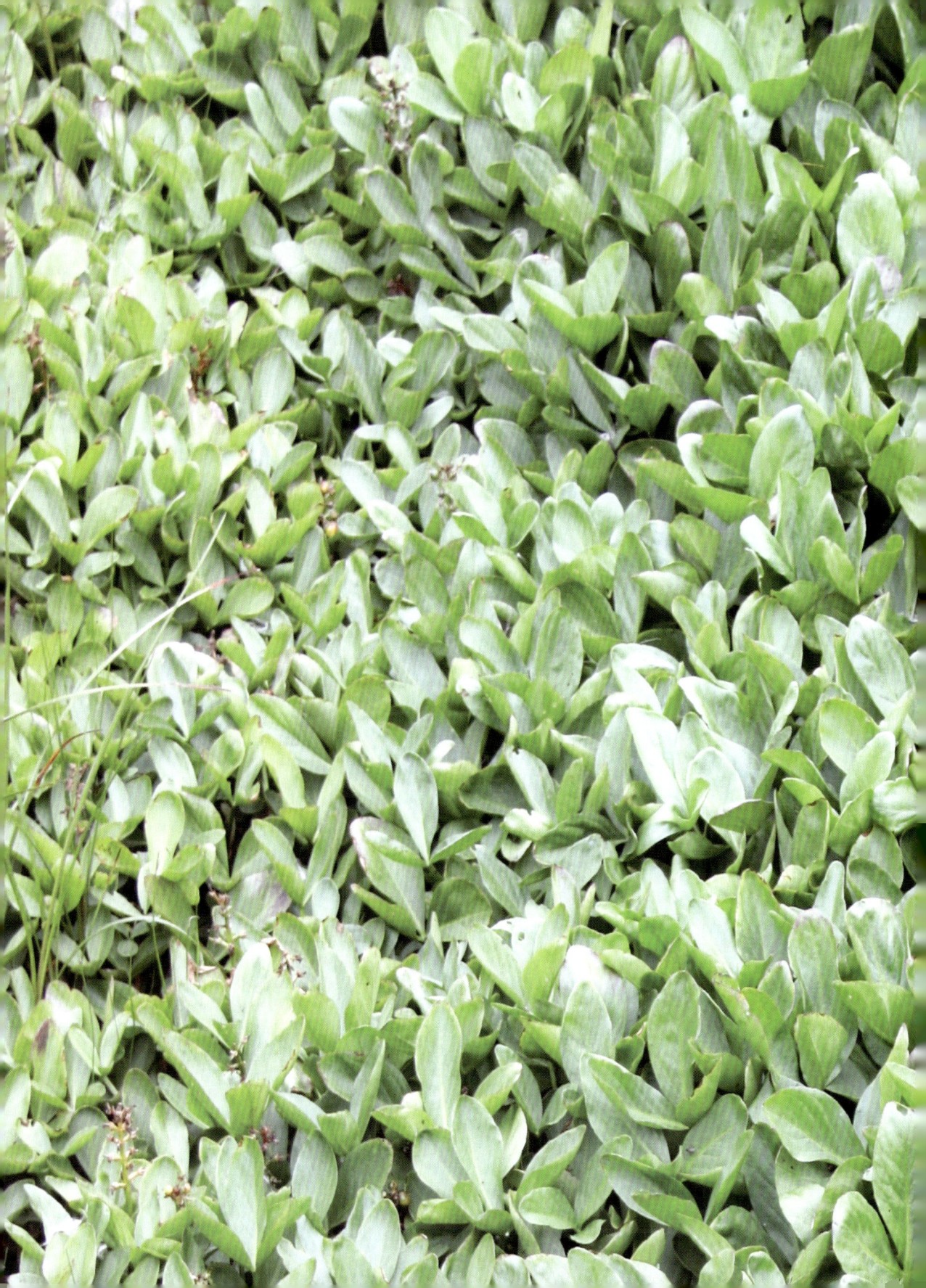

Butterwort

Pinguicula vulgaris
Lentibulariaceae—*Lyfjagras*

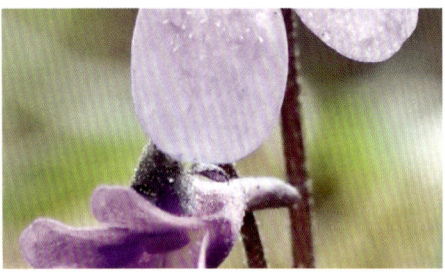

Habitat

Butterwort is common all over Iceland and grows mainly on dry heaths.

Parts Used

Leaves.

Harvesting

The leaves are collected just before bloom in June. Butterwort is rare and is endangered in many countries. Although common in Iceland, it is small and grows sparsely and not in wide expanses, so collection of Butterwort for medicinal purposes is not recommended.

Constituents

Mucilage, tannins, cinnamic, benzoic and valeric acids.

History

The Icelandic name "Lyfjagras" (rennet grass) refers to its use for curdling milk, as this type of rennet used to be called "lyf." Butterwort was used in the past in Welsh herbal medicine for its laxative properties. In Scandinavia, Butterwort was associated with witchcraft and was believed to protect both people and their dwellings, especially livestock, milk, and butter. Canadian Inuits believed that Butterwort brought good luck, and they preserved the dry root so they could enjoy this luck when needed. Butterwort is one of the few herbs in Iceland that is insectivorous: insects stick to its slimy leaves, where they eventually dissolve and are then used for nourishment by the plant.

Action

Antitussive, expectorant, vulnerary, and demulcent.

Uses

Butterwort is not used much in Western herbal medicine nowadays. It was used in the past for coughs and lung diseases and was thought to have similar properties to Sundew, which is still used today for these purposes. Both of these herbs were considered to be very powerful against whooping cough. The fresh leaves were thought to heal chapped skin and sores.

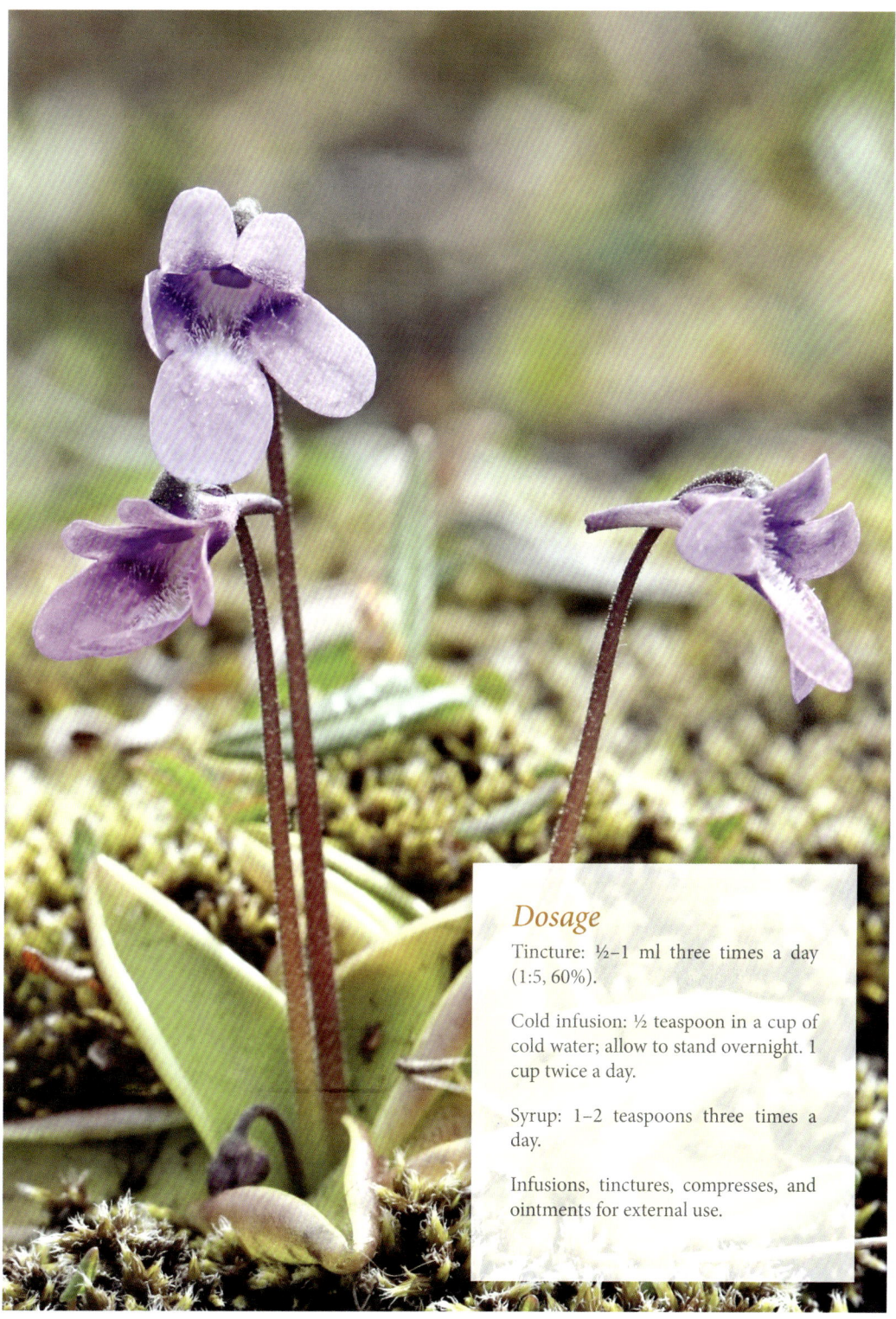

Dosage

Tincture: ½–1 ml three times a day (1:5, 60%).

Cold infusion: ½ teaspoon in a cup of cold water; allow to stand overnight. 1 cup twice a day.

Syrup: 1–2 teaspoons three times a day.

Infusions, tinctures, compresses, and ointments for external use.

Caraway

Carum carvi
Apiaceae—Kúmen

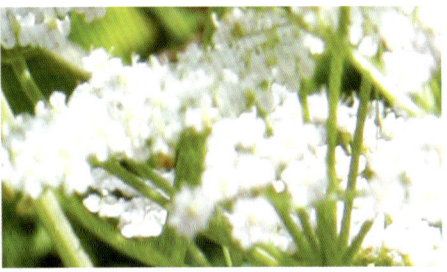

Habitat

Caraway is found mainly in fields in South Iceland and is rather rare in other areas of the country.

Parts Used

Seeds.

Harvesting

Caraway seeds are collected in August.

Constituents

Essential oils, flavonoids (quercitrin), polysaccharides, and oils.

History

Caraway seeds have been used for medicinal purposes for over 5,000 years. The seeds have always been used as a spice (e.g., in soup, bread, cakes, cheese, and wine). In Iceland it was customary to drink Caraway coffee by adding Caraway seeds to coffee before making it. In the past, the roots of Caraway were also used as a vegetable and the leaves were boiled in soups.

The seeds of this herb strengthen the stomach, spread and loosen mucus where it has collected, cure gripe, and thin and cleanse the blood. Spirits, wherein Caraway seeds have lain overnight or longer, have proved good medicine for jaundice, a small sip taken in the mornings. Caraway, a small amount eaten in the morning, is good for stitches, flatulence and also halitosis. It is said to increase the milk in women's breasts and also cure fevers, steeped and drunk in hot ale. For hearing problems, sourdough bread shall be baked with plenty of Caraway and laid warm over the ear or the steam allowed to go through a funnel into the ear.

Björn Halldórsson, Uses of Herbs, 1783

Action

Carminative, expectorant, diuretic, antispasmodic, antibacterial, galactagogue, and emmenagogue.

Uses

For centuries, Caraway seeds have been considered good for stomach cramps, bloating and flatulence. They have traditionally been used to stimulate breast milk and are thought to be good for colic in infants. Caraway seeds are also reputed to work well against respiratory diseases, laryngitis, throat infections, bronchitis, asthma, and coughs. They are used for menstrual pain and to stimulate menstruation. The seeds increase appetite and reduce both edema and diarrhea. In Tibet, Caraway seeds are thought to lower fever, aid digestion, increase appetite, and strengthen eyesight. In India, the seeds are used in a similar way to Western herbalism, but they are also reported effective for eliminating worms. The seeds are also considered good as a diuretic and astringent and, externally, for pain caused by rheumatism and gout. In Morocco, it is

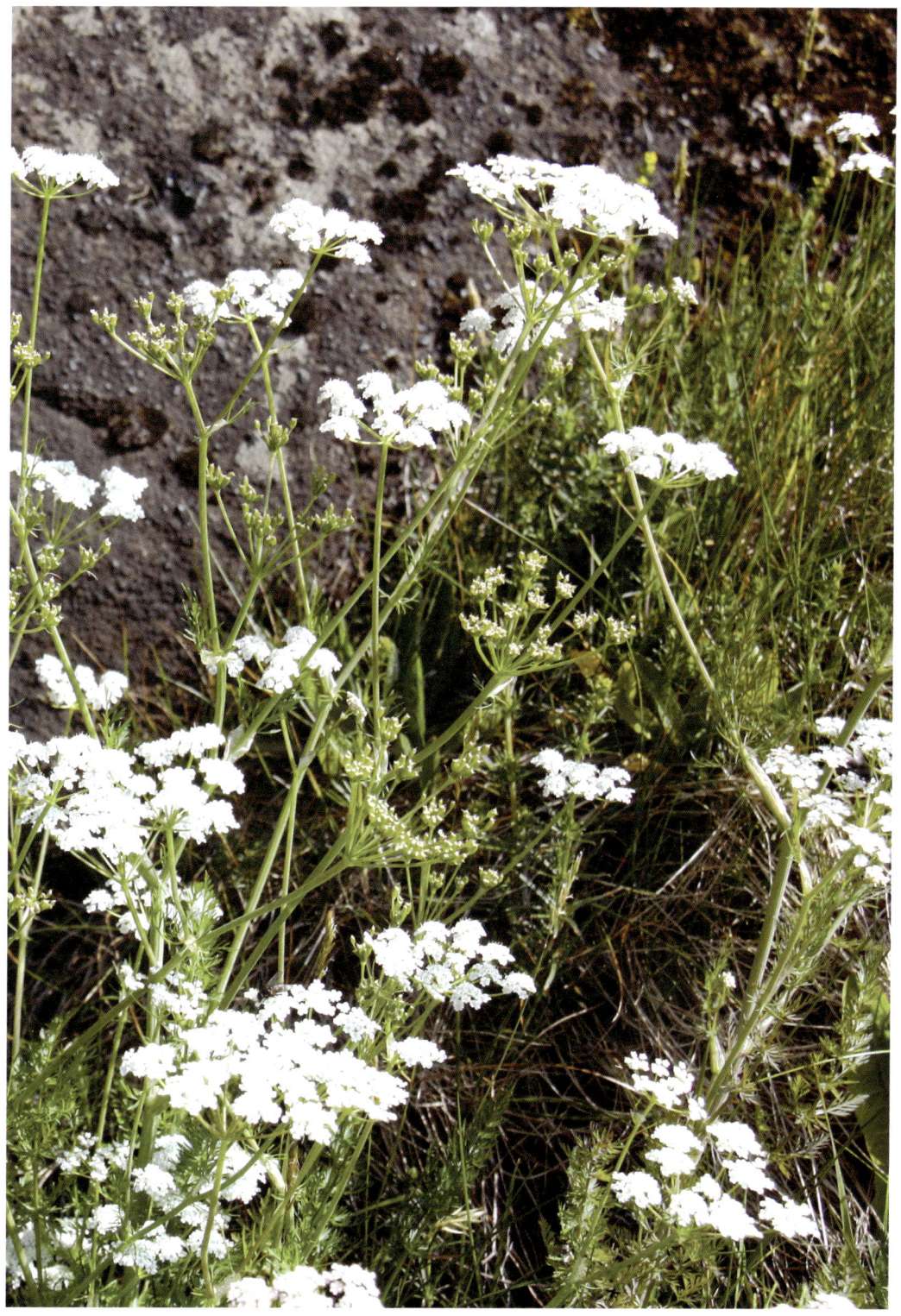

customary to use Caraway seeds for edema, high blood pressure, and diabetes.

Research

In vitro testing on Caraway seeds has revealed their antibacterial properties[1–4] (e.g., on *Helicobacter pylori*, which causes gastritis and stomach ulcers,[5] and on many other bacteria in the digestive system).[6] Caraway seeds are also antifungal,[1,7] and insecticidal[8] (e.g., against Japanese termites[9] and mosquito larvae).[10,11] One study showed the enhanced action of anti-tubercular drugs if an isolated constituent from Caraway was given simultaneously with the drugs, thus allowing the dosage to be lowered by 40%.[12] Research has also shown that Caraway seeds are diuretic,[13] hypoglycemic,[15] lower cholesterol,[14] and heal stomach ulcers.[16]

The antioxidant properties of Caraway seeds have been significantly researched,[1,17–20] especially their use as a preservative in food products.[1–3,17] *In vitro* tests show that Caraway seeds inhibit cancer cell growth[19,21–23] and research with respect to colon cancer[19,24,25] has also been done on the seeds. Research from the country Georgia, where meat consumption is substantial, showed a possible connection between low incidence of colon cancer and the amount of spices used in meat, one of which was Caraway seed.[19]

Dosage

Tincture: 1–3 ml three times a day (1:5, 40%).

Infusion: ½-1 teaspoon in a cup three times a day.

Warning

The use of Caraway seeds is not recommended during pregnancy.

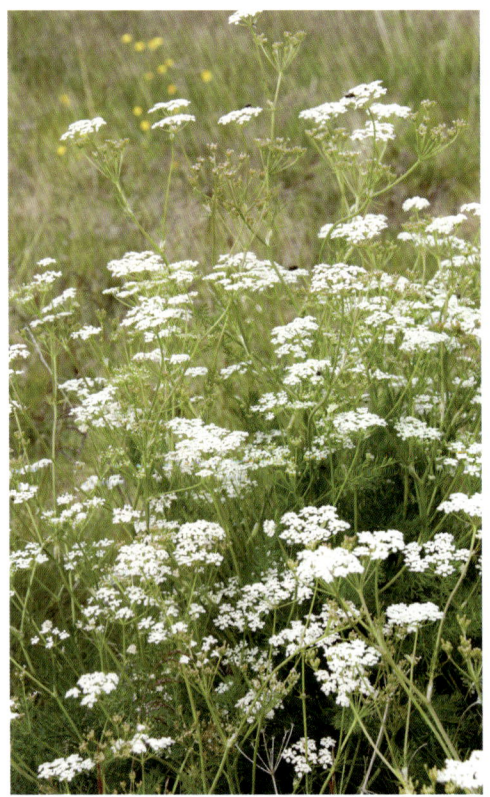

Tea for Flatulence

1 part Caraway seeds

1 part Creeping Thyme

1 part Angelica seeds

Put 3–4 tablespoons of the blend into a 750 ml vacuum flask and pour boiling water into it. Strain the tea into cups and then put the herbs back into the flask and allow to stand the whole day. Drink from the flask throughout the day.

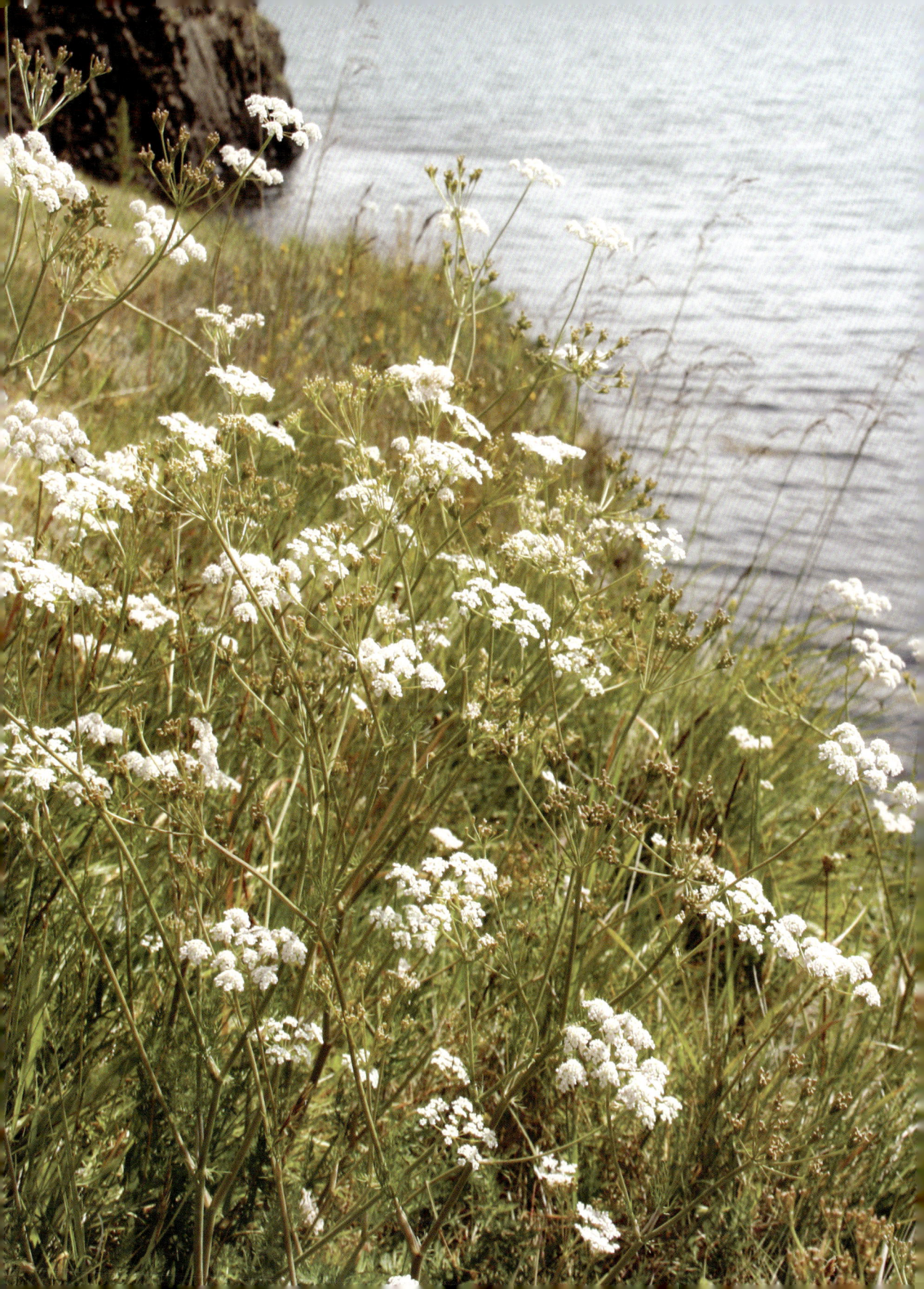

Chickweed

Stellaria media
Caryophyllaceae—*Haugarfi*

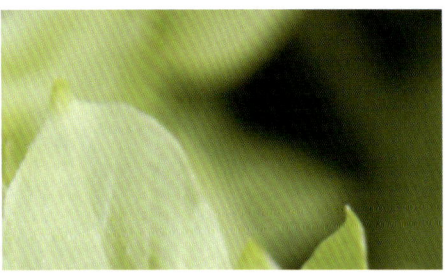

Habitat

Chickweed is a common weed all over Iceland.

Parts Used

The entire plant is used, except for the root.

Harvesting

It is collected all summer.

Constituents

Saponin, coumarin, flavonoids (rutin), carboxylic acid, and vitamin C.

History

The Latin name *Stellaria* is derived from "stella", meaning star, and refers to the star-shaped flowers of Chickweed. The English name indicates the centuries-old use of the weed as chicken feed. In Iceland it was used to keep food cool (e.g., fresh fish was wrapped in Chickweed as it was thought to keep better that way). Arthritis sufferers were thought to benefit by lying in a patch of Chickweed as it would cool and reduce swelling.

Action

Vulnerary, demulcent, cooling, anti-inflammatory, and relieves itching.

Uses

Chickweed is mainly used externally. It is excellent against itchiness and skin rashes and has long been used for eczema, psoriasis, inflammations and boils. It is also healing for wounds, such as those caused by varicose veins and burns. Chickweed is used for joint pain and mastitis. It is not used much internally in Western herbal medicine nowadays, but can be used in small amounts to stimulate digestion and for respiratory diseases and arthritis. In China, Chickweed taken internally is thought to stimulate menstruation, increase lactation, and stimulate blood circulation.

Research

In vitro testing on Chickweed demonstrated its antioxidant properties[1-3] and its inhibiting effect on cancer cell growth.[1]

Dosage

Tincture: 1–3 ml three times a day (1:5, 40%).

Infusion: 1 teaspoon in a cup three times a day.

Infusions, tinctures, compresses, and ointments for external use.

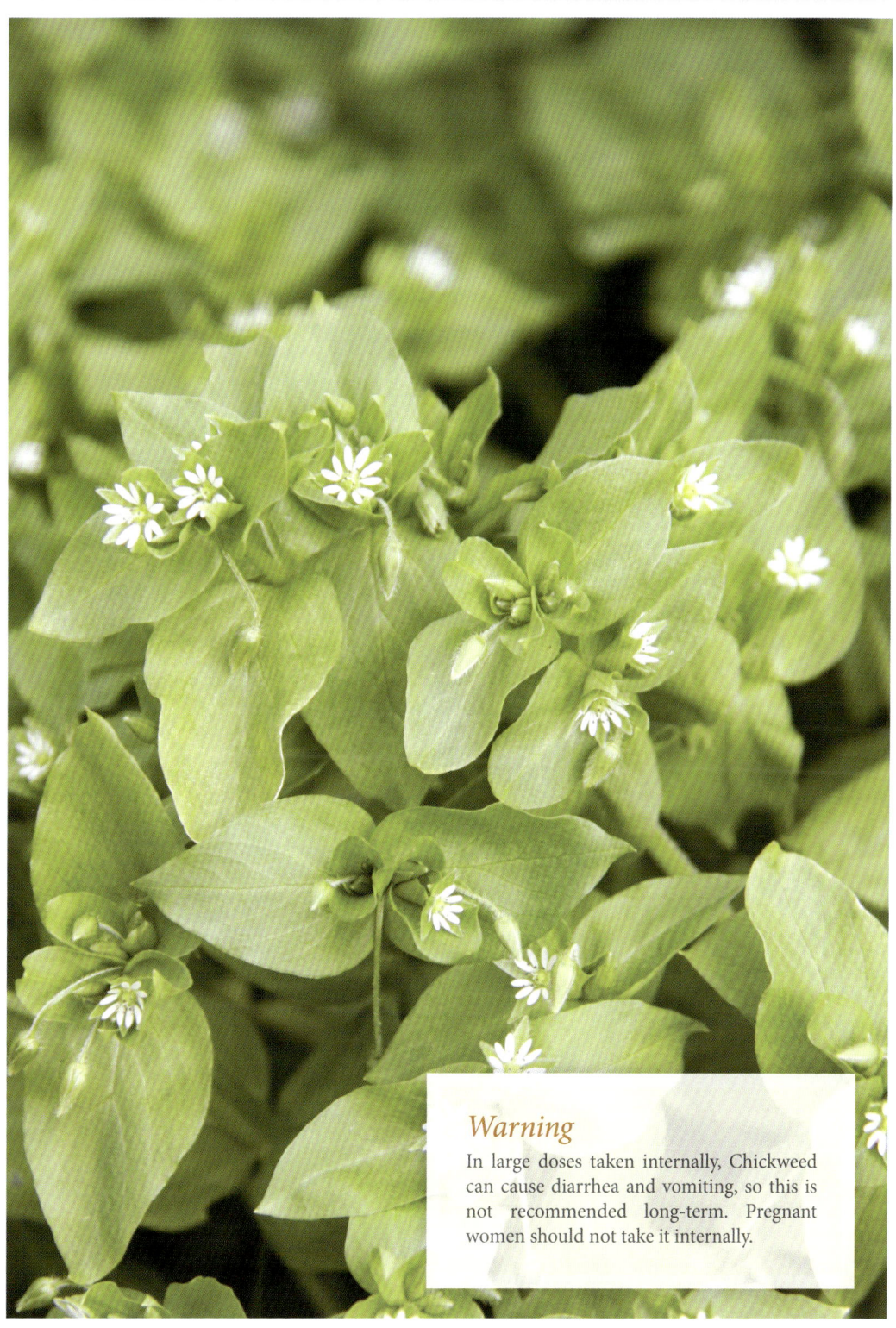

Warning

In large doses taken internally, Chickweed can cause diarrhea and vomiting, so this is not recommended long-term. Pregnant women should not take it internally.

Cold-weather Eyebright

Euphrasia frigida
Scrophulariaceae—*Augnfró*

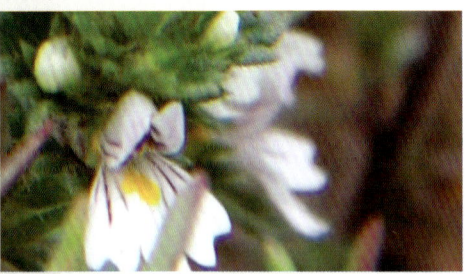

Habitat

Cold-weather Eyebright is a small plant that is common throughout Iceland. It grows in dry pastures and heaths.

Parts Used

The entire plant, except for the root.

Harvesting

Collected during bloom in July and August.

Constituents

Iridoid glycosides (aucubin), tannins, phenolic acids (gallic acid, caffeic acid), essential oils, and flavonoids.

History

The best-known medicinal herb of the *Euphrasia* genus is *E. officinalis*, but there are many other species (e.g., Cold-weather Eyebright, *E. frigida*). Cold-weather Eyebright is smaller than *E. officinalis* but sources reveal they have similar healing powers. Two other Euphrasia plants grow in Iceland: *E. stricta*, which is rather rare,

This herb is one of those that distributes and disintegrates and has a bitter taste. Specifically, this herb claims the power to heal swollen and cloudy eyes. The herb is bruised and the juice thereof is put in the eyes morning and night. Another way is to steep the herb in wine and drink it, which is believed to give it the same power to heal the eyes. It may be placed, bruised, over the eyes. Mr. Von Linné is the only man who claims it has less power in this respect, which now has been mentioned. But I hereby, with many others, claim its greatness against sore and stiff or sad eyes. This herb may be substituted for hops in beer-making and it will still have the same effect on eye weakness. This particular beer is said to taste good, and will strengthen the mind and memory, clean the brain and cure dizziness and scotomy.

Björn Halldórsson, Uses of Herbs, 1783

and *E. calida,* which is protected. The word *Euphrasia* comes from the Greek word "euphrosyne," meaning joy. The name is attributed to the healing power of Eyebright for eye diseases and the great joy that improved eyesight gives people. Eyebright has a long history as a medicinal herb, and sources revealing its effects on eye disease date back to the 13th century. In Britain, where there is a tradition of smoking herbal cigarettes for lung diseases, Eyebright is one of the herbs used for this purpose.

Action

Astringent, anti-inflammatory, anti-catarrhal, and strengthens mucous membranes.

Uses

As the name itself indicates, Cold-weather Eyebright has been associated with its special

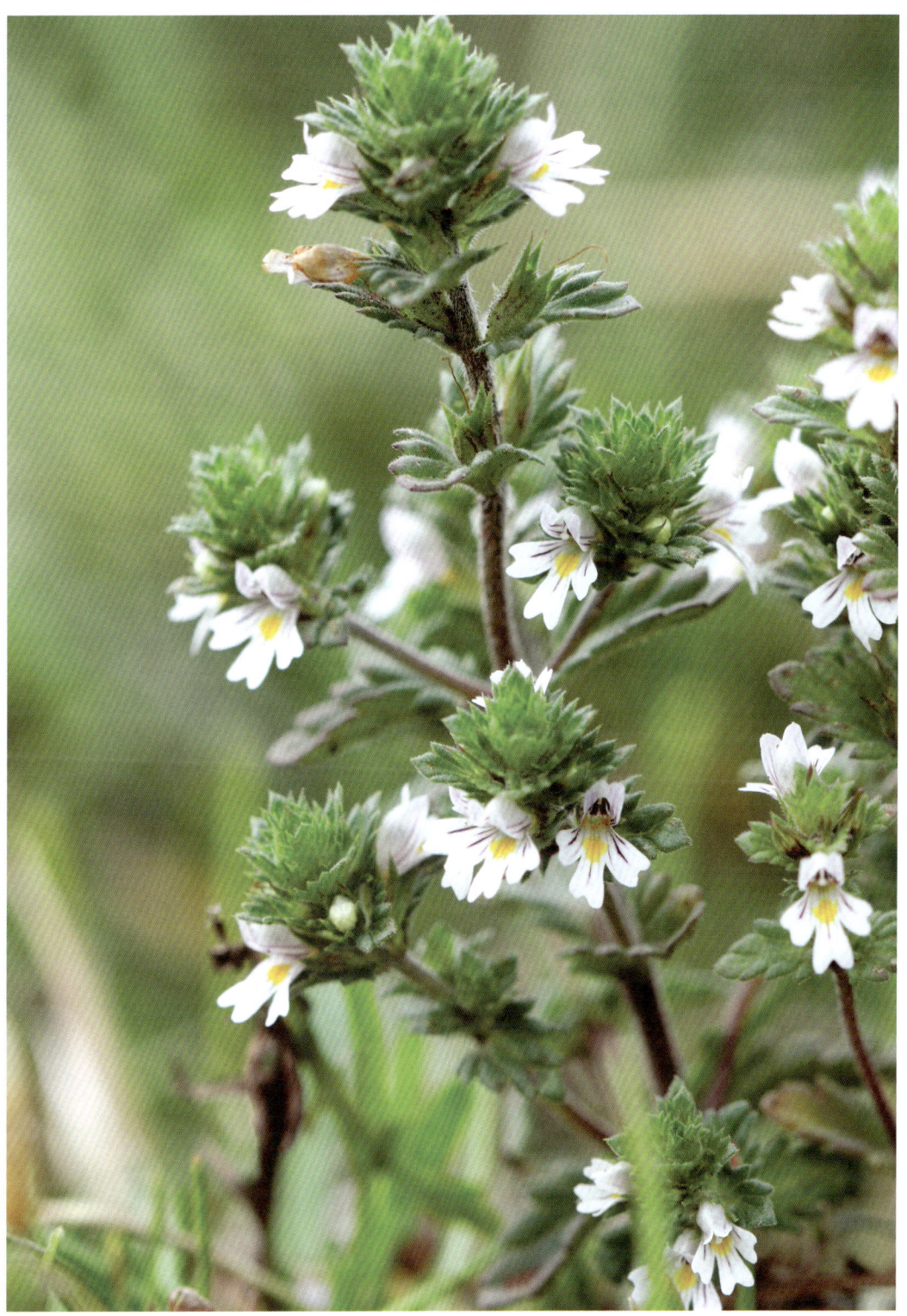

effect on eye diseases. It is considered to be a powerful anti-inflammatory for mucous membranes and for the lower and upper eyelids, while it is also believed to reduce itching. It is used both as an eyewash and internally for eye diseases. It is reputed to be effective against infections and allergies in the eyes, middle ear, sinuses, nose, and throat. Eyebright is astringent and dries up excess mucus, and is also good for eyes that are sensitive to light. It is effective as a gargle for gum and throat infections. Cold-weather Eyebright is well known for strengthening eyesight and poor memory, together with increasing blood flow to the brain. In Tibet, Eyebright is used for eye diseases but is also deemed to be diuretic and to counteract cystitis.

Research

Clinical research has been done with eye drops from *E. roskoviana* against conjunctivitis. Out of the 65 participants, 81.5% fully recovered, good results were felt by 17%, but 1.5% got worse.[1] Eyebright contains an active compound called aucubin, which has undergone intensive *in vitro* testing. Results show that aucubin works against various bacteria, fungi, and viruses, while the research also shows that it inhibits cancer cell growth, is anti-inflammatory, and protects against liver damage.[2,3] Eyebright lowers blood sugar in animals with high blood-sugar levels, but has no effect on animals with normal blood-sugar levels.[4]

Dosage

Tincture: 2–6 ml three times a day (1:5, 40%).

Infusion: 1–2 teaspoons in a cup three times a day.

Infusions, tinctures, and compresses for external use.

Warning

Long-term use of Eyebright eyewash for eye infections is not recommended if no improvements are seen after a few days.

Recipe for Eyewash

Put 1 teaspoon of Cold-weather Eyebright in a cup and steep in boiling water. Let it stand for 10 minutes. Pour through a coffee filter so that no sediment is left in the tea. Wait until the tea is cold and then pour into an eye cup (available from pharmacies). Put the cup to the eye, tilt the head backward, and blink a few times. Rinse both eyes this way. Drink the leftover tea. Repeat two to four times a day. It is also possible to fill the eye cup with boiling water and then add 2–3 drops of Eyebright tincture. Let it stand until cold and then rinse eyes as described above. Also, a cotton ball can be soaked in Eyebright tea and placed over swollen eyes.

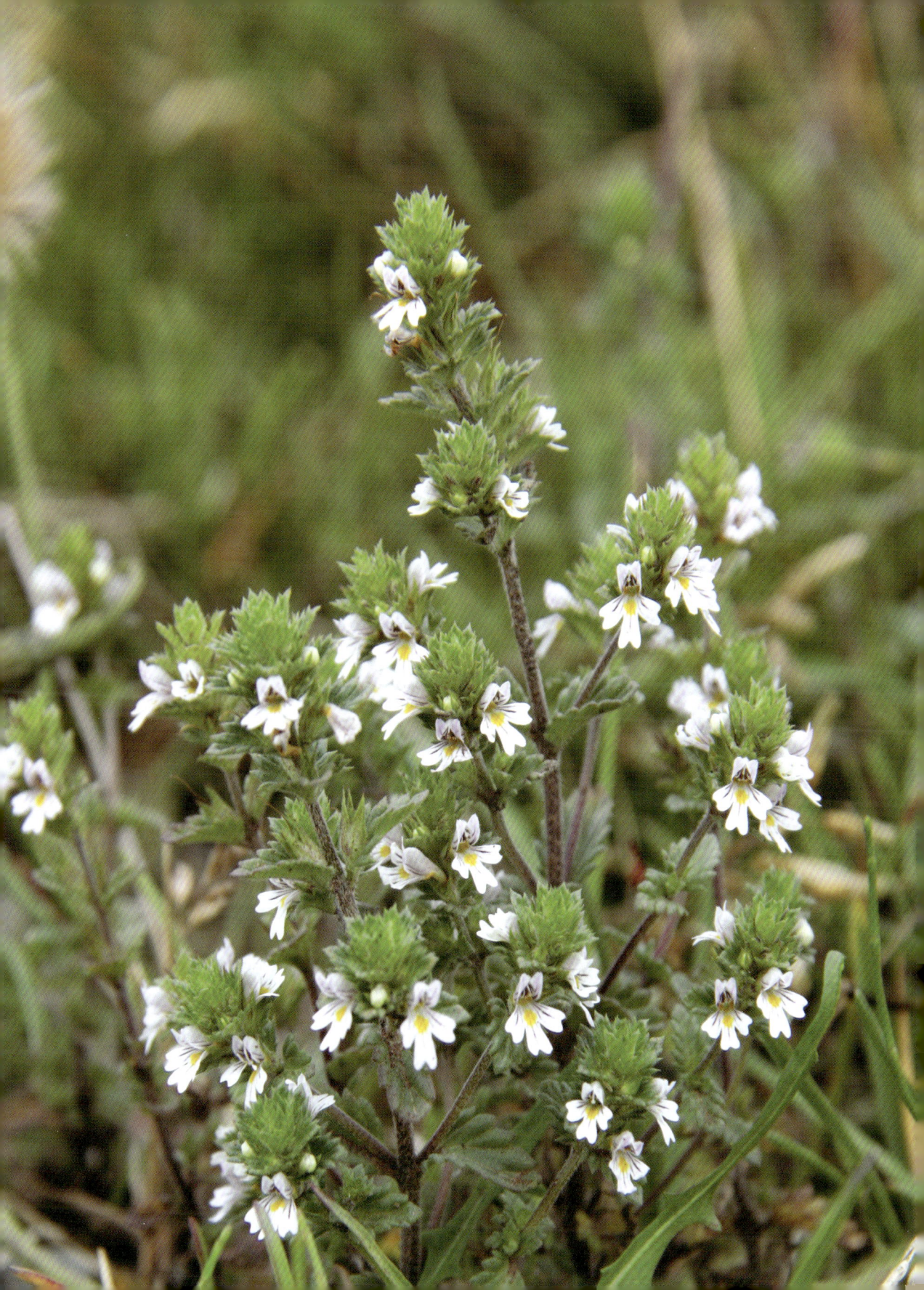

Coltsfoot

Tussilago farfara
Asteraceae—*Hófífill*

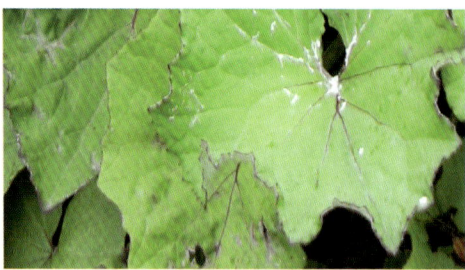

Habitat

Coltsfoot grows mainly around Reykjavík and in Southwest and North Iceland.

Parts Used

Leaves and flowers.

Harvesting

The flowers are picked in April–May and the leaves in June–July.

Constituents

Mucilage, flavonoids, pyrrolizidine alkaloids, triterpenes, sterols, vitamin C, and zinc.

History

The literal meaning of the Latin genus name *Tussilago* is antitussive and Coltfoot has been used for coughs for centuries. The leaves of Coltsfoot are thought to resemble the hoof of a horse, which explains the Icelandic name "Hófífill" (Hoof Daisy), the Latin name *farfara,* and the English Coltsfoot. It is customary in England to use Coltsfoot in herbal cigarettes intended for asthma patients.

Action

Expectorant, antitussive, antispasmodic, anti-inflammatory, demulcent, and mild diuretic.

Uses

For centuries, Coltsfoot has been considered exceptionally good for easing coughs and loosening mucus, as well as for soothing the respiratory tract. It works well for dry coughs, spasmodic coughing, whooping cough, throat infections, bronchitis, emphysema, and asthma. Coltsfoot is thought to be a mild diuretic as well and has been used for cystitis. Fresh, bruised leaves are used topically for abscesses and weeping wounds. In China, there is a centuries-old tradition of using Coltsfoot flowers for coughs of all kinds, and no evidence can be found in any old sources that long-term use of the flowers could be dangerous, as modern research indicates.

Research

The following research mostly discusses the isolated compound tussilagone from Coltsfoot and not the entire herb itself. *In vitro* tests show that Coltsfoot is anti-inflammatory,[1-3] anti-bacterial,[4,5] antispasmodic, and an immune stimulant,[2] and has antioxidant action as well.[6,7] It is also thought that Coltsfoot could possibly be used in treatments for obesity, diabetes type 2, Alzheimer's, and Parkinson's disease.[8,9]

Dosage

Tincture: 2–4 ml three times a day (1:5, 25%).

Infusion: 1–2 teaspoons in a cup three times a day.

Infusions, tinctures, compresses, and ointments for external use.

Syrup: 1–2 teaspoons three times a day.

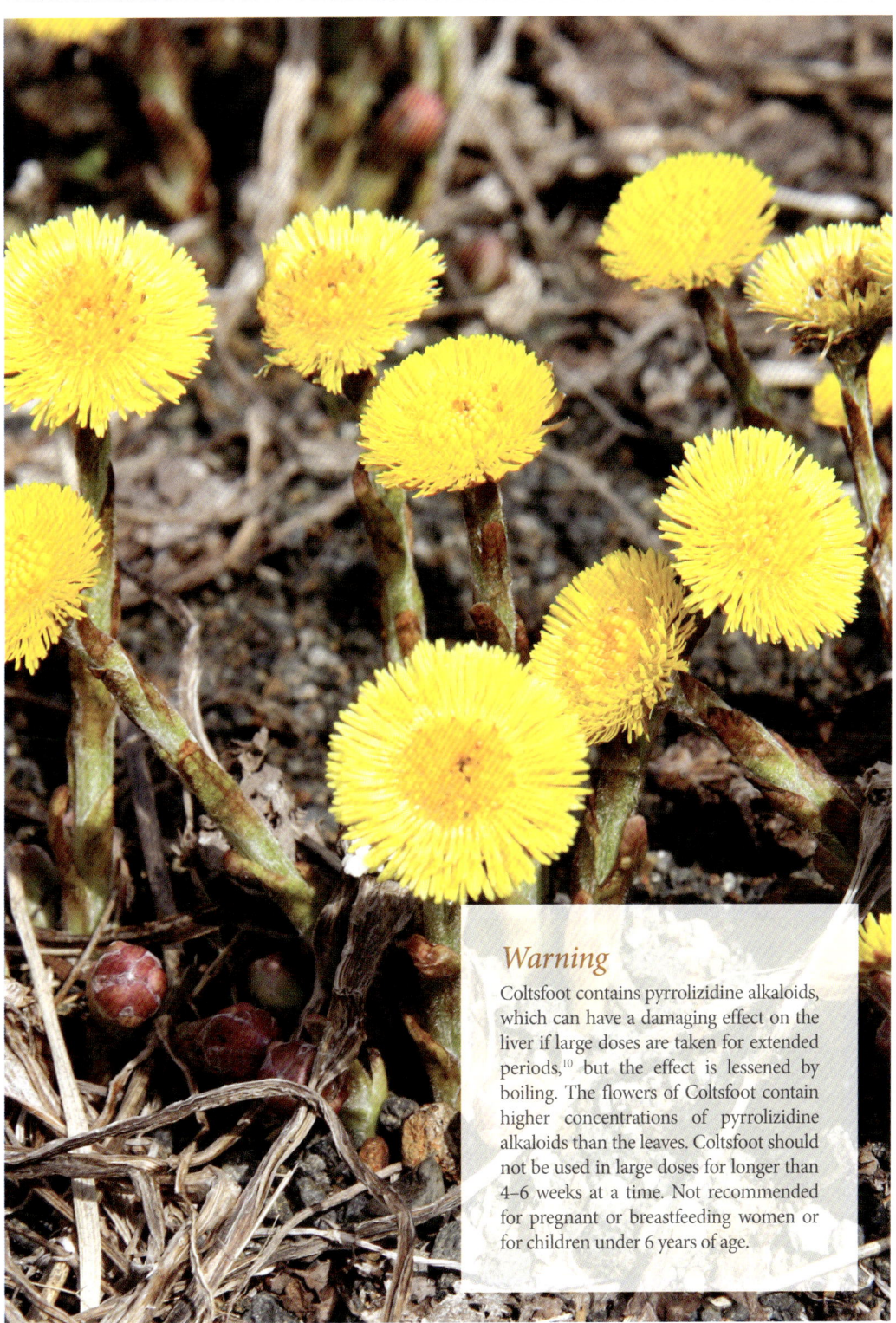

Warning

Coltsfoot contains pyrrolizidine alkaloids, which can have a damaging effect on the liver if large doses are taken for extended periods,[10] but the effect is lessened by boiling. The flowers of Coltsfoot contain higher concentrations of pyrrolizidine alkaloids than the leaves. Coltsfoot should not be used in large doses for longer than 4–6 weeks at a time. Not recommended for pregnant or breastfeeding women or for children under 6 years of age.

Common Sea-thrift

Armeria maritima
Plumbaginaceae—*Geldingahnappur*

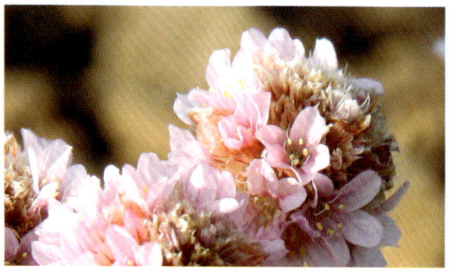

Habitat
It is common all over Iceland and grows mainly in sandy and stony ground.

Parts Used
The entire plant is used, including the root.

Harvesting
It is collected in bloom in June.

Constituents
Phenolic acid, tannins, iodine, and bromine.

History
Sources from Ireland and Britain reveal the use of Common Sea-thrift for tuberculosis. The root was boiled in sweet milk and was a popular remedy for tuberculosis up to the 18th century. It was also well known among sailors as a hangover remedy: they boiled the plant with the root and drank it cold. In the past, Common Sea-thrift was used for cystitis, obesity, wounds, epilepsy, and problems with the nervous system. However, it is known that if Common Sea-thrift is used to treat cystitis, it might cause inflammation of the kidneys and if it is used topically, it might cause swelling and skin irritation. No recent research supports the use of Common Sea-thrift for obesity, although the herb does contain iodine, like Bladderwrack (*Fucus vesiculosus*). Iodine is known for its effect on hypothyroidism, one symptom of which is abnormal weight gain.

Action
Antibacterial and antispasmodic.

Uses
It is not known if Common Sea-thrift is used in Western herbal medicine today.

Warning
Common Sea-thrift is not recommended for use as a medicinal herb, either externally or internally.

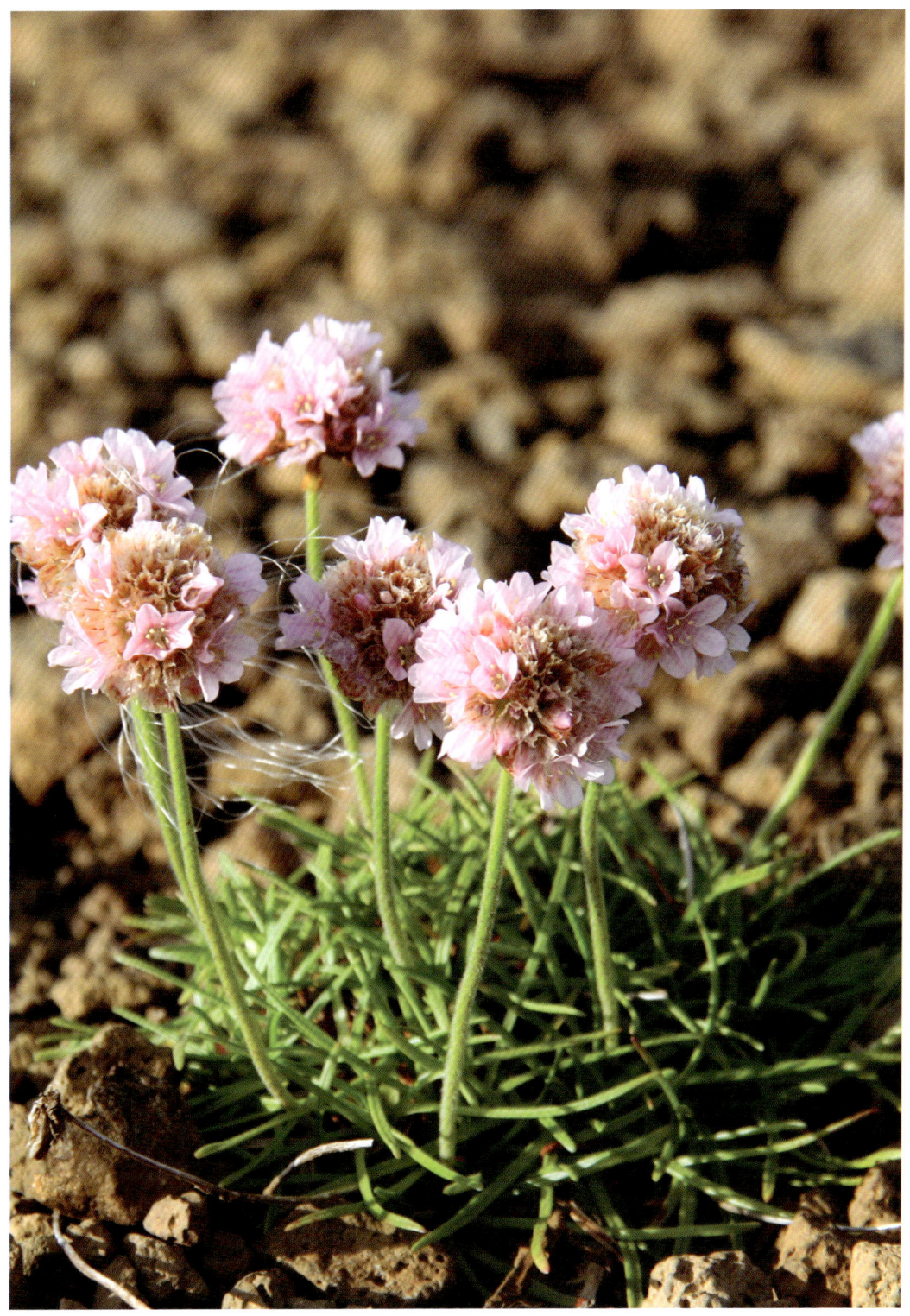

Couch Grass

Elytrigia repens
Poaceae—Húsapuntur

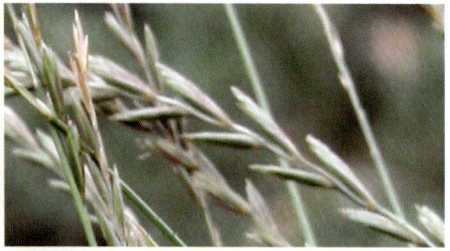

Habitat

Couch Grass is common all over Iceland near farmhouses and in uncultivated areas.

Parts Used

Rhizomes and seeds.

Harvesting

The seeds are collected in June–July and the rhizomes harvested in autumn or spring.

Constituents

Carbohydrates (triticin), mucilage, phenolic acids, essential oils, silicic acid, and iron.

History

The former English name for this plant is Dog Grass and refers to the fact that dogs look for it when they are sick and then eat it to induce vomiting. In past centuries, the British deemed Couch Grass to be good for liver and gallstone diseases and the decoction thereof was a popular drink in spring to cleanse the blood. The Native Americans used Couch Grass for bladder and kidney stones, for incontinence, and as a vermifuge, but also rubbed a decoction of Couch Grass on swollen feet. The rhizomes were formerly used as a coffee substitute, in flour for bread-making, to brew beer, and to dye yarn.

Action

Diuretic, demulcent, mild laxative, mild anti-inflammatory, and antibacterial.

Uses

For centuries, rhizomes of Couch Grass have been considered effective against various infections and irritations in the urinary system and are also regarded as diuretic. The grass is used for cystitis and urethritis and is deemed to work well against kidney diseases and kidney stones, particularly when combined with other herbs. Couch Grass is also a conventional medicinal herb against benign prostate enlargement and infections in the prostate gland. It is considered good for both gout and osteoarthritis and also for chronic skin diseases. In Germany, the seeds are used as hot compresses for stomach ulcers. Couch Grass is considered effective for jaundice and other liver problems, as well as being a mild laxative.

Research

Couch Grass was given to 313 patients with cystitis, prostatitis, or urethritis and the results were good or very good in 84% of the patients after 12 days. It was well tolerated and no side effects were shown.[1] *In vivo* testing revealed the diuretic effects[2,3] of Couch Grass and the mild anti-inflammatory[2] effect, but no effect was seen on kidney stones.[3]

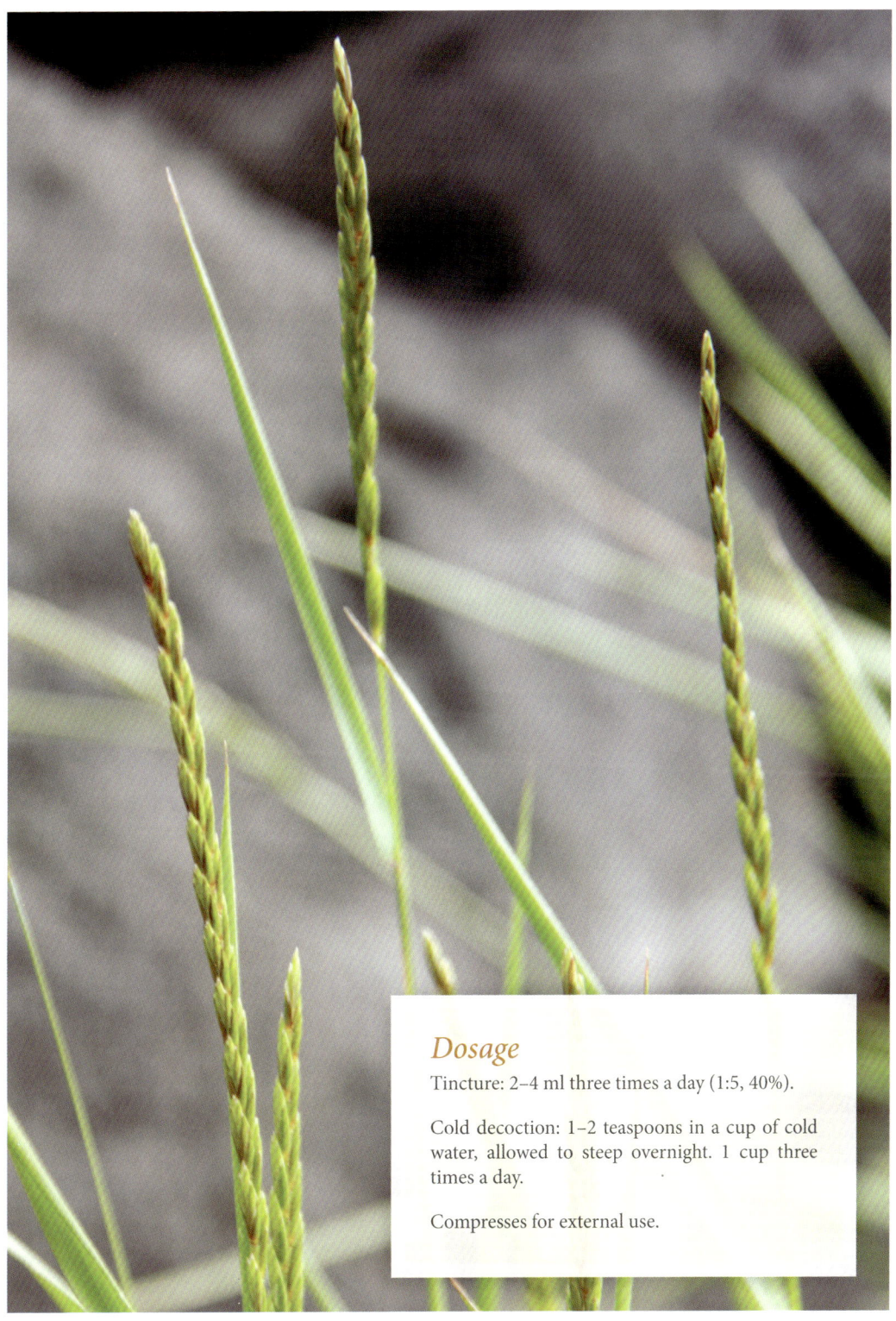

Dosage

Tincture: 2–4 ml three times a day (1:5, 40%).

Cold decoction: 1–2 teaspoons in a cup of cold water, allowed to steep overnight. 1 cup three times a day.

Compresses for external use.

Cow Parsley

Anthriscus sylvestris
Apiaceae—*Skógarkerfill*

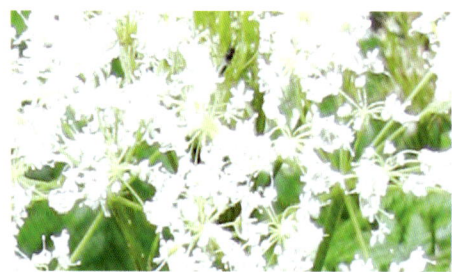

Habitat

Cow Parsley is an imported species that spreads rapidly and forms large swaths. It is common all over Iceland.

Parts Used

The entire plant is used, including the root.

Harvesting

The leaves are collected before bloom in June, the seeds in August, and the root in the autumn.

Constituents

Essential oils, polyphenols (deoxypodophyllotoxin), and flavonoids.

History

There are references to the use of Cow Parsley in Europe for cancer (e.g., lymphoma, as well as for warts and corns). The juice of Cow Parsley has also been used for skin problems. Both the leaves and the roots of Cow Parsley have been boiled for food, but it is debatable as to how tasty they are. The leaves are also used in salads and to dye yarn.

Action

Mild diuretic.

Uses

Cow Parsley is not used in Western herbal medicine nowadays and very few modern references exist to its use as a medicinal herb. In the past, Cow Parsley was used for edema and digestive problems, and to heal wounds. It was also considered to stimulate both metabolism and contractions during childbirth.

Research

Cow Parsley has been researched recently in Korea, Japan, and Italy. The active ingredient, deoxypodophyllotoxin, has been the main focus of *in vitro* tests as it is said to inhibit the growth of cancer cells.[1–9] The same constituent is also thought to have a positive effect on allergies.[10]

Dosage

Not known.

Warning

Cow Parsley should not be used in pregnancy.

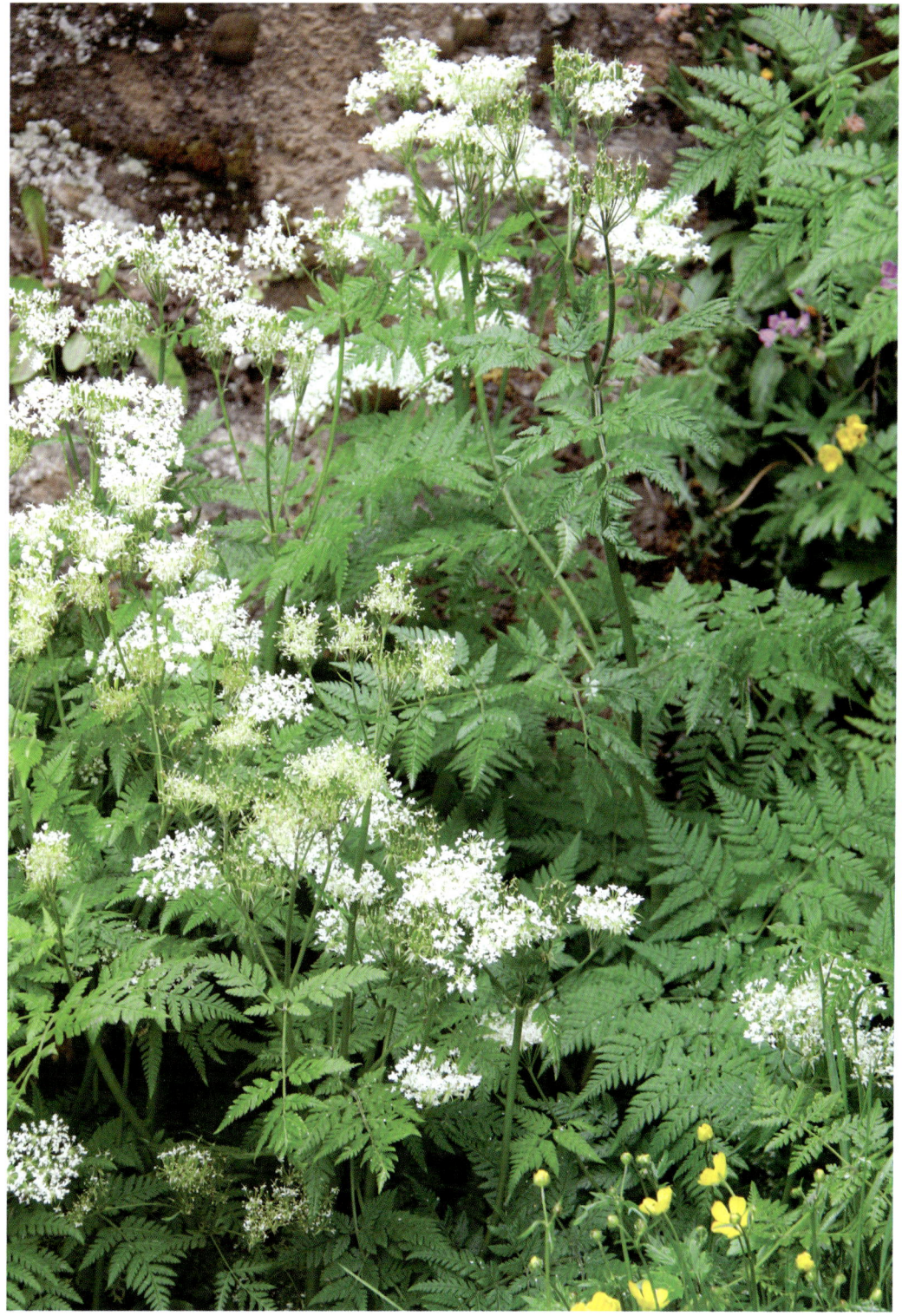

Creeping Thyme

Thymus praecox
Labiatae—Blóðberg

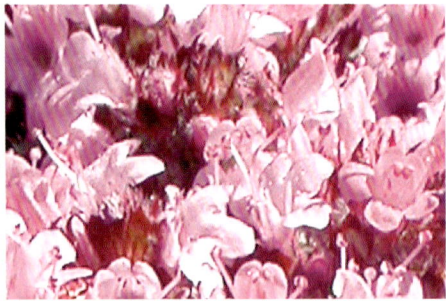

Habitat

Creeping Thyme is found all over Iceland and grows best in gravelly ground and on dry heaths.

Parts Used

The entire plant is used, except for the root.

Harvesting

Creeping Thyme is collected in bloom in June–July.

Constituents

Essential oils, flavonoids, phenolic acids, tannins, and resins.

History

Creeping Thyme is closely related to Thyme (*T. vulgaris*), which has a very long history as both a medicinal and culinary herb and has been extensively researched. The properties of Creeping Thyme and Thyme are similar, but the essential oil from Creeping Thyme is considered to be milder than that from Thyme. The genus name *Thymus* means "smoke cleanser" and refers to the use of Creeping Thyme as incense, both for its aroma and as a purifier. The word can also mean "brave" and in the old days it was believed that Creeping Thyme gave men more courage. It has always been a popular tea and culinary herb in Iceland and is reputed to be good for hangovers. It was also a symbol for submission and loyalty, and in the past it was customary for German brides to put Creeping Thyme in their shoes.

Action

Antispasmodic, analgesic, carminative, antitussive, expectorant, antibacterial, antifungal, diuretic, vulnerary, and emmenagogue.

Uses

Creeping Thyme has been used for centuries to treat colds, influenza, throat infections, coughs, asthma, and bronchitis. It loosens and dries up mucus in the respiratory tract as well as being good for stuffy noses and sinusitis. It is also used

> This herb has good power to strengthen tendons. The wine in which this herb has been steeped heals leg cramps when drunk. It also cures colds, clears and strengthens the head, thins the blood, and cures flatulence and constipation in those who have eaten too much solid food. It warms cold stomachs and also strengthens them. Compresses, moistened with this wine and laid on the head, improve fainting and dizziness, headaches and fevers. A decoction of this herb is good for coughs and cures hangovers in the morning for those who have overindulged the night before. The decoction also stimulates sweating and is good for chest pains. [...] Creeping Thyme, bruised and placed over the temples, relieves headaches and improves insomnia.
>
> *Björn Halldorsson,* Uses of Herbs, *1783*

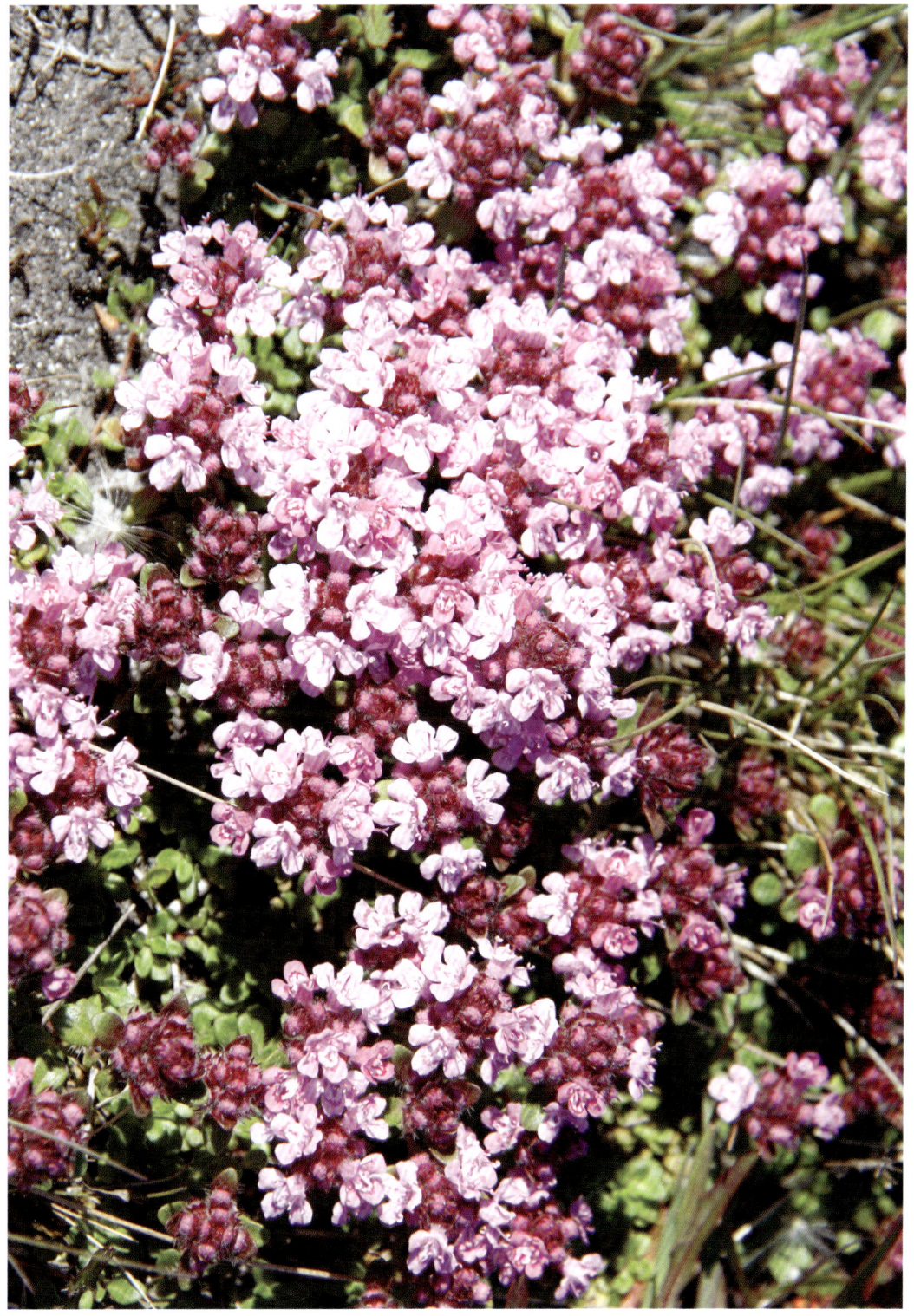

for ear infections, both externally and taken internally. It is considered a good rinse for gingivitis and throat infections. Creeping Thyme is also effective against colic, flatulence, and bloating and has been used to eliminate worms. It is used externally to heal and disinfect wounds, and for arthritic pain, muscle pain, and neuritis, (e.g., sciatica). It is also considered good for menstrual pain and delayed menstruation, and externally for mastitis, vaginal discharge, and candida.

Research

Many *in vitro* tests have shown the antioxidant properties of Creeping Thyme.[1-4] It also kills *Bacillus subtilis, Staphylococcus aureus,* and other bacteria,[5,6] and is a good insecticide.[7] The antibacterial properties of Creeping Thyme were also shown in tests performed on the shelf life of fresh fish. Fresh fish that was kept on ice with Creeping Thyme, instead of just plain ice, showed a shelf life 15–20 days longer than normal.[8]

Dosage

Tincture: 2–6 ml three times a day (1:5, 40%).

Infusion: 1–2 teaspoons in a cup three times a day.

Syrup: 1–2 teaspoons three times a day.

Infusions, tinctures, compresses, and ointments used externally.

Warning

Creeping Thyme is not recommended during pregnancy.

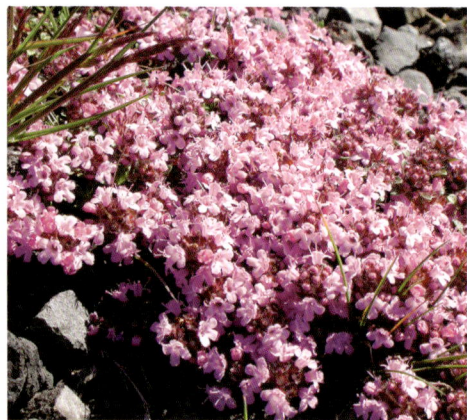

Infusion for Sore Throats and Colds

1 part Creeping Thyme

1 part Angelica seed

1 part Yarrow

Put 3–4 tablespoons of the blend into a 750 ml vacuum flask and pour boiling water into it. Sieve the infusion into cups and then put the herbs back into the flask and allow to stand the whole day. Drink from the flask throughout the day.

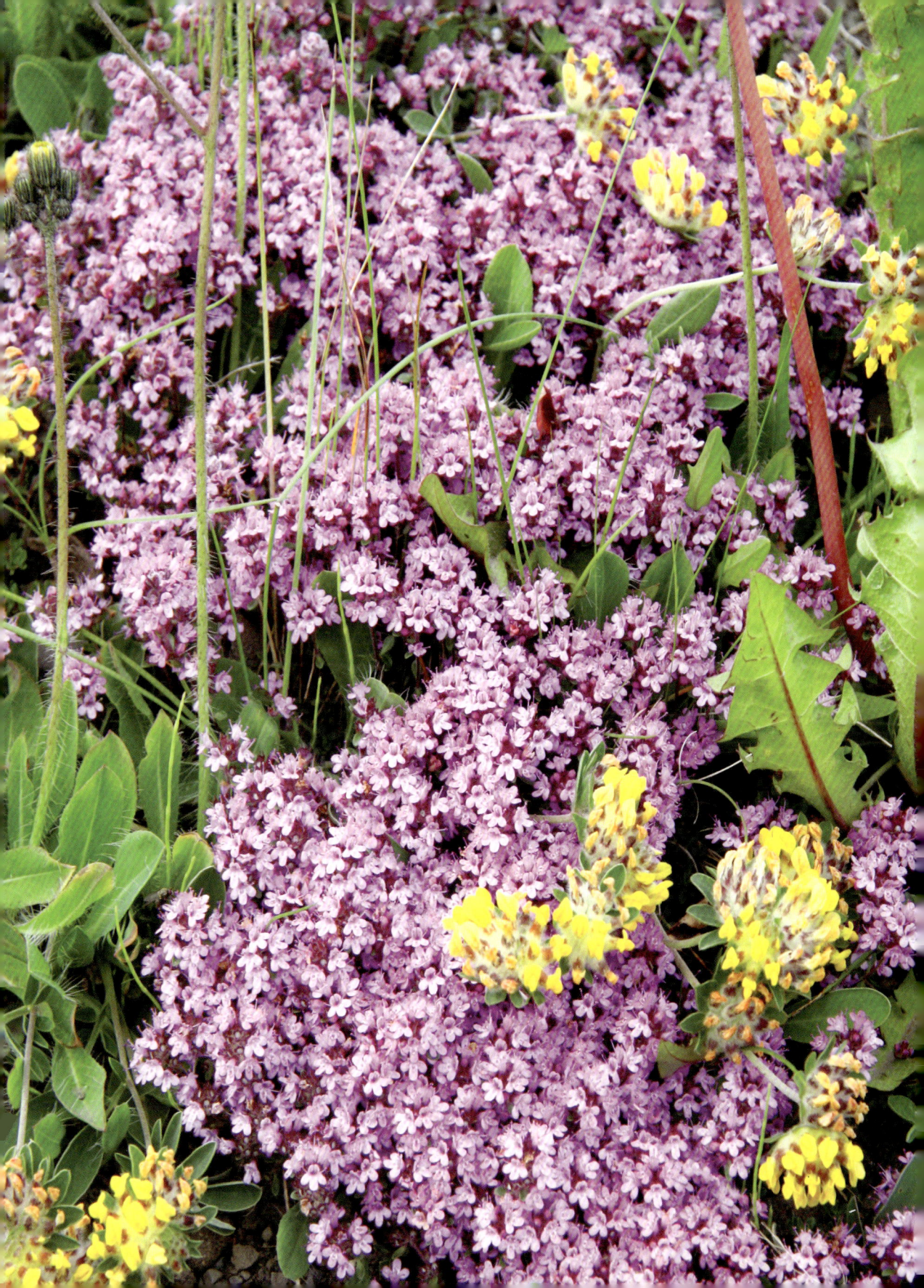

Crowberry

Empetrum nigrum
Ericaceae—*Krækiber*

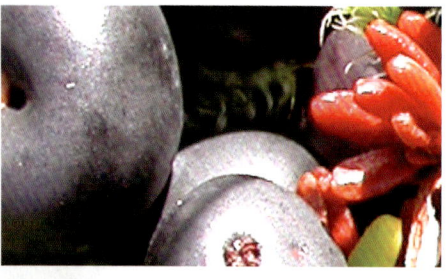

The berries of this herb are cooling, and slightly astringent. Liquid of the boiled berry is good against diarrhea, when 2 tablespoons are taken every two hours. Jam from the berries, mixed with water, is a good drink for thirst and epidemic fevers.

Oddur Jónsson Hjaltalín,
Icelandic Botany, 1830

Habitat

Crowberry is very common all over Iceland and grows on moors and heaths.

Parts Used

The entire shrub is used, except for the root.

Harvesting

The leaves are collected in early summer, just before bloom, and the berries are picked in autumn.

Constituents

Berries: Polyphenols (anthocyanin, procyanidin), vitamins, iron, and fiber. Leaves: Phenols and tannins.

History

The Latin name *Empetrum* is derived from the Greek "en petros," meaning up on the rocks, and *nigrum*, which means black. Crowberries have been used for centuries in northern hemisphere cuisine. Picking berries and making juice used to be an essential activity in autumn for Icelanders, and for many it still is. Crowberry leaves have also been used as fuel and chicken feed, and to make wine and dye yarn. In the past it was called "lúsalyng" (lice heather), as it was believed that it killed fleas and other pests when placed in the bed. The Native Americans also made good use of the berries as food and used them either boiled or dried for diarrhea. They used the leaves for medicinal purposes: the decoction was thought to be diuretic, to lower fevers, and to be good for diarrhea, like the berries. A decoction from the leaves was also used for colds and kidney problems, while a decoction from the roots was used as an eyewash.

Action

Astringent, diuretic, nourishing and antibacterial.

Uses

Neither the leaves nor the berries of this shrub are used much in Western herbal medicine nowadays. In the past, an infusion or decoction from the leaves was considered to be diuretic and good for kidney diseases. Boiled and dried berries are well known for their beneficial effect on diarrhea, especially for children, and the leaves have also been used for this purpose. Fresh berries, however, have a laxative effect, especially if too many are eaten at once. The decoction from the leaves was considered effective against influenza and was also used to wash swollen eyelids. Crowberries are rich in vitamins and iron, and the berry juice is considered to be good for anemia.

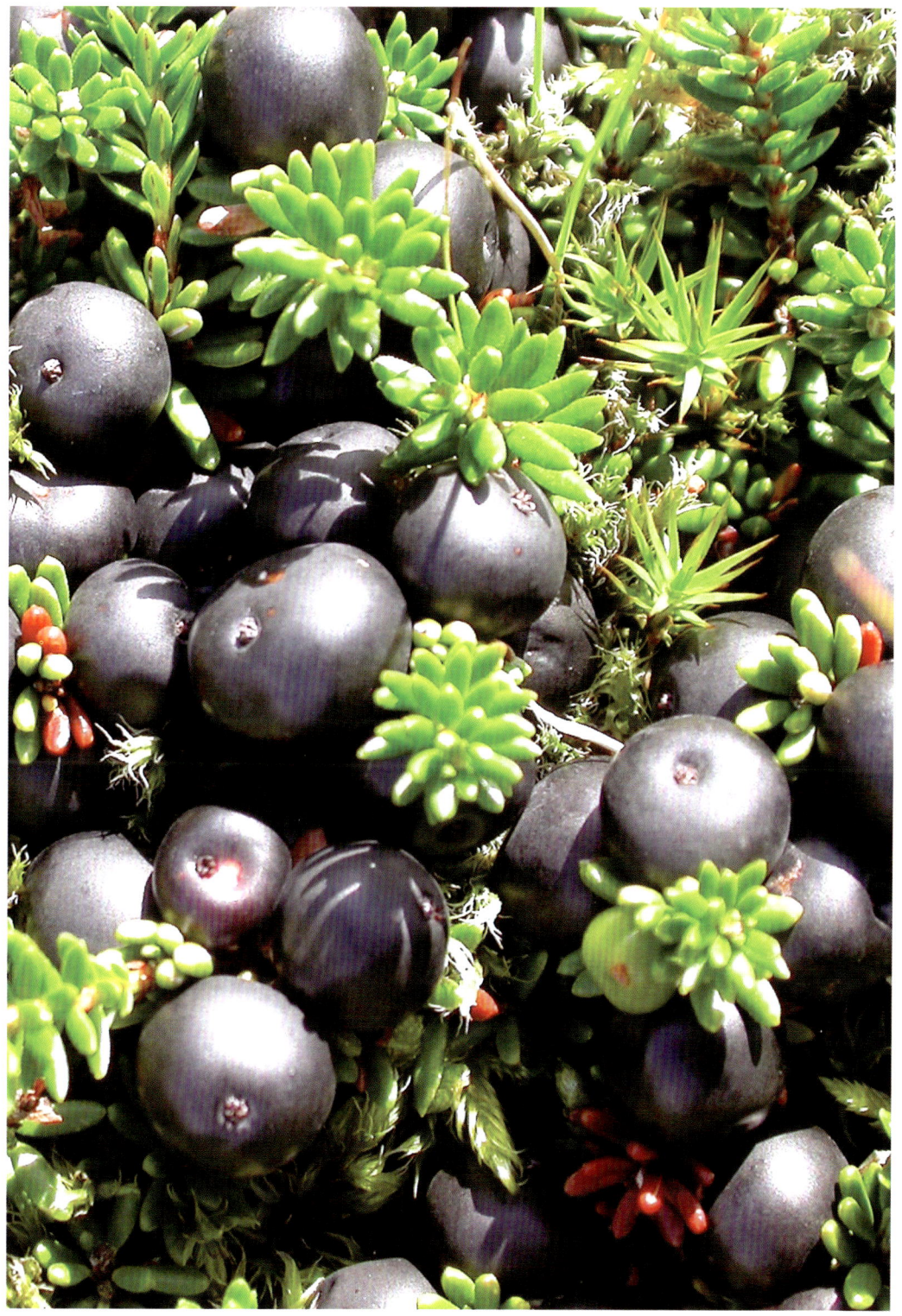

Research

Recent research in Japan revealed that Crowberry contains 13 different antioxidants totaling 41.8 mg/g, which is more than many other berries, and thus it is considered to be a strong antioxidant. The antioxidant effect of Crowberry is also deemed to reduce the risk of chronic illnesses.[1,2] Crowberry leaves showed an inhibiting effect on the tuberculosis bacteria *Mycobacterium tuberculosis*[3,6] and in Canadian research it was shown that the tincture of Crowberry leaves has antifungal properties.[4] Crowberry juice has also demonstrated possible inhibiting effects on the *Streptococcus pneumoniae* bacteria, which causes pneumonia, meningitis, and otitis.[5] In Icelandic research, both the berries and the leaves have shown antibacterial properties (e.g., against specific strains of *staphylococci* that are known for their resistance to antibiotics).[7]

Dosage

Tincture: 2–4 ml three times a day (1:5, 40%).

Infusion: 1–2 teaspoons in a cup three times a day.

Decoction: 1–2 teaspoons in a cup three times a day.

Fresh berries: 1–2 tablespoons three times a day.

Raw Juice

Juice from pressed Crowberries is called raw juice and is extracted using a mincing machine or a juice extractor. It is best to use a muslin cloth in the sieve to obtain the pulp, then squeeze the cloth to extract all of the liquid. The raw juice can be stored in plastic bottles and frozen without using any sweeteners. Another good idea is to pour the juice into ice-cube bags and freeze it.

Crowberry Juice

1 liter raw juice

400-500 g sugar or raw sugar

Place the raw juice and sugar in a pot and bring to a boil, or until the sugar is dissolved. Allow to cool slightly and pour into sterilized bottles. The juice keeps for 6–12 months. Less sugar can be used, but then the shelf life is shortened.

Crowberry Juice from the Pulp

The pulp formed while making raw juice is ideal for juice. Place 350 g of well-squeezed pulp in a pot with 1 liter of water. Boil for 20 minutes, allow to cool, then sieve the pulp. Use the same method for bottling as in the raw juice recipe.

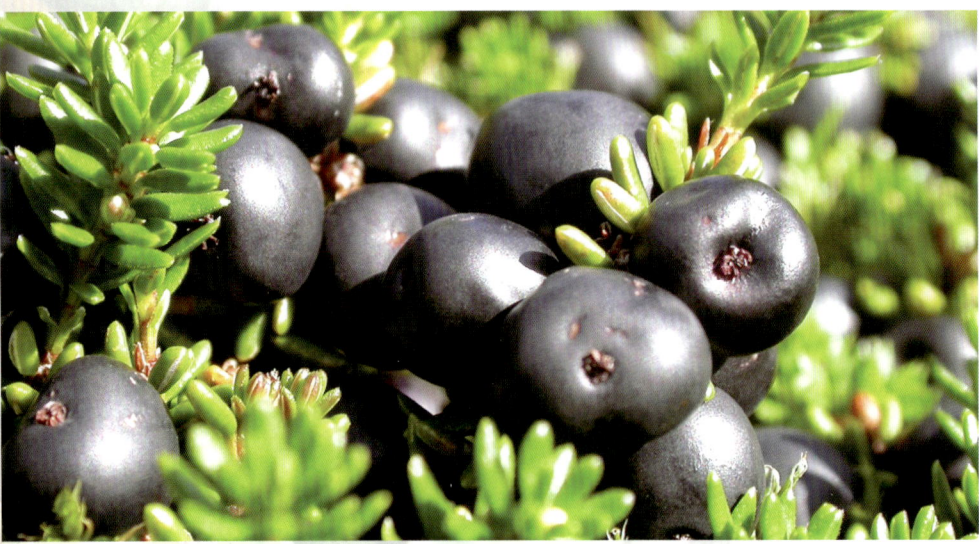

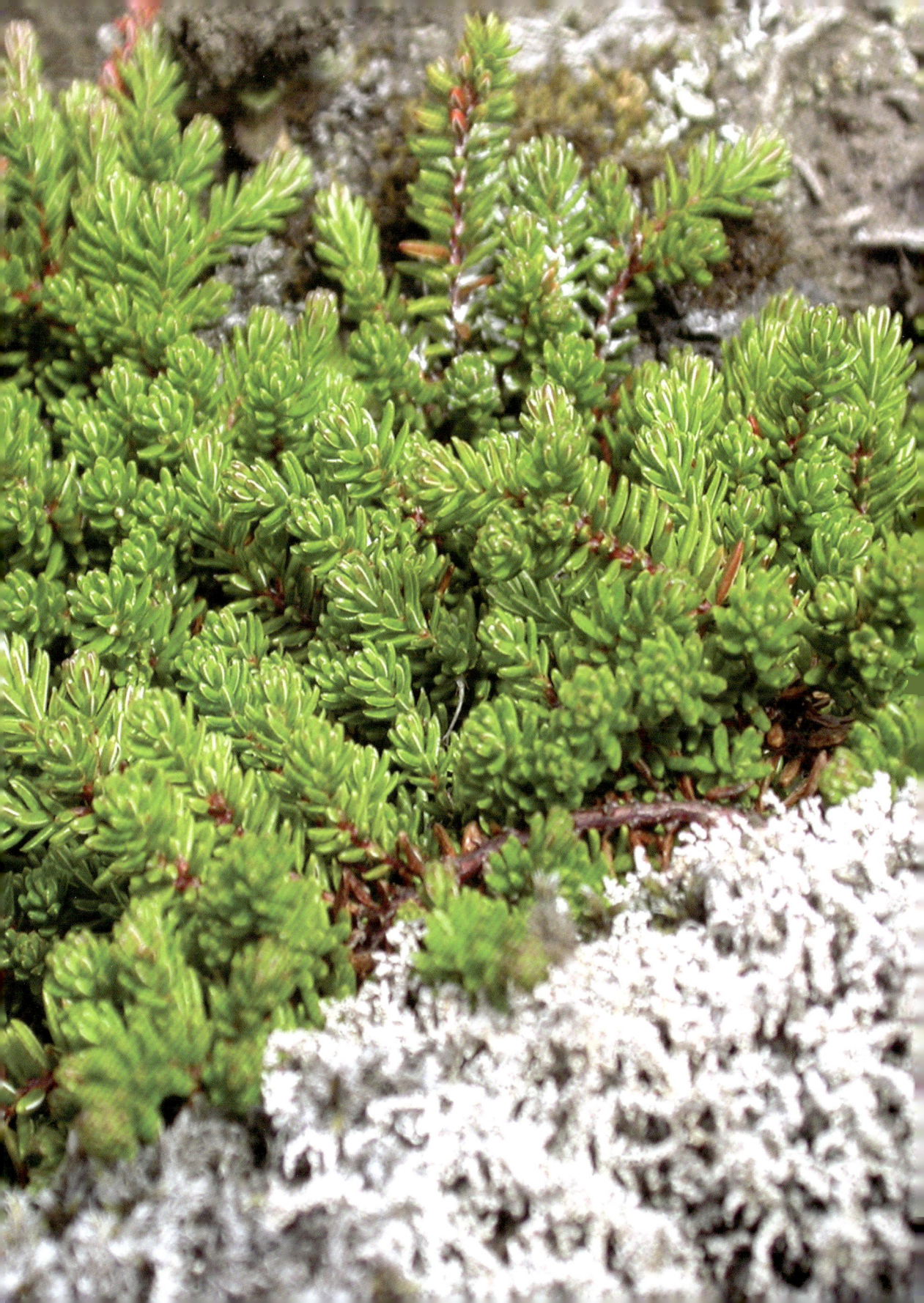

Cuckooflower

Cardamine pratensis subsp. *angustifolia*
Cruciferae—*Hrafnaklukka*

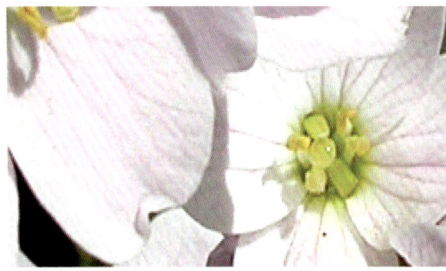

Habitat

Common all over Iceland.

Parts Used

The entire plant, except for the root.

Harvesting

Cuckooflower is collected while blossoming in May and June.

Constituents

Glucosinolates, vitamin C, and minerals.

History

The Latin name *Cardamine* is the old Greek word for Cress and refers to the strengthening effect of Cuckooflower on the heart. The Old English name for Cuckooflower was Lady's Smock, which referred to the possible aphrodisiacal properties of the herb. The flowers were considered to be nervines, febrifugal, and good for headaches. It was also considered to be antispasmodic and effective against epilepsy, hysteria, and St. Vitus Dance. In old Icelandic folklore it was believed that tea from the purple flowers worked well for insomnia and that tea from the white flowers was good if one wanted to keep awake. Cuckooflower is used in food, and is particularly good in sandwiches, salads, and soups. It has a similar taste to Watercress, being of the same family. In the past, Cuckooflower was grown as a vegetable and was sold in markets in Britain.

Action

Diuretic, antispasmodic, carminative, scurvy preventive, and stomachic.

Uses

Cuckooflower is not used much in Western herbal medicine today. In the past it was used for edema, spasms, flatulence, skin disorders, and scurvy. It was also used to increase appetite and stimulate sluggish digestion, as well as for anaemia. Cuckooflower was thought to hasten recuperation after a long illness, as it is rich in both vitamins and minerals.

Dosage

Tincture: 1–4 ml three times a day (1:5, 40%).

Infusion: 1–2 teaspoons in a cup three times a day.

Warning

Cuckooflower should not be used during pregnancy.

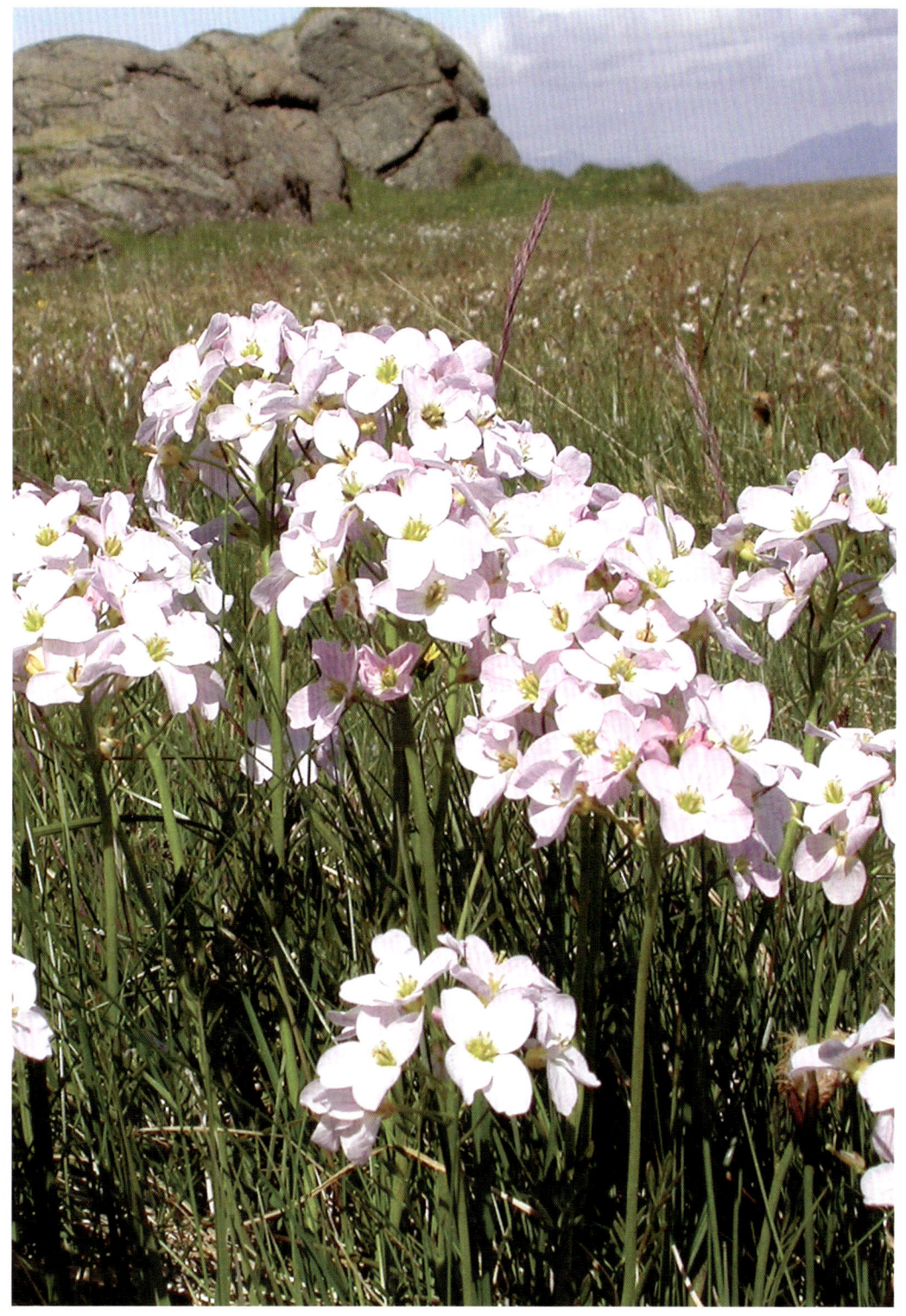

Daisy

Bellis perennis
Asteraceae—Fagurfífill

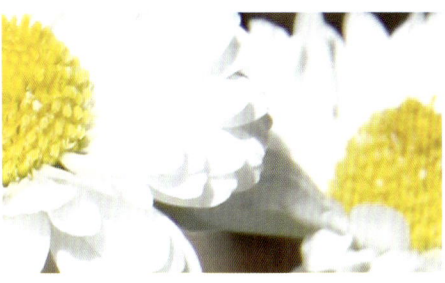

Habitat

Daisy is a rare imported Asteraceae species that grows sparsely in grassy patches in the East and West Fjords as well as in Siglufjörður and the Westman Islands. Daisy is common in other countries and is easy to grow.

Parts Used

Flowers.

Harvesting

Daisy is collected while in bloom in June and July.

Constituents

Saponins, phenolic acids, flavonoids, and essential oils.

History

Daisy used to be a popular medicinal herb and was considered excellent for healing wounds. It was also used in cases of hepatitis. The Old English name for Daisy is "Bruisewort." It was considered good for fevers, and in 14th-century England Daisy was used in ointments for wounds, painful joints, gout, and fever. Historical sources reveal that Daisy root was good for scurvy if taken long-term and superstition had it that puppies that drink the root boiled in milk would not grow bigger. Daisy leaves have been used in salads and soups and the flower buds steeped in vinegar. Daisy has been used in North America for stomach pain.

Action

Astringent, vulnerary, expectorant, and anti-inflammatory.

Uses

Daisy is not used much as a medicinal herb nowadays. It is considered good as a topical application for wounds, inflammations, bruises, and skin problems. Internally, it is used for coughs and bronchitis as well as being effective for inflammation in the digestive system. In the Czech Republic, Daisy is viewed as being both a diuretic and an expectorant.

Research

In vitro tests indicate mild antioxidant properties[1,2] and isolated compounds have shown antibacterial and antifungal properties.[3,4] *In vitro* tests also point toward active constituents of Daisy being effective against obesity.[5,6]

Dosage

Infusion: 1 teaspoon in a cup three times a day.

Infusions, tinctures, compresses, and ointments used externally.

Warning

It is not recommended to drink Daisy in large doses or for long periods of time.

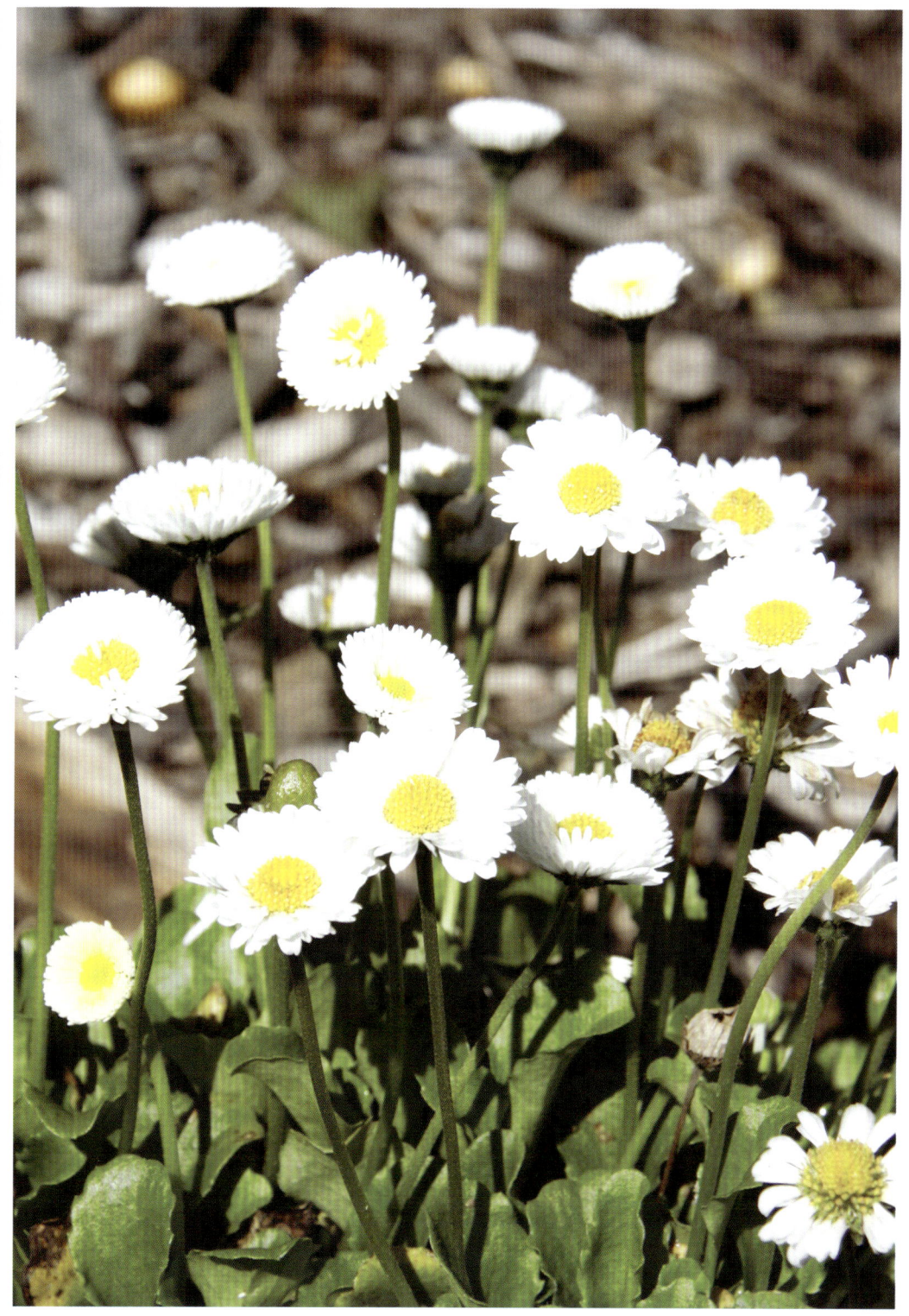

Dandelion

Taraxacum officinale
Asteraceae—*Túnfífill*

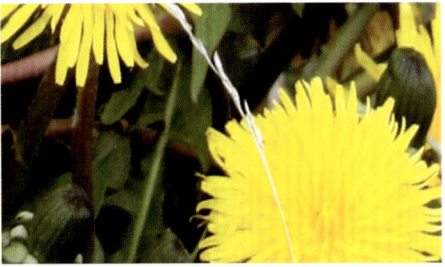

Habitat

Dandelion is very common all over Iceland and is found both in towns and in the mountains.

Parts Used

Leaves and roots.

Harvesting

Dandelion leaves are collected in early spring before bloom and the roots are harvested in autumn.

Constituents

Leaves: Sesquiterpenes, triterpenes, phytosterols, flavonoids, coumarin, fatty acids, carotene, minerals (3.5–4.5% potassium), vitamins A, B, C, and D. Roots: Sesquiterpenes, triterpenes, benzyl glucosides, phenylpropanoids, phytosterols, phenolic acids, 1.8–2.6% potassium, vitamins A, B, C, and D, amino acids, and inulin.

History

The Latin name *Taraxacum* is from the Greek "taraxos," meaning disorder, and "akos," meaning medication, and Dandelion has been a popular medicinal herb for millennia. Dandelion leaves

If a cloth is soaked in the liquid of this herb and placed over infected lesions or other inflammation, it cools down the burning thereof. This herb alone can regulate blood and open the liver and spleen well. It is also good for arthritis and jaundice. For all hot and serious internal diseases, wine is put with Dandelion and then drunk. The decoction of the herb gives the face some color, even if it was blackish or darkish before. The milk of this herb, or the juice, removes warts from the body, and clears the eyes when such juice is applied to them. [...] The leaves, which make a salad, reduce blood heat of angry men and are good for insomnia; eaten in the evening, they soften stools. They are also good for young men who live solitary lives: they dampen lust, but rejuvenate, and help with good digestion of food, both cold and boiled. [...] This herb may be bruised and used for headaches, also for burns, and this improves both of these as it cools and reduces overheating, both externally and internally.

Björn Halldórsson, Uses of Herbs, *1783*.

are rich in vitamins and minerals and have long been used in food (e.g., in salads and sauces). It is a tradition in Europe to make Dandelion wine and Dandelion syrup with the flowers and in England they are deep-fried as fritters and eaten. The roots are also roasted in the oven and used as a coffee supplement. They were also used for brewing beer at one stage. In past times in Iceland, the roots were harvested in spring, roasted on a fire, and eaten hot with butter.

The Native Americans used Dandelion a great deal, both as food and medicine. It was considered effective for anemia, digestive disturbances, constipation, back pain, inflamed eyes, edema, kidney disease, menstrual cramps, heartburn, and as a blood cleanser. Externally, poultices of the leaves were thought to be good

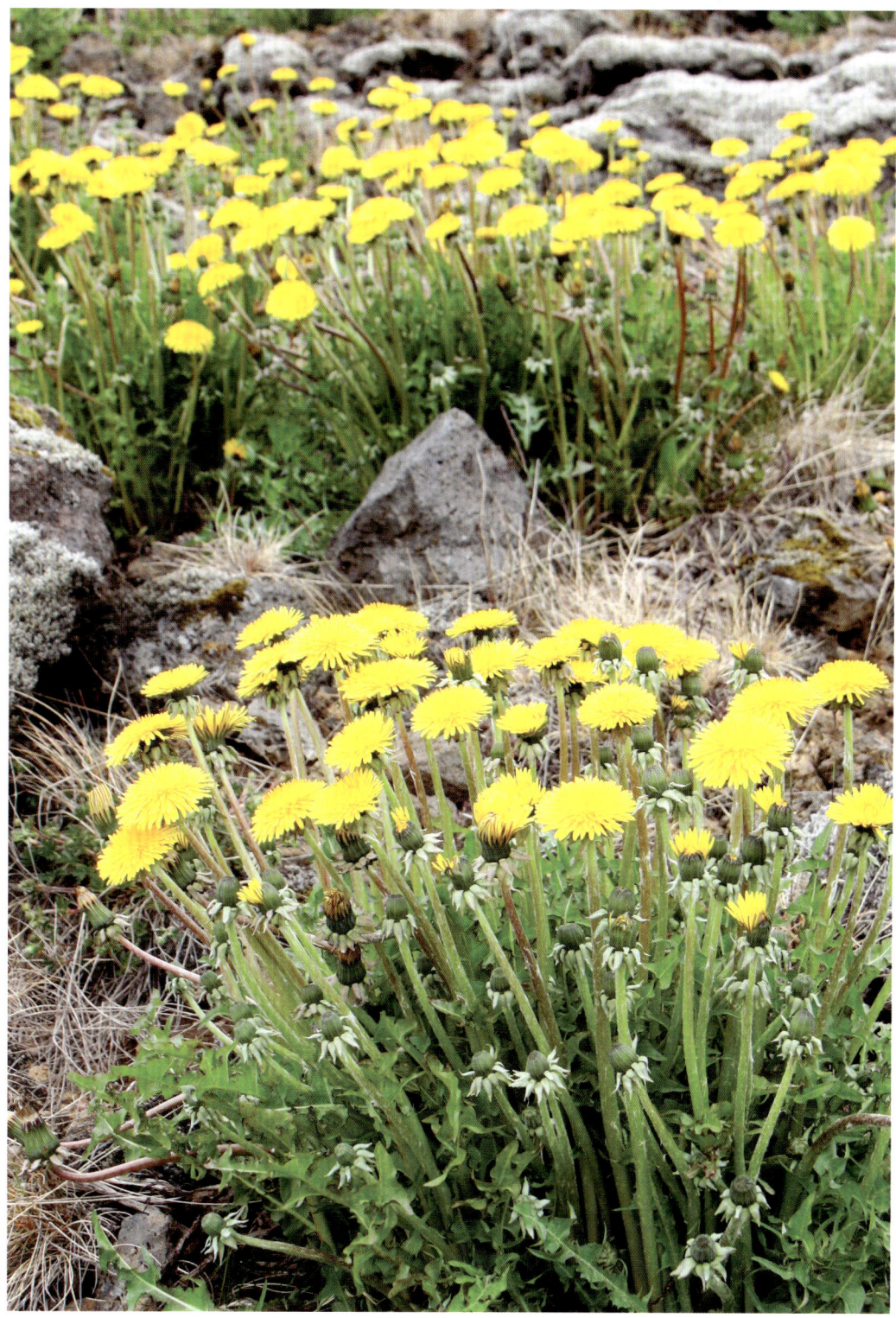

for gastritis, sore throats, wounds, inflammations, bruises, and broken bones, and poultices of the flowers were placed over inflamed testicles. The roots were chewed for toothache and to increase breast milk, but were also used in a wash against evil spirits and as a love potion.

Action

Diuretic, hepatic, cholagogue, carminative, and laxative.

. . . .

Uses

Since time immemorial, Dandelion has been seen as one of the best diuretic herbs available. The leaves are thought to be the most diuretic part of the plant, although some action is seen in the roots. When kidney function is stimulated, potassium is released on urination and this could have an effect on heart function. Dandelion leaves, however, contain large amounts of natural potassium, and thus are a very good way to increase urination. Dandelion root, on the other hand, has a stimulating effect on liver and gallbladder function, and has long been regarded as a good herb for hepatitis, jaundice, gallstones, bloating, flatulence, and constipation. It has also been used to strengthen the liver after long periods of medication or alcohol use. The root is also considered to be good internally for skin diseases and disorders such as eczema, psoriasis, and acne. There is a long tradition of using Dandelion root for rheumatism, gout, and osteoarthritis. Both the leaves and the roots have a stimulating effect on the gallbladder and they are thought to be useful in preventing gallstones. Dandelion milk, present in the stems, is frequently used externally to remove warts. The fresh milk is rubbed onto the wart twice a day and covered with a plaster. This is repeated for 1–2 weeks.

Research

In vivo research has shown the diuretic effect of Dandelion, but it is stronger in the leaves than in the roots.[1] Research has also shown that the amount of potassium in Dandelion leaves is enough to replenish that which is lost with urination.[2] *In vivo* tests have also revealed a 40% increase in bile flow with the use of Dandelion root.[1,2] Both the root and the leaves have shown antioxidant properties in *in vitro* tests, but the leaves more so than the roots.[2,3] *In vitro* and *in vivo* tests have also indicated that Dandelion root is anti-inflammatory,[2] inhibits cancer cell growth,[4] lowers blood sugar, heals wounds, and stimulates the immune system.[5]

Dosage

Tincture: 2–5 ml three times a day (1:5, 25%).

Infusion: 1–2 teaspoons in a cup three times a day.

Decoction: 1–2 teaspoons in a cup three times a day.

Warning

Dandelion milk from the stems can be irritating and caution should be taken that it does not come into contact with the eyes or mouth. The use of Dandelion is not recommended in known cases of bile duct blockage, infections, or acute gallbladder inflammation. It is also known that plants from Asteraceae can cause allergic reactions.

Diuretic Tea

2 parts Dandelion leaves

1 part Downy Birch

1 part Horsetail

Put 3–4 tablespoons of the blend into a 750 ml vacuum flask and pour boiling water into it. Strain the tea into cups and then return the herbs to the flask and allow to stand the whole day. Drink from the flask throughout the day.

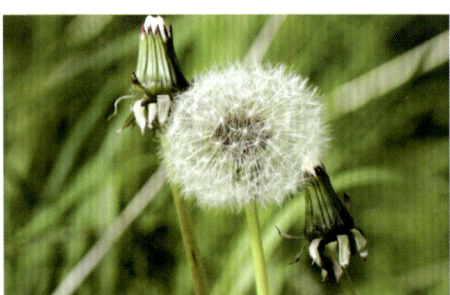

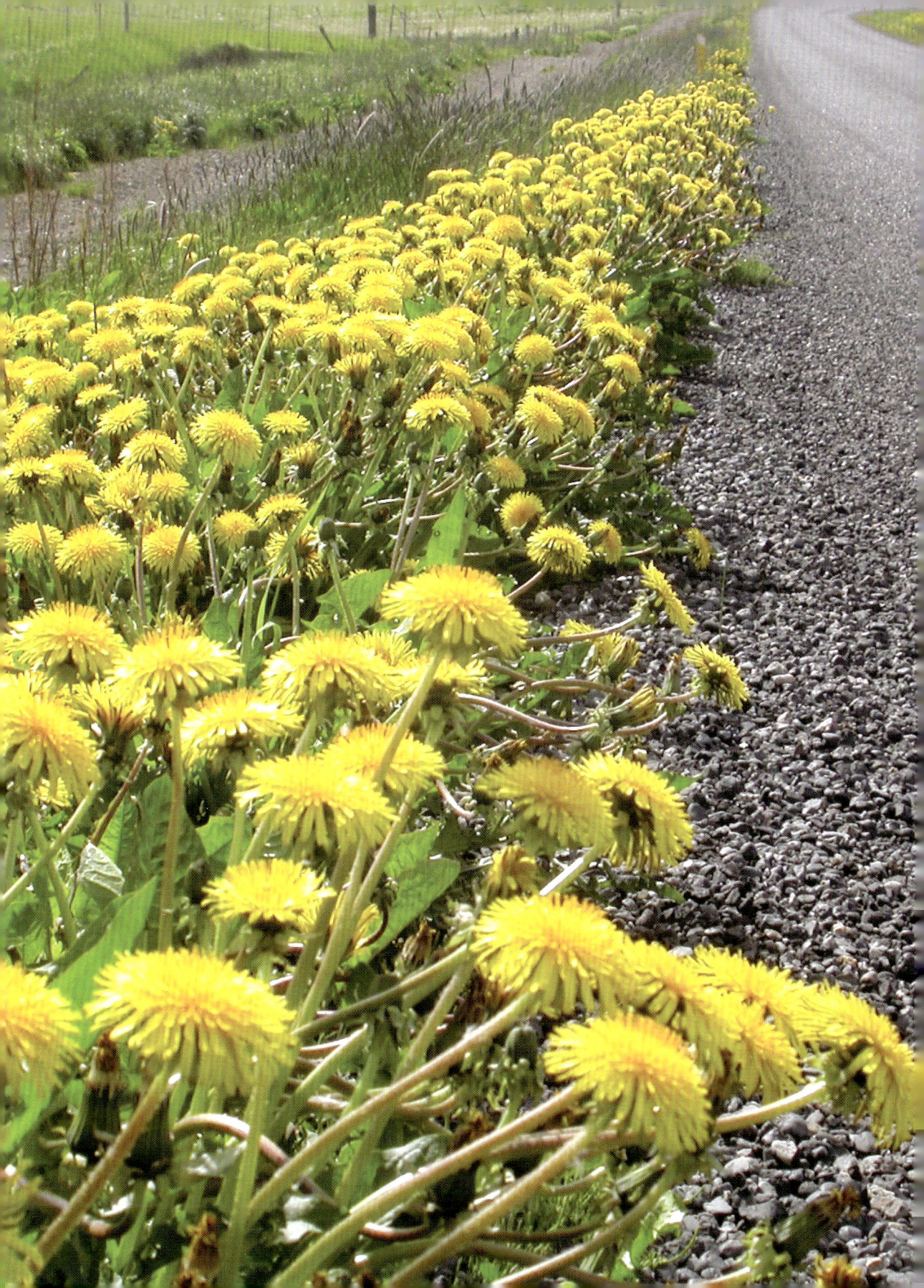

Devil's Bit Scabious

Succisa pratensis
Dipsacaceae—*Stúfa*

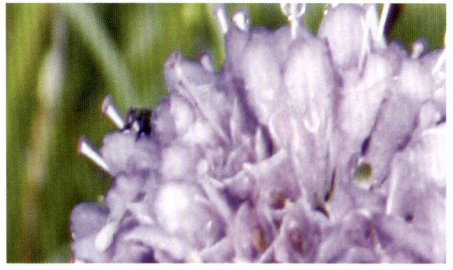

Habitat

Devil's Bit Scabious grows on slopes facing the sun. It is found only in Southwest Iceland and in the Westman Islands.

Parts Used

The entire plant is used, including the root.

Harvesting

Devil's Bit Scabious is collected in bloom in July–August.

Constituents

Iridoids.

History

The name Devil's Bit Scabious and the Icelandic "Stúfa" (stump) both refer to how the root ends suddenly, as if it had been bitten off. Legend tells that even the Devil himself did not like how the plant was revered so much for its medicinal properties and all the good it did for humans, so he bit off a piece of the root. The Old Icelandic name is actually "púkabit," meaning demon's bite. The name Scabious refers to the fact that this herb was thought to work well against scabies, which fits with the old Latin name for this species, *Scabiosa succisa*. Devil's Bit Scabious has been used to dye yarn.

Action

Diaphoretic, demulcent, febrifuge, and mild expectorant.

Uses

Devil's Bit Scabious is not used in Western herbal medicine nowadays but it was used for coughs, fevers, and internal inflammation in the past. It was also thought to work well externally for all sorts of rashes and dandruff. It was considered effective for bruises and itching of the skin and as a gargle for sore throats.

Dosage

Tincture: 2–4 ml three times a day (1:5, 25%).

Infusion: 1–2 teaspoons in a cup three times a day.

Decoction: 1–2 teaspoons in a cup three times a day.

Infusions, decoctions, tinctures, compresses, and ointments for external use.

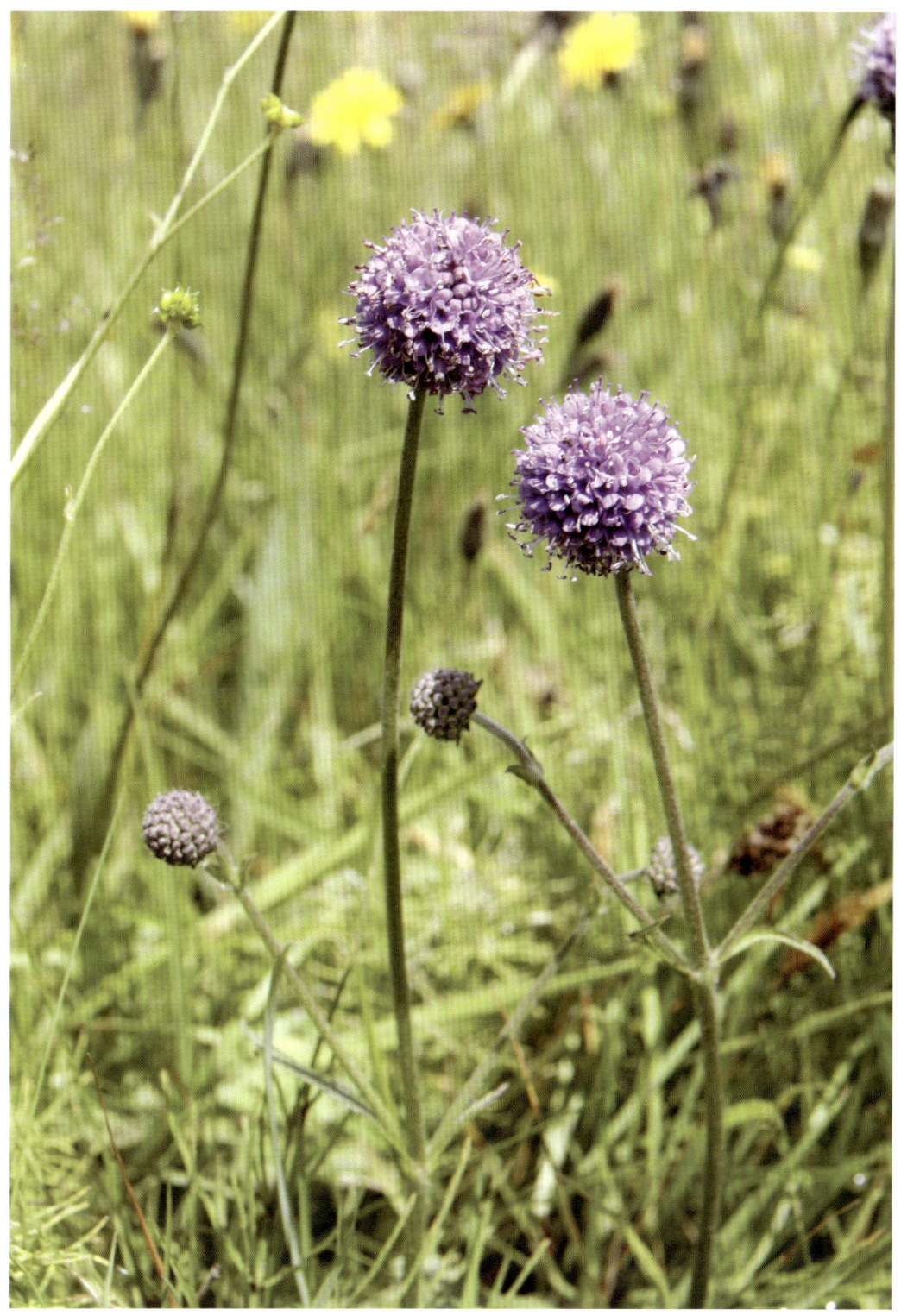

Downy Birch

Betula pubescens
Betulaceae—*Birki*

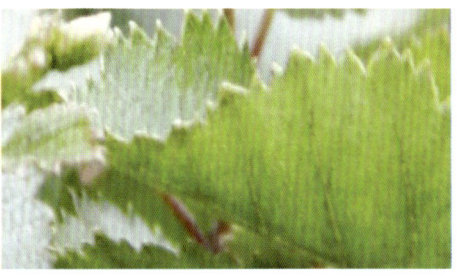

This tree has strengthening, diuretic, blood cleansing and astringent powers. Tea is made from the young shoots and dried leaves. A decoction is made from the bark which is fitting when taken 2 tablespoons at a time and powder from the bark is good against weakness, fatigue and loss of appetite. A teaspoonful mixed with whey, to be taken three times a day.

Oddur Jónsson Hjaltalín,
Icelandic Botany, 1830

Habitat

Common all over Iceland.

Parts Used

Leaves, bark, sap, and the tips of young twigs.

Harvesting

Leaves and the tips of the young shoots are picked in May and June. Leaves, bark, and sap are collected during the spring.

Constituents

Bark: Triterpenes (betulinic acid). Leaves: Flavonoids (quercetin), phenolic acids (chlorogenic acid), tannins, terpenes, and essential oil (methyl salicylate).

History

Birch has been used as a medicinal herb for centuries. Many species of Birch have been used for healing, the most well known being Silver Birch, *B. pendula,* which does not grow in Iceland. However, according to source materials the Icelandic species has very similar effects. The origin of the name goes back to the Old English word "beohrt," meaning bright, shiny.

An essential oil that primarily contains methyl salicylate is distilled from the bark of Sweet Birch, *B. lenta.* It is a very strong oil so caution should be taken when using it and it should always be blended with a base oil. This oil is mainly used as a pain reliever for muscular and joint pain. In Russia, Birch tar oil from the wood and the bark is traditionally used: this is usually mixed in an ointment or soap and used for skin problems such as eczema and psoriasis. Tar oil was also used to protect leather and for developing photographs. Birch bark was used to cure leather in Europe and both the leaves and the bark have been used as dyes. It is also common practice in many countries to tap the sap off the plant and use it for medicinal and culinary purposes.

Dwarf Birch (*B. nana*) is closely related to Birch and is also used for healing, but this has not been well documented.

Action

Diuretic, anti-inflammatory, antibacterial, astringent, diaphoretic, and mildly analgesic.

Uses

Downy Birch leaves are excellent for healing as they have diuretic properties and have been used in cases of arthritic conditions, especially rheumatoid arthritis, psoriatic arthritis, and gout. The leaves are also effective in the treatment of

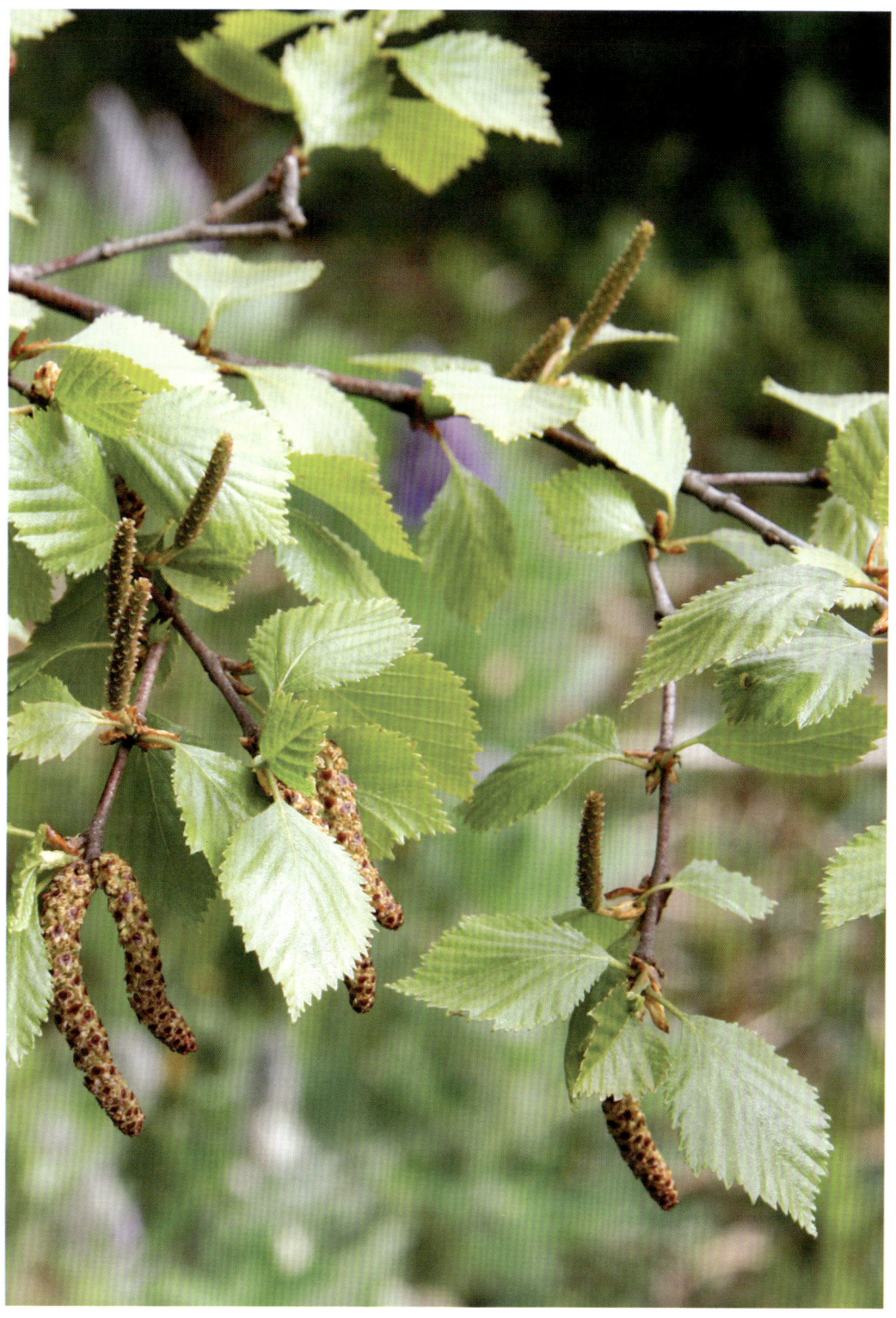

kidney stones, edema, cystitis, and other urinary infections. They are also reputed to be excellent, both internally and externally, for skin diseases such as eczema and psoriasis. The decoction or tincture of the bark is effective in the treatment of muscular and joint pain: soak a cloth in the liquid and put it on the painful area. Birch is used in hair products as it is reported to stimulate hair growth. It is considered healing and is often used in ointments to heal wounds and various kinds of rashes. In India, *B.utilis* is used for cramp, dysentery, bleeding, and skin diseases.

Research

Some of the following research refers to components that have been isolated from Birch bark. Although many of these research studies have been done on Silver Birch (*B. pendula*), which does not grow in Iceland, sources show that Downy Birch and other species have all been used in a similar way to Silver Birch. Open clinical trials without a placebo were undertaken using Birch leaf on 1,066 individuals with urinary inflammations or infections. More than half of the group received antibiotics. At the end of the trial, the results showed that 80% of those who took the antibiotics had no symptoms and 75% of those who received only Birch were also symptom-free. Over 90% of both doctors and patients believed that the effect of the Birch was good or very good. Less than 1% of participants showed mild side effects. In a small double-blind clinical study using a placebo, patients with urinary infections were given Birch tea for 20 days. Microbes in the urine decreased by 39% in those who received Birch but only by 18% in those who received the placebo. Results showed that three out of seven patients who received the Birch were free of symptoms whereas only one out of six were symptom-free in the placebo group. In a trial where animals were given Birch tea, a significant increase in the volume of urine and the excretion of chloride was detected; another trial showed no increase in urine volume but an increase in both the excretion of chloride and urea. In a third *in vivo* test, new leaves were shown to have no diuretic effects at all. Further *in vivo* research has shown both positive and negative diuretic effects of the Birch leaf. There is also evidence that the potassium content in Birch leaves causes their diuretic properties.[1]

Active ingredients of Birch bark have proved successful in the treatment of sores (e.g., cold sores[2,3]), and skin problems.[4-7] It is said that the active ingredients of certain Birch species inhibit cancer cells (e.g., in the stomach, lungs, and pancreas).[8-16] Research on Manchuria Birch (*B. platyphylla* var. *japonica*) points strongly to evidence that the bark stimulates the immune system,[17] is anti-inflammatory, and protects the cartilage in cases of osteoarthritis,[18,19] has anti-oxidant properties, and has a protective effect on the liver.[14,20] Birch tar oil has also been shown to inhibit the bacteria that causes pneumonia, *Legionella pneumophilia*,[21] while the bark works on the tuberculosis bacteria.[22] Scientific research on Downy Birch has shown its inhibiting effects on *Staphylococcus aureus*.[23] Other research has revealed the antibacterial and antifungal properties as well as anti-inflammatory properties of Birch.[24-26] There is also evidence that Birch has a beneficial effect on arthritic diseases.[27]

Dosage

Tincture: 1-5 ml three times a day (1:5, 25%).

Infusion: 1–2 cups three times a day.

Decoction: 1–2 teaspoons in a cup three times a day.

Infusions, decoctions, tinctures, compresses, and ointments for external use.

It is thought that by adding a pinch of baking soda to the infusion, it will increase the potency.

Warning

Research indicates that Birch leaves are contraindicated for those with edema due to dysfunction of the heart or kidneys.

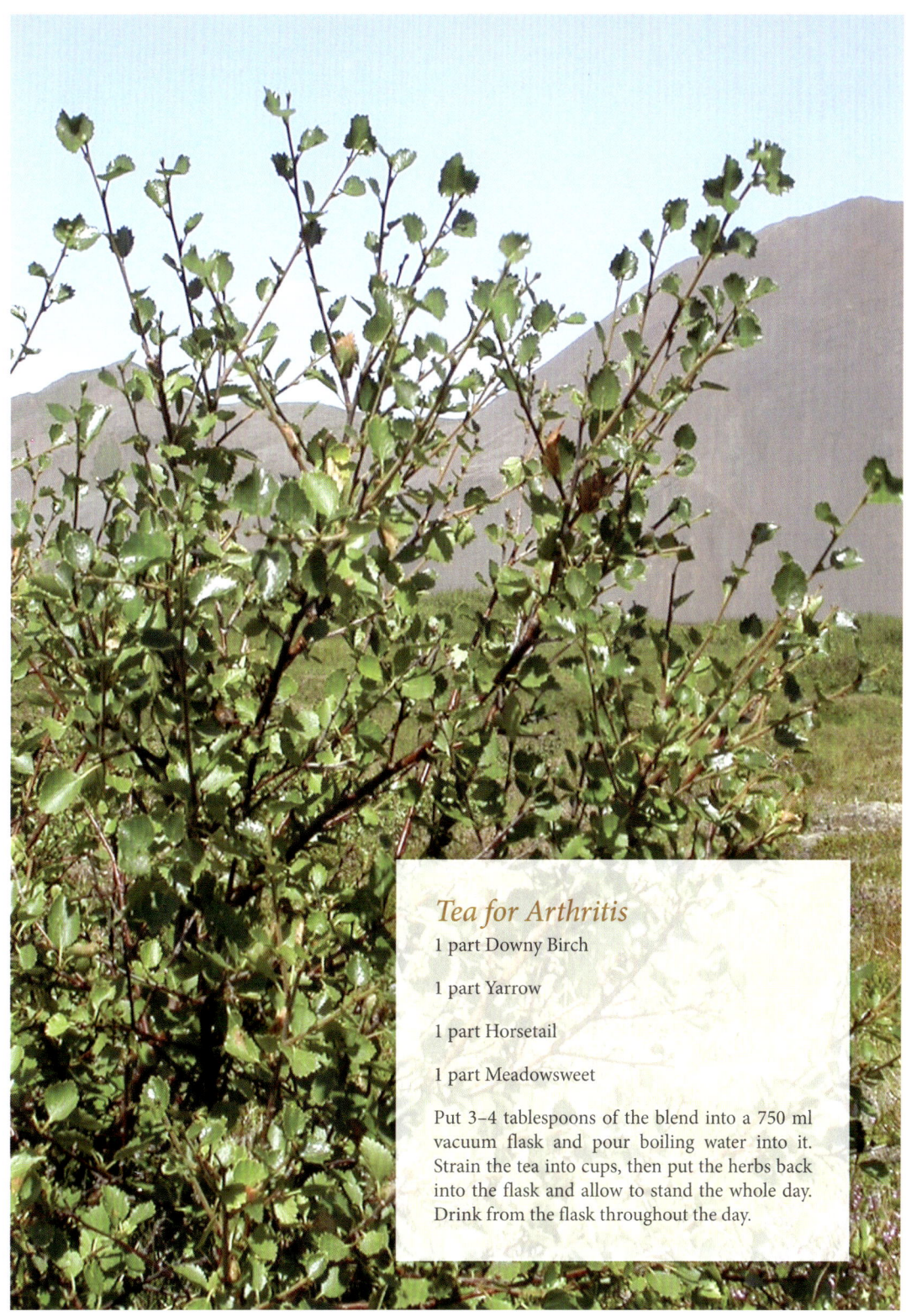

Tea for Arthritis

1 part Downy Birch

1 part Yarrow

1 part Horsetail

1 part Meadowsweet

Put 3–4 tablespoons of the blend into a 750 ml vacuum flask and pour boiling water into it. Strain the tea into cups, then put the herbs back into the flask and allow to stand the whole day. Drink from the flask throughout the day.

Dulse

Palmaria palmata
Palmariaceae—*Söl*

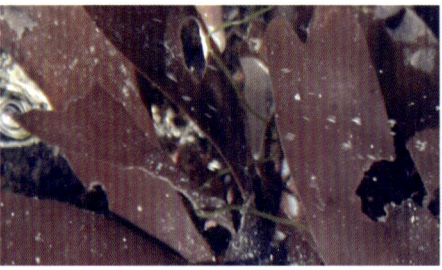

Dulse is stimulating to the digestion and nourishing, has a pleasant taste, is healthy and provides nourishment very quickly, even if there is sickness or exhaustion. Dulse is high in salt and is good for cold diseases. It stimulates both appetite and thirst, heals nausea and protects against sea sickness, bloating and constipation. It takes care of all the natural functions of the body, it fattens and strengthens both men and women for childbearing. Those who have overindulged and spoiled the rule of the stomach and blood regulation will do well to use Dulse for a meal and as a spice the next day.

Björn Halldórsson, Uses of Herbs, 1783

Habitat

Dulse grows on beaches all over Iceland, but is most common in South and West Iceland.

Parts Used

The entire seaweed.

Harvesting

It is possible to collect Dulse all summer, but usually it is collected between August and November.

Constituents

Protein, vitamins A and B, calcium, iodine, iron, potassium, phosphorus, magnesium, zinc, and various other minerals.

History

The collection of Dulse in Iceland is part of a rich tradition dating back to settlement times, although it is not as common today as it was in the past. One famous story concerns Egill Skallagrimsson, a well-known figure of the Icelandic Sagas who went on a hunger strike but ended it by eating Dulse on the insistence of his daughter Þorgerður. Dulse was valuable currency, similar to Iceland Moss, and many references concern the collection of Dulse. In addition, a number of place names in Iceland contain the word "Söl" (Icelandic for Dulse) (e.g., Sölvamannagötur, which ran along the Saurbæjar beaches in Gilsfjord where the most Dulse could be found and to which seventeen parishes had access). Dulse was also a common food in Ireland, Scotland, and North America.

In Scotland there is a saying about the healing properties of Dulse: "He who eats the Dulse will escape all maladies except Black Death." In Iceland a number of sayings concern Dulse (e.g., "The sick are not offered Dulse" and "Heartache is calmed by eating raw Dulse"). These examples show that there was a difference of opinion about the goodness of Dulse. In Scotland and Ireland, Dulse was considered a cure-all and thought to be good for scurvy, worms, poor eyesight, migraines, gastritis, kidney and bladder stones, fevers, throat infections, and stomach pain, and for making placental birth easier.

Dulse has been used in different ways for centuries: Dulse soup was, for example, common in Scotland while in Iceland it was boiled and eaten with butter, cod liver oil, or dried fish, usually accompanied by milk or a soured drink. Dulse was also

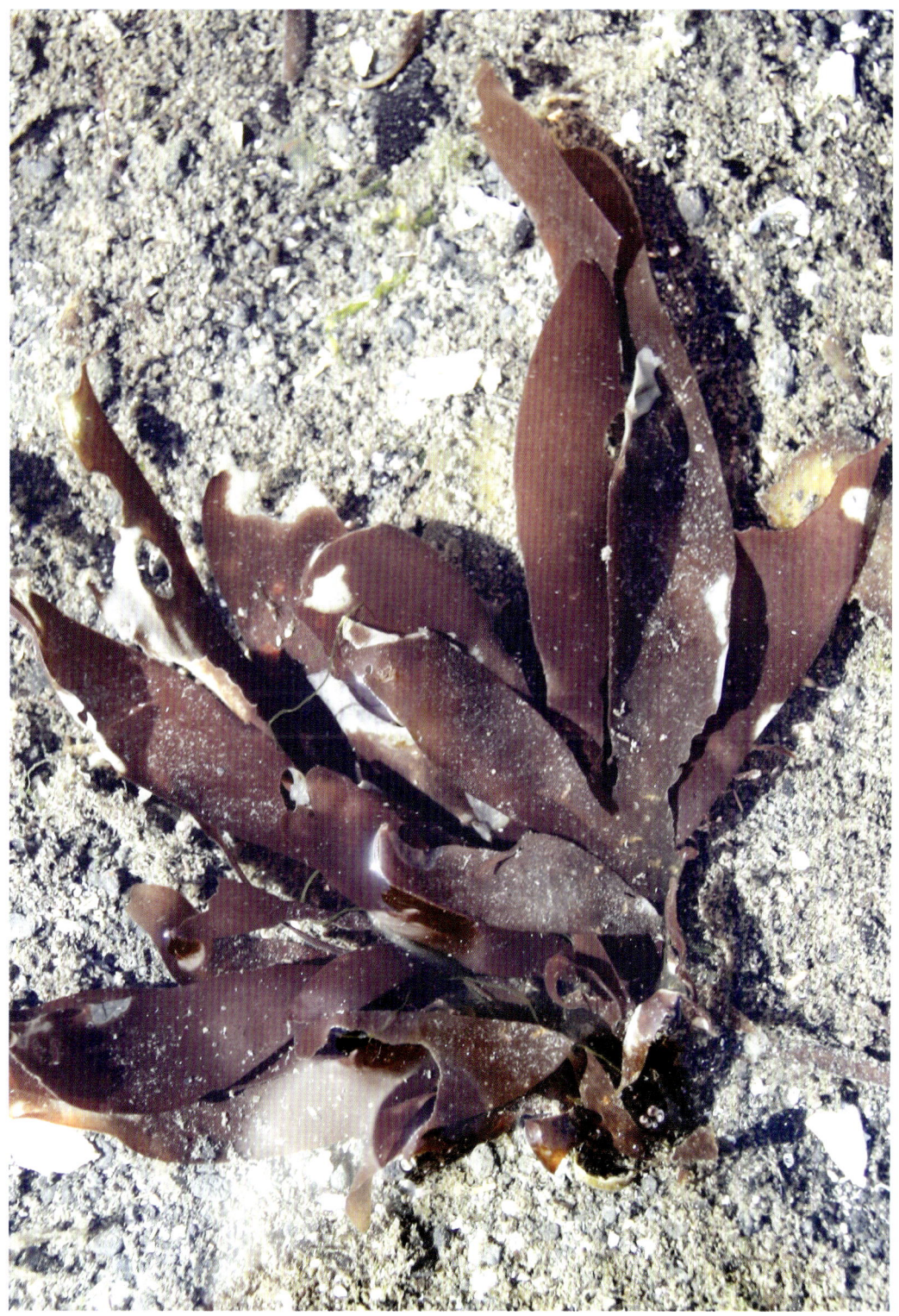

chopped and eaten with bread, porridge, or blood pudding, but nowadays Dulse is usually eaten as it is, and then usually as a snack. Dulse works very well in soups, salads, or with fish.

Action

Mild laxative and nourishing.

. . . .

Uses

Dulse is rarely used in Western herbal medicine nowadays. Due to its high content of iodine, it was thought to be good for hypothyroidism. Dulse is also rich in iron and is therefore good for those who suffer from anemia, besides being frequently recommended for menstruating and breastfeeding women. It is also thought to be good as a digestive stimulant and for colds and influenza. As Dulse is rich in minerals, it is also said to be good for stimulating hair growth and strengthening nails.

Research

Dulse contains about 34 times more potassium than bananas. A patient with diabetes and chronic kidney disease complained of nausea, vomiting, and general malaise and was diagnosed with too much potassium in his blood. This was traced back to his having eaten about 200 g of Dulse the same day as the above symptoms appeared.[1] *In vitro* research on Dulse revealed that it may have antioxidant properties and an inhibiting effect on the growth of cervical cancer cells.[2,3]

Dosage

Dulse is mainly eaten dried, either on its own or with other food.

Infusion: 1 teaspoon in a cup three times a day.

Warning

Dulse should not be used by people with hyperthyroidism, those who are taking medication for thyroid diseases, or those with disturbed kidney function. Eating Dulse in large amounts for extended periods of time is not recommended.

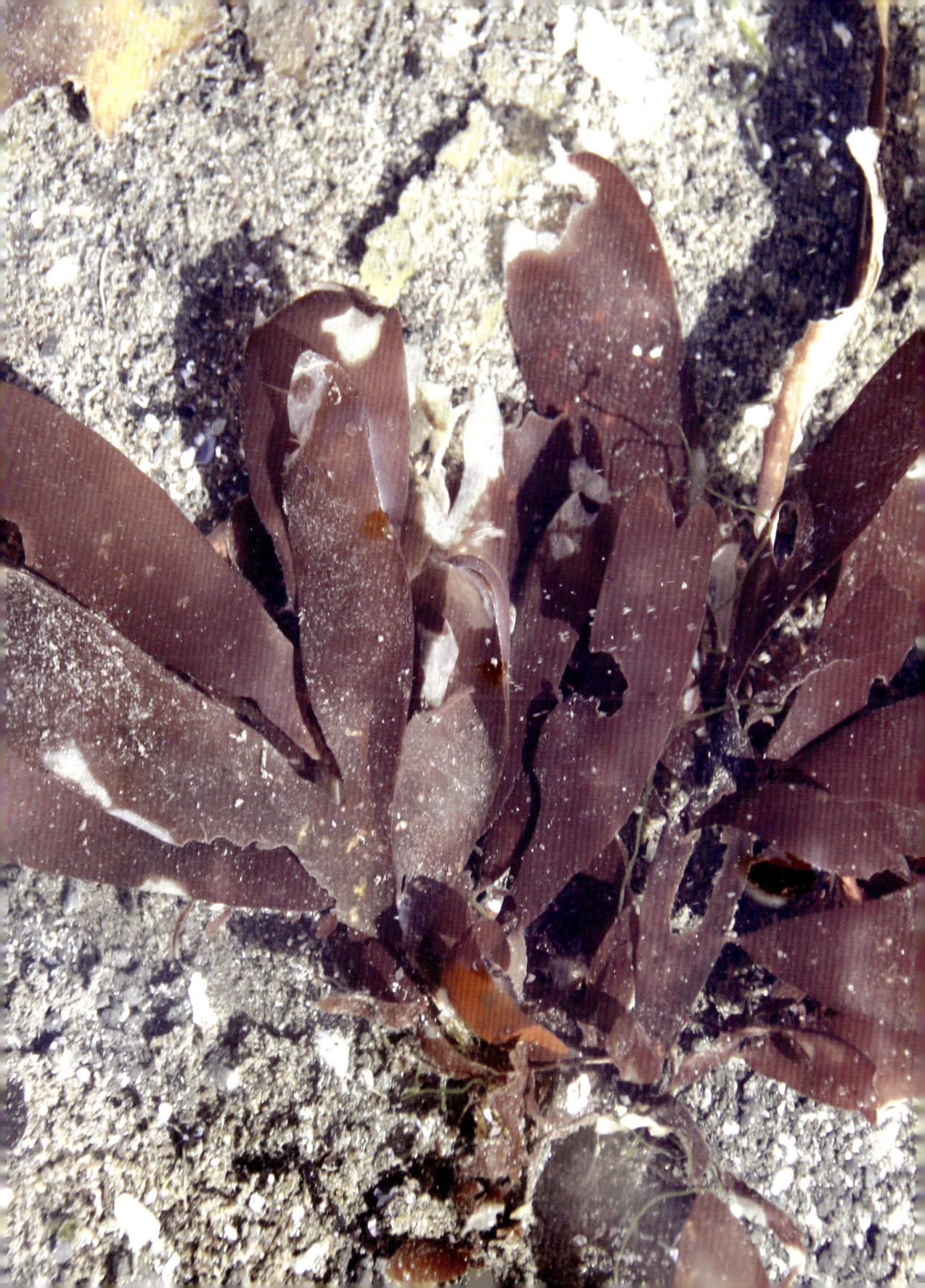

Field Gentian

Gentianella campestris
Gentianaceae—*Maríuvöndur*

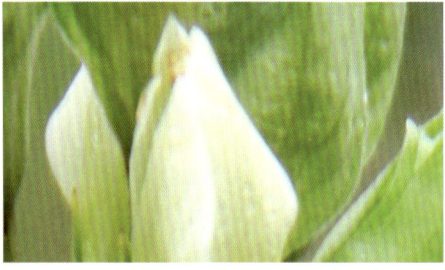

Habitat

Field Gentian is common all over Iceland and grows mainly in dry grasslands.

Parts Used

The entire plant is used, including the root.

Harvesting

Field Gentian is collected in bloom in July–August. The roots are harvested in autumn.

Constituents

Not known.

History

There are many medicinal herbs in the Gentian family and all of them are bitter. The best-known medicinal herb in this family is *Gentiana lutea,* which does not grow in Iceland, but references to its medicinal properties can be found dating back to the second century BC.

The genus name for Field Gentian is either *Gentiana* or *Gentianella*, both of which have their roots in the name of the King of Illyria, Gentius (180–167 BC), who was said to have discovered the healing powers of *Gentianella*. In Iceland, there are two species of *Gentianella*, Field Gentian and *G. amarella*, which are referred to as having been used as medicinal herbs in the past. These are both said to have similar action to *Gentiana lutea*. The old name for Field Gentian is "kveisu-gras," meaning colic grass, and refers to its uses as a medicinal herb for colic.

Action

Hepatic, cholagogue, carminative, and anthelmintic.

Uses

Field Gentian is rarely used in Western herbalism nowadays. Bitter herbs have the quality of stimulating digestive juices, which aids the assimilation of nutrients from the digestive system. Field Gentian is thought to strengthen and stimulate digestion and help with flatulence, loss of appetite, digestive disturbances, and worms. In Tibet, herbs from the *Gentianella* genus are considered to be good for lowering fevers, reducing inflammation, and stimulating the gallbladder. They are used for jaundice and inflammation of the eyes, liver, and kidneys.

Dosage

Tincture: 1–2 ml three times a day (1:5, 40%).

Infusion: ½ teaspoon in a cup three times a day.

Decoction: ½ teaspoon in a cup three times a day.

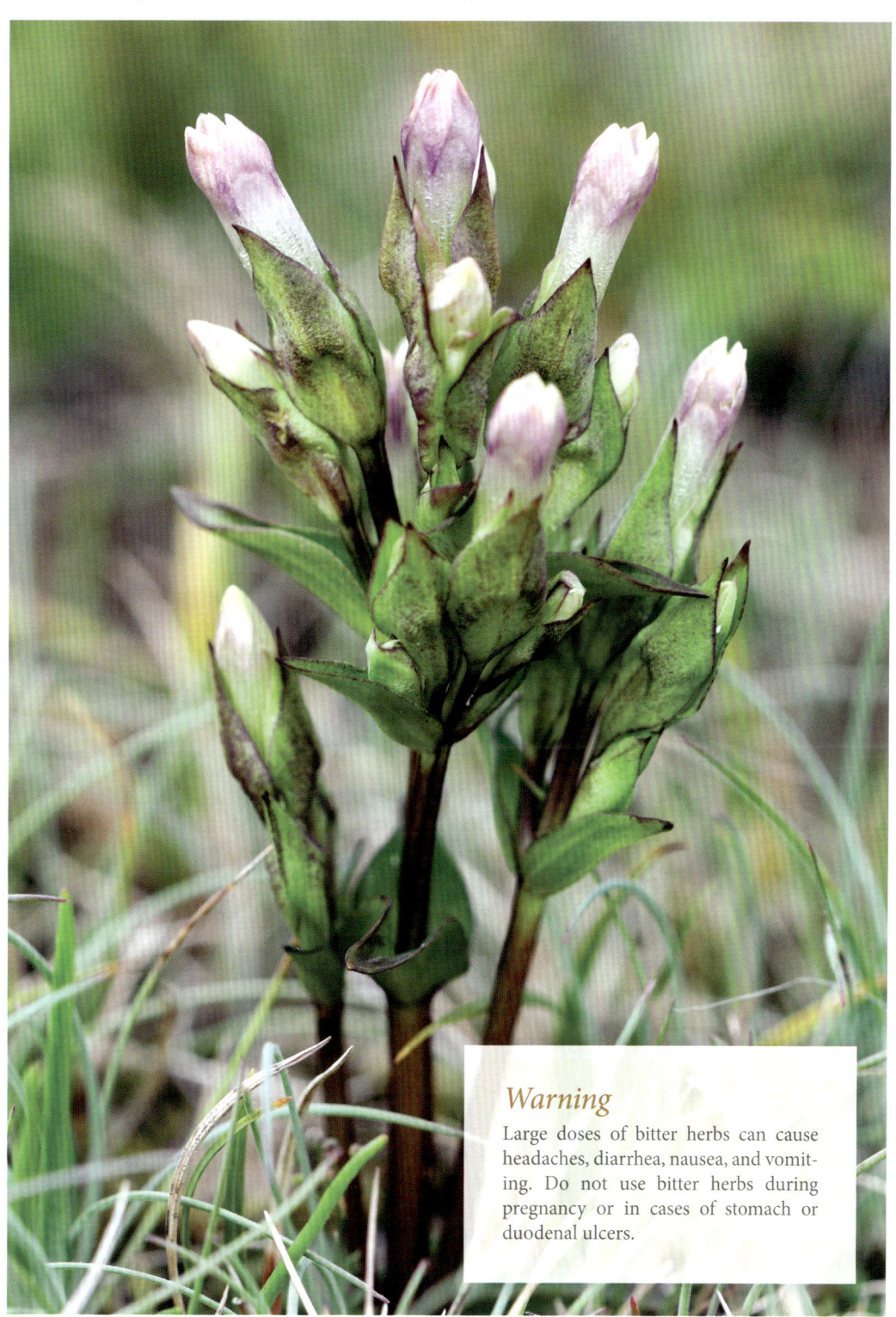

Warning

Large doses of bitter herbs can cause headaches, diarrhea, nausea, and vomiting. Do not use bitter herbs during pregnancy or in cases of stomach or duodenal ulcers.

Fir Clubmoss

Huperzia selago
Huperziaceae—*Skollafingur*

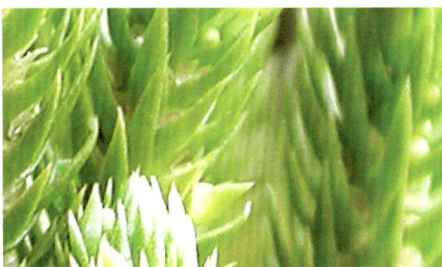

Habitat

Fir Clubmoss is common all over Iceland except in the South.

Parts Used

The entire plant is used, except for the root.

Constituents

Lycopodium alkaloids and resins.

History

Fir Clubmoss used to be classified under the genus *Lycopodium,* which means fox or wolf paw. References from the Canadian Inuits report that Fir Clubmoss was used to induce vomiting and diarrhea, and externally was used as a compress to ease headaches. They also used it to achieve altered states of mind, as sources say that only 8 stalks of the plant needed to be ingested to cause loss of consciousness. In these references, it is also mentioned that Wolf's Foot (*L. clavatum*) was used in a similar way to Fir Clubmoss. *L. clavatum* is a protected plant in Iceland, but is a well-known medicinal herb elsewhere and is similar to Fir Clubmoss in appearance.

Stiff Clubmoss (*L. annotinum*) has also been used as a medicinal herb in Iceland and is thought to be good for bloating, intense pain, dysentery, and diarrhea. Fir Clubmoss has also been used as a fixative for dyeing yarn.

Action

Laxative and emetic.

Uses

It is not known whether Fir Clubmoss is used in Western herbal medicine today, but it was used in the past for constipation and to induce vomiting.

Research

In recent German research it is shown that all Lycopodium are safe to use except for Fir Clubmoss. There have been two reported incidents where an infusion of Fir Clubmoss was taken by mistake and caused sweating, vomiting, diarrhea, dizziness, cramps, and slurred speech.[1] At the University of Iceland, a few of the Huperziaceae species have been researched, including Fir Clubmoss, Stiff Clubmoss (*L. annotinum*), and Alpine Clubmoss (*Diphasiastrum alpinum*). Isolated alkaloids in the Huperziaceae have been researched by *in vitro* testing and have aroused attention because of their inhibiting effect on the breakdown of an enzyme called acetylcholinesterase. This research indicates a possible effect on memory loss and stimulation of the immune system.[1–4]

Warning

Fir Clubmoss is poisonous and is not recommended for medicinal use under any circumstances.

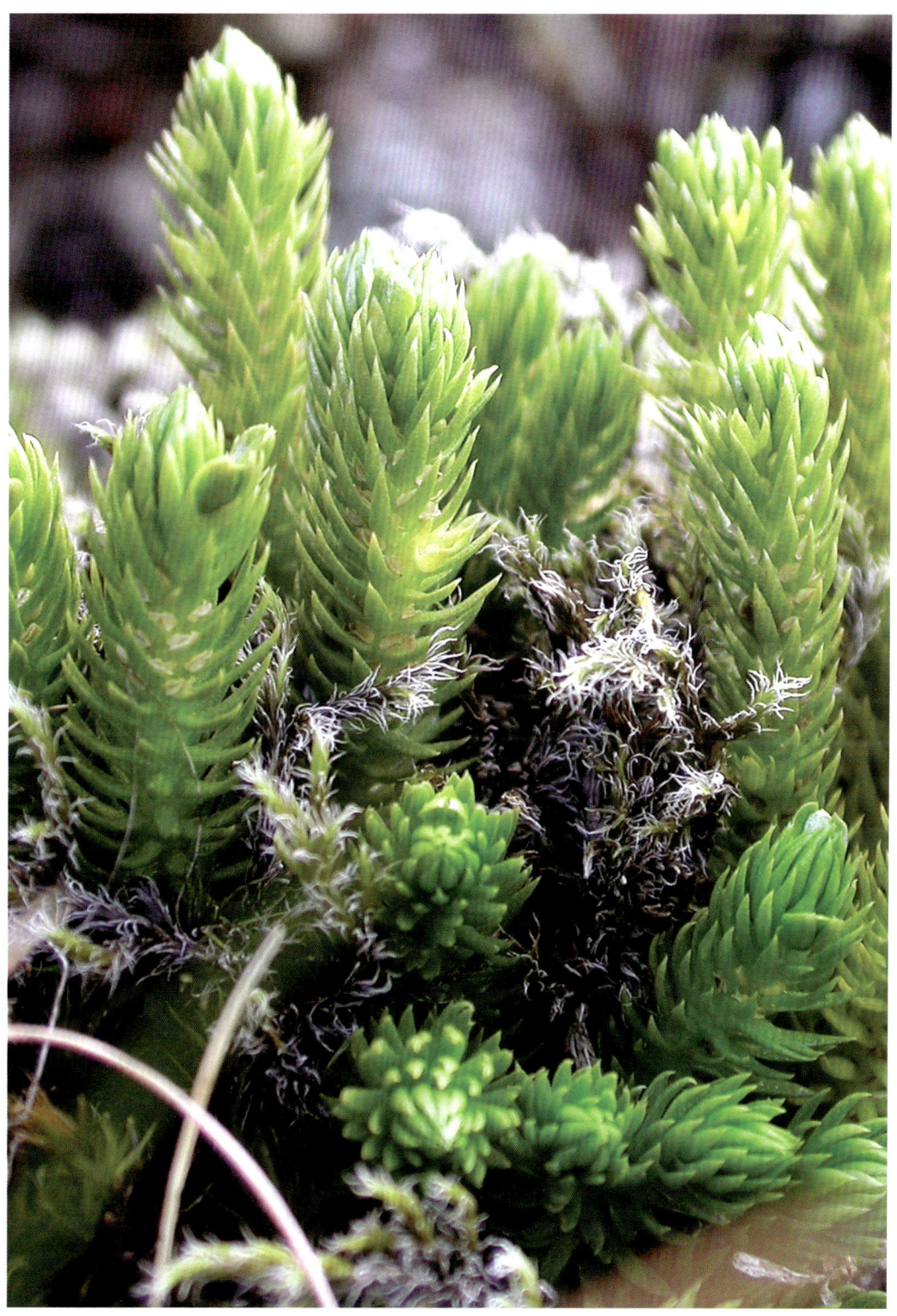

Grass of Parnassus

Parnassia palustris

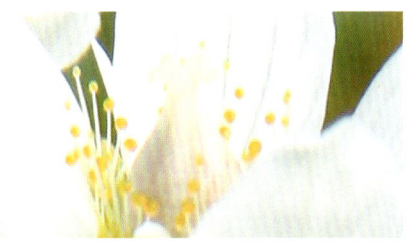

Celastraceae—*Mýrasóley*

Habitat

Grass of Parnassus is common all over Iceland and grows only in wetlands and heaths.

Parts Used

The entire plant is used, except for the root.

Harvesting

Grass of Parnassus is collected in bloom in June–July.

Constituents

Tannins, resin, and mucilage.

History

In old Icelandic references, Grass of Parnassus is called "liver herb with white blossoms" as it was thought to cure liver problems. In Spanish, it has been called "Hepática blanca," meaning "liver herb with white blossoms", which is still the name in use today.

Action

Astringent, sedative, mild diuretic, and vulnerary.

Uses

It is not known if Grass of Parnassus is used much in Western herbalism nowadays. It was thought to be good for diarrhea, restlessness, and irregular heartbeat, and was reputed to be a tonic for the nerves and heart. The infusion of the herb was thought to be good for conjunctivitis, gingivitis, and mouth ulcers, but there is differing opinion about whether it is effective or damaging to eyes. Grass of Parnassus has also been used externally to heal wounds. In Tibet, the closely related *P. cabulica* is used medicinally. This is considered to be anti-inflammatory and stimulating for the liver and gallbladder and is used for inflammation, fevers, and various infections. In Nepal, another closely related species, *P. nubicola*, is used to clean wounds, using both the decoction of the root and the fresh juice from the leaves.

Research

There is no known research on the medicinal properties of Grass of Parnassus, but *in vitro* testing shows that the decoction of the root of *P. nubicola* could have an anti-inflammatory effect and inhibit cancer cell growth.[1,2]

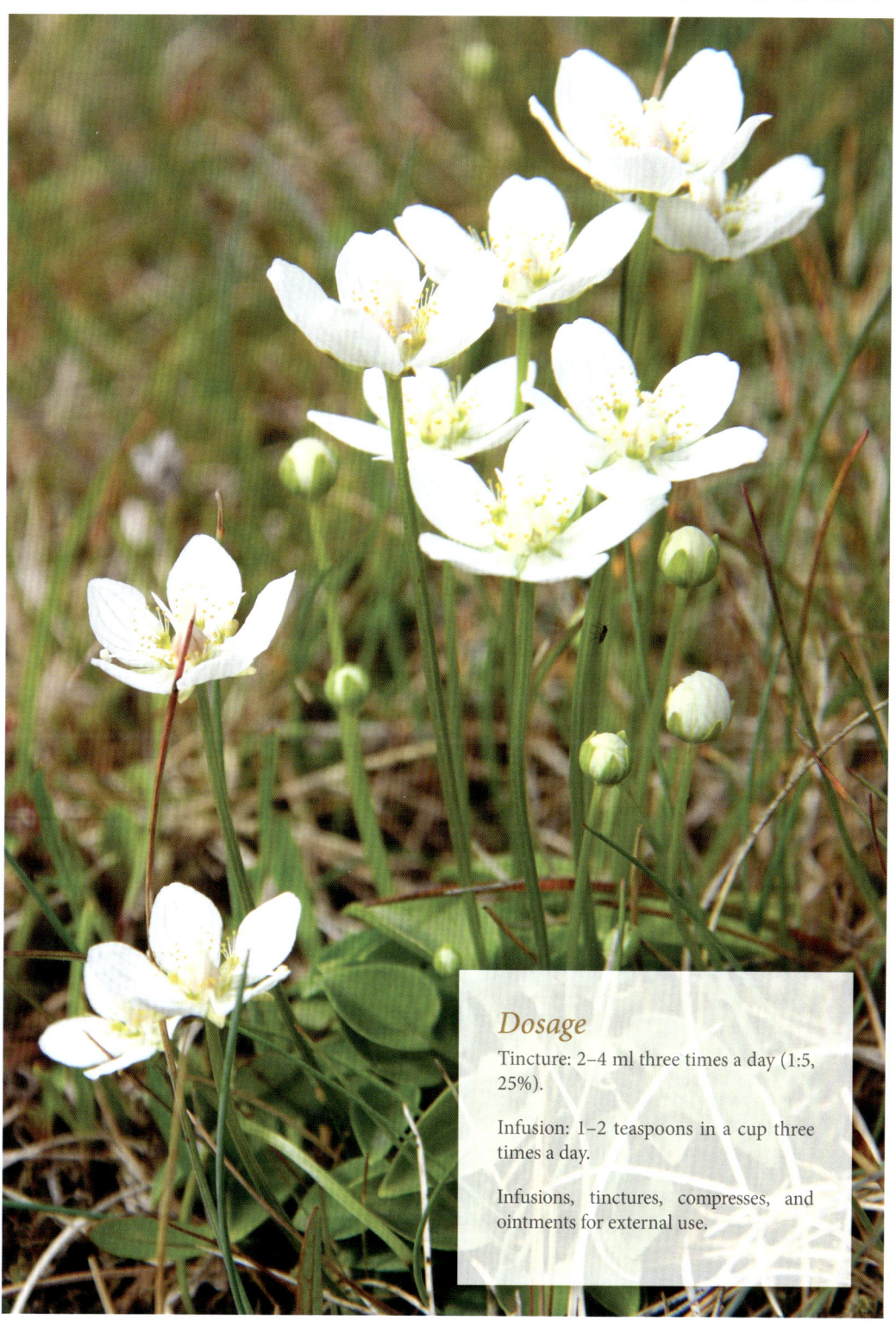

Dosage

Tincture: 2–4 ml three times a day (1:5, 25%).

Infusion: 1–2 teaspoons in a cup three times a day.

Infusions, tinctures, compresses, and ointments for external use.

Greater Burnet

Sanguisorba officinalis
Rosaceae—Blóðkollur

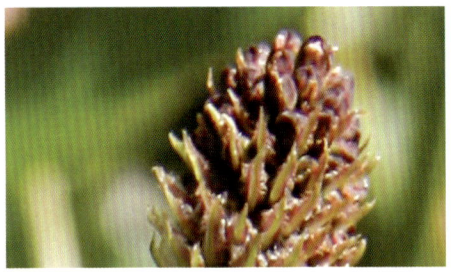

Habitat

Greater Burnet is rare in Iceland, but is found in the South and on the Snæfellsnes Peninsula.

Parts Used

The entire plant is used, including the root.

Harvesting

Due to its rarity, harvesting is not recommended.

Constituents

Tannins, triterpenes (ursolic acid), and flavonoids (rutin).

History

The genus name *Sanguisorba* indicates its medicinal properties, as "sanguis" means blood and "sorbere" means suck up or swallow in Latin, thus perhaps explaining the long tradition of using Greater Burnet to stop bleeding. As an example, American soldiers in the 18th century were given Greater Burnet to drink as a preventive for losing blood should they be wounded. Culpepper, a respected English herbalist in the 17th century, recommended putting two to three stems with leaves of the plant in a glass of white wine, to lift the spirits and strengthen the heart. It is also customary to use the leaves of Greater Burnet in salads or boiled as a vegetable. It has also been used as animal fodder and for brewing beer. The roots were used to tan leather, because of the high tannin content.

Action

Astringent, hemostatic, antibacterial, antifungal, antiviral, vulnerary, anti-inflammatory, and antiemetic.

Uses

It is traditionally used for digestive disorders, being especially effective for diarrhea, colitis, and ulcerative colitis. In both Western and Chinese herbal medicine, it is traditionally used to treat heavy menstrual bleeding. Externally it is used for hemorrhoids, varicose veins, vasculitis, burns, eczema and sores, vaginal discharges, and as a gargle for sore throats. In China, Greater Burnet has been used for centuries. There, leaves are used to reduce fever. Roots are used more often in China and are thought to be analgesic, to stop internal and external bleeding, and to reduce fever, as well as being good for bacterial dysentery, hemorrhoids, eczema, tumors, nausea, itching, snake bites, and inflammation of the womb. In China, Greater Burnet ranks 19th out of 250 plants that are reputed to be contraceptive. In Korea, this plant has long been considered as anti-inflammatory, analgesic, and antibacterial.

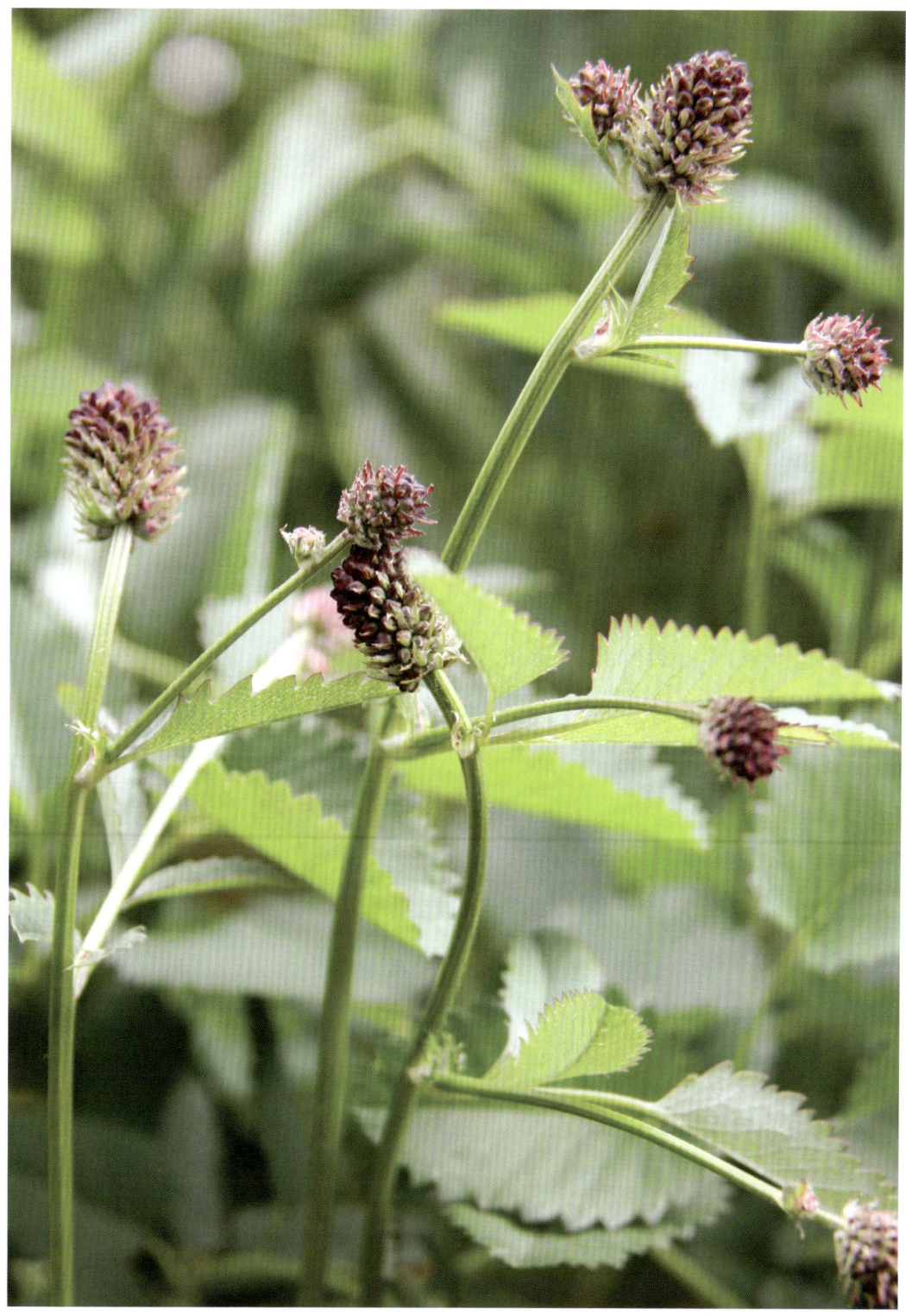

Research

Some clinical research has been done in China on Greater Burnet. This has revealed that it is effective against bleeding in the stomach and duodenum, heavy menstrual bleeding, bacterial dysentery, and pulmonary tuberculosis with hemoptysis, as well as an ointment for eczema. In some of these studies, Greater Burnet was combined with other herbs.[1]

Other *in vitro* and *in vivo* tests indicate that Greater Burnet acts against viral infections (e.g., hepatitis B,[2] bacterial infections,[1,3] and athero-sclerosis),[4] while also having antioxidant properties.[5–7] It is also thought to be good for the skin; it heals burn wounds[1] and is reputed to prevent wrinkles[8,9] as well as being a skin lightener.[10] Greater Burnet is also anti-inflammatory,[11] stops bleeding,[1] lessens vomiting,[1] and minimizes allergic reactions.[12,13] It is thought to inhibit cancer cell growth[1,14,15] and shows properties that could be used in the treatment of strokes.[16,17]

Dosage

Tincture: 2–6 ml three times a day (1:5, 40%).

Infusion: 1–2 teaspoons in a cup three times a day.

Decoction: 1–2 teaspoons three times a day.

Infusions, tinctures, compresses, and ointments used externally.

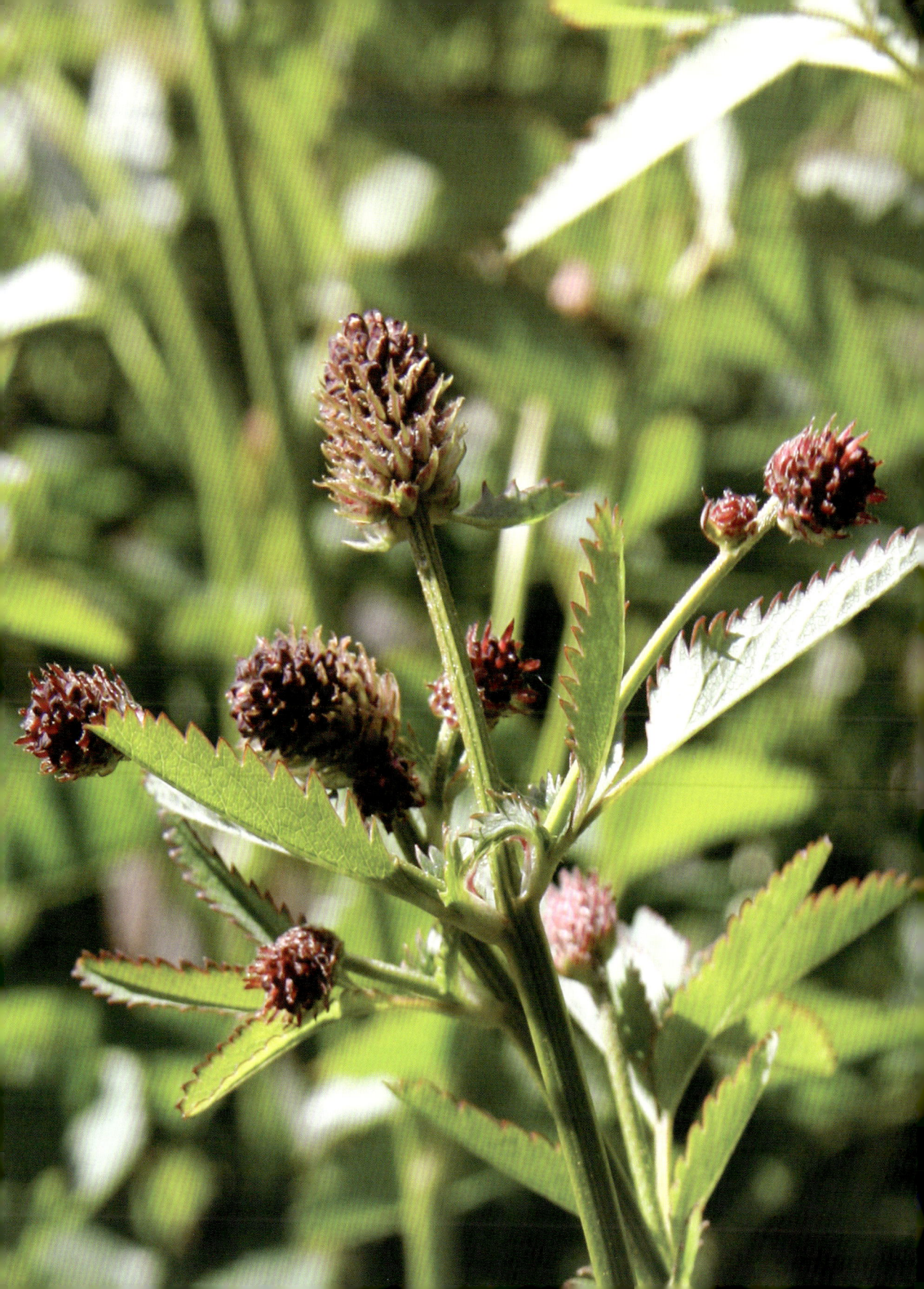

Greater Plantain

Plantago major
Plantaginaceae—*Græðisúra*

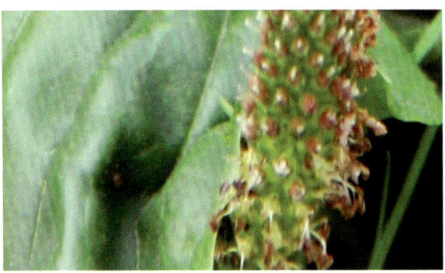

Habitat

Greater Plantain grows mainly in South and West Iceland and can be found close to farmhouses and geothermal areas.

Parts Used

The entire plant is used, including the root.

Harvesting

The leaves and flowers are gathered in bloom in June–July. The seeds are collected in late summer and the roots harvested in autumn.

Constituents

Mucilage, iridoids (aucubin), triterpenes (ursolic acid), flavonoids, and tannins.

History

Greater Plantain is a vulnerary, as the Icelandic name indicates, and has a long history as a medicinal herb, for both topical and internal use. The Old Icelandic names include "græðablaðka" (vulnerary leaves), "læknisblað" (doctor's leaf), and "vogsúra" (sour pus). "Vogur" means pus and Greater Plantain is thought to be good for drawing out pus from wounds. The Latin name

Plantago means sole; leaves of the plant were traditionally put in shoes to protect feet from sores and blisters.

Plantain has a long traditional history as a medicinal herb among the Native Americans. It was used topically to heal wounds, boils, blisters, insect bites, and skin rashes as well as for easing arthritic pains, swelling, and bruises. Taken internally, it was considered good for coughs, fevers, stomach pains, constipation, vaginal discharges, and dysentery. In early spring, the plants were used as food. Sea Plantain (*P. maritima*) is said to have similar action to Greater Plantain. The seeds of *P. ovata* and *P. psyllium* are well-known laxatives; both types are closely related to Greater Plantain but do not grow in Iceland.

Action

Astringent, vulnerary, anti-inflammatory, analgesic, hemostatic, expectorant, antibacterial, antifungal, and antiviral.

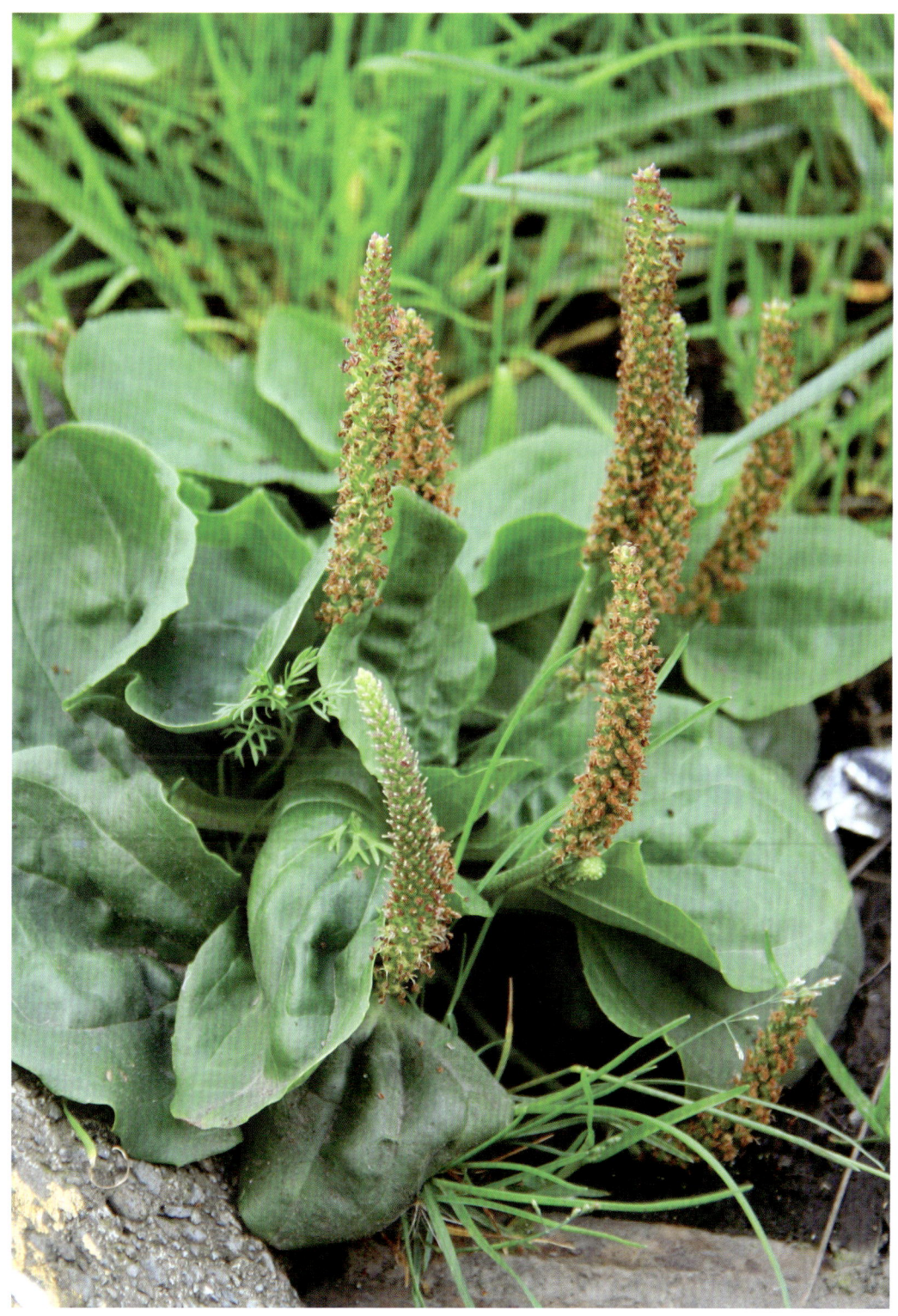

Uses

There is a long tradition for using Greater Plantain to heal wounds both internally and externally, as well as for healing insect bites and fungal infections and for stopping bleeding. Sources state that it is also useful for broken bones and bruises. It is used topically for hemorrhoids and inflamed eyelids. When taken internally, Greater Plantain is considered good for drying up mucus in colds, influenza, coughs, and allergies, besides being useful for laryngitis. It is found to be healing for the mucous membrane of the digestive tract and thus is used for gastritis, stomach ulcers, diarrhea, and colitis. It is also traditionally used for cystitis where there is bleeding. The seeds of the plant have a laxative effect. In China, Greater Plantain is used for urinary tract diseases, tuberculosis wounds, dysentery, and hepatitis. In Asia, Mexico, and Spain, Greater Plantain is used to treat cancer. In China, *P. asiatica*, a close relative of Greater Plantain, is used for various infections in the respiratory, digestive, and urinary systems.

Research

Clinical research showed positive results using Greater Plantain on patients with chronic bronchitis, acute hepatitis, bacterial dysentery, digestive disturbances, and kidney disease.[1] Research studies on the plant show that it has an inhibiting effect on *Streptococcus pneumoniae*[2] and other bacteria.[1,3-6] Greater Plantain has also been shown to have a positive effect on the mucous lining of the stomach and stomach ulcers[1,7] and works well for diarrhea[8] as it has an inhibiting effect on *Escherichia coli*[3] and *Giardia duodenalis*,[9] both of which can cause diarrhea. It also has anti-inflammatory properties[11-13] and an inhibiting effect on viral and fungal infections.[4,5,14,15] Greater Plantain works well for pain[16] and has been shown to protect the liver[10,17] and strengthen the womb.[18]

Research studies on Greater Plantain show that it is an expectorant and antitussive[1] while also being beneficial for asthma and allergies.[19] It has shown antioxidant properties,[6,20] has a balancing effect on the immune system,[15,21] and inhibits the growth of cancer cells.[4,17,21-24] In other research it was reported that Greater Plantain does not inhibit cancer cell growth[25] and does not have diuretic properties.[26]

Dosage

Tincture: 2–5 ml three times a day (1:5, 25%).

Cold infusion: 1–2 teaspoons in a cup of cold water, allowed to steep overnight. 1 cup three times a day.

Decoction: 1–2 teaspoons in a cup three times a day.

Infusions, decoctions, tinctures, compresses, and ointments for external use.

Syrup: 1–2 teaspoons, three times a day.

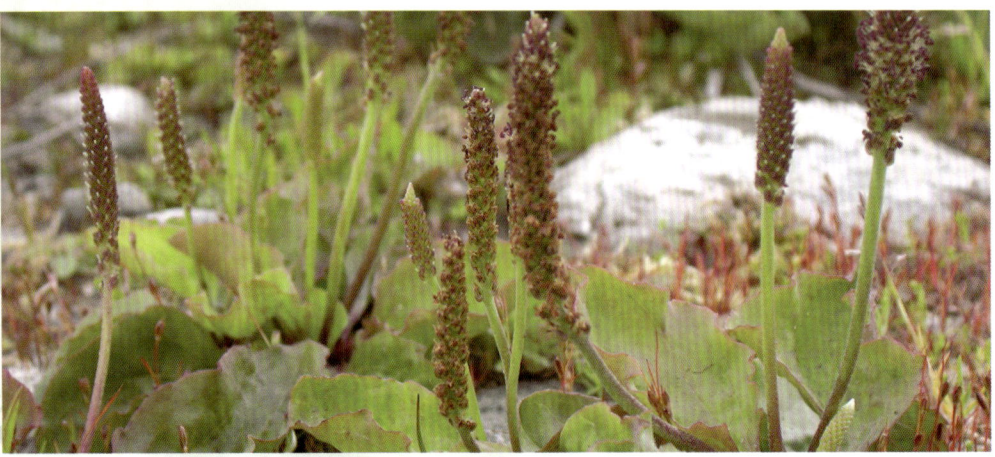

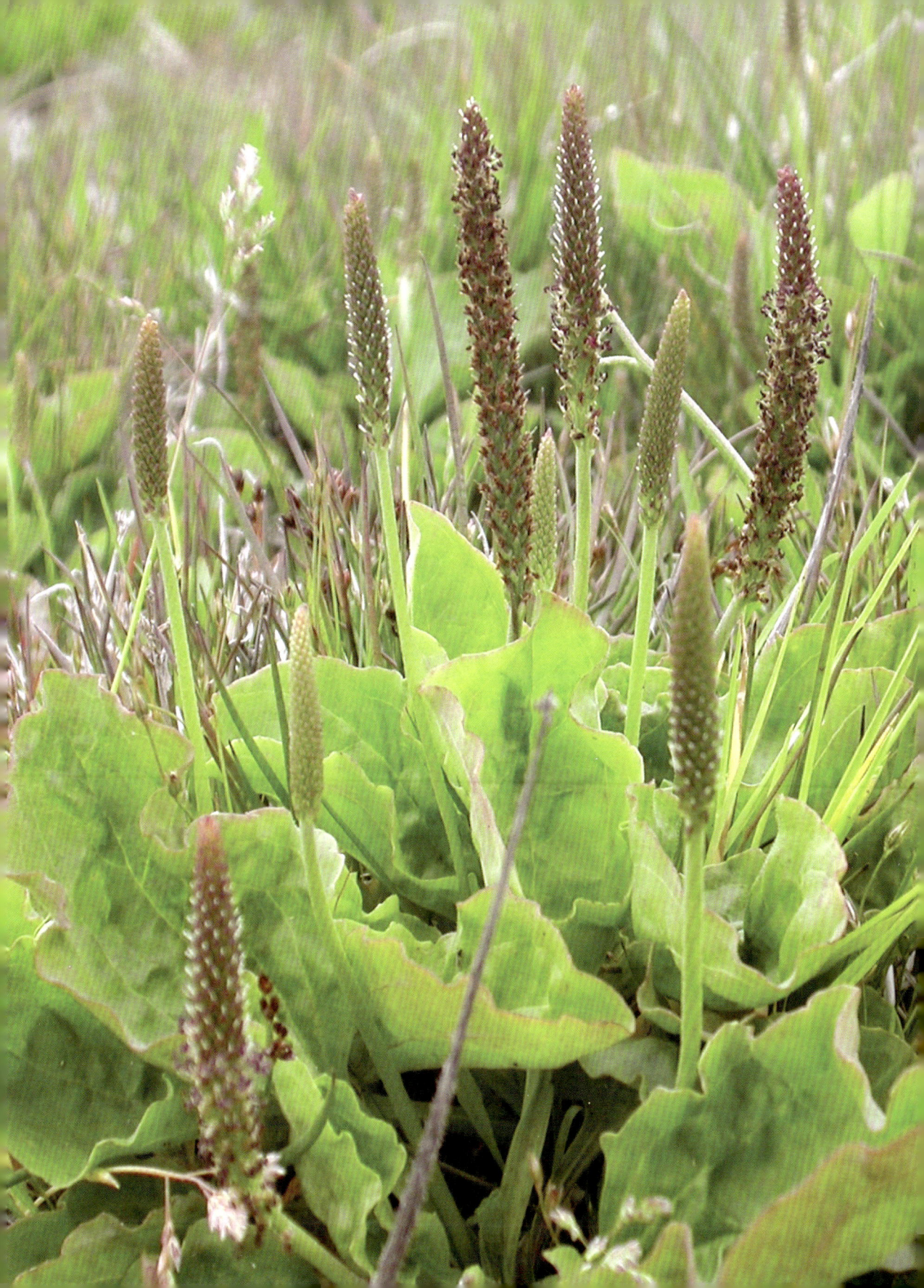

Groundsel

Senecio vulgaris
Asteraceae—*Krossfífill*

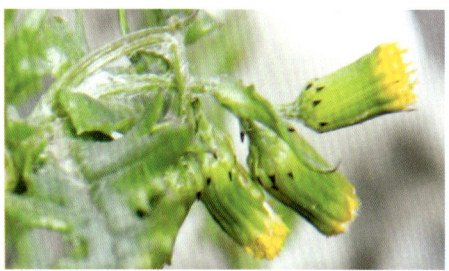

Habitat

Groundsel is a common weed in gardens, in industrial areas, and on pavements in South Iceland. In other parts of Iceland it is found only in built-up areas and is rather rare.

Parts Used

The entire plant is used, except for the root.

Harvesting

Groundsel is collected in early summer, just before bloom in June.

Constituents

Pyrrolizidine alkaloids, essential oils, and flavonoids.

History

The English name literally means "ground swallower," which indicates the tenacity of this weed. Many other related species are used for medicinal purposes, the most common in Europe being *S. aureus, S. cineraria,* and *S. jacobaea.* In the USA, there are references to the use of *S. flaccidus, S. multicapitatus,* and *S. ambrosiodes.*

All of these species have one thing in common: in most cases they are recommended for external use only, mainly for arthritis. The seeds of Groundsel were traditionally used as parrot food.

Action

Laxative, diuretic, diaphoretic, emmenagogue, anthelmintic, and cholagogue.

Uses

Groundsel is not used much in Western herbal medicine nowadays. It was used internally in the past as a diuretic and diaphoretic herb as well as to stimulate bile. It was also used to stimulate menstruation, for balancing the menstrual cycle, and for menstrual pain. Externally, it was conventionally used in compresses for digestive disturbances and arthritis. A weak infusion of Groundsel was considered to be laxative, but a strong tea would bring on vomiting. Groundsel is traditionally used in Europe to purge the body of worms.

Research

Venous blockage in the liver was traced to the patient's use of Groundsel for constipation. There is strong circumstantial evidence that pyrrolizidine alkaloids caused the blockage.[1] Another example of liver damage in patients was attributed to the use of a Groundsel infusion for a two-year period.[2] *In vitro* tests have also revealed the antibacterial properties of Groundsel.[3,4]

Dosage

Compresses for external short-term use.

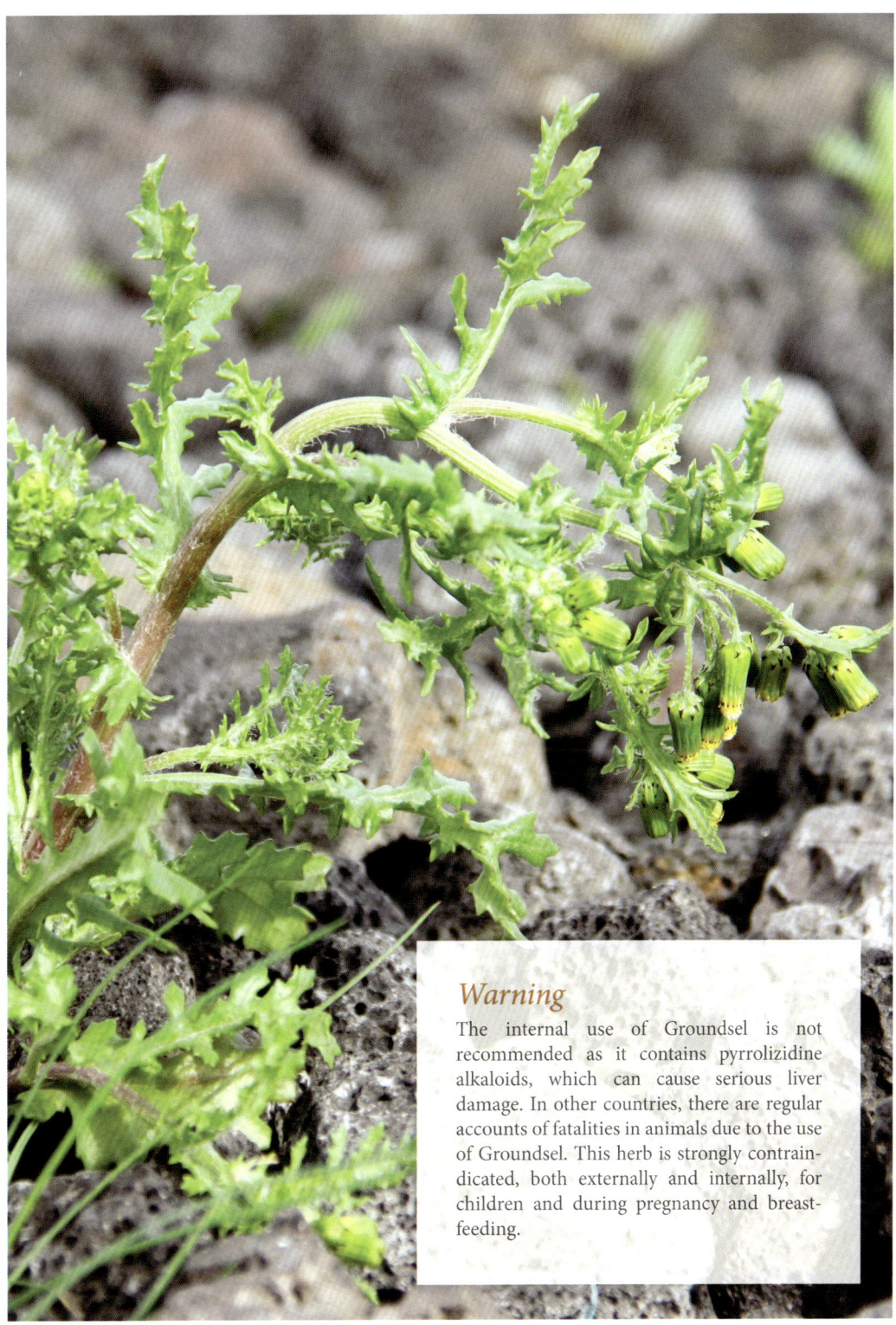

Warning

The internal use of Groundsel is not recommended as it contains pyrrolizidine alkaloids, which can cause serious liver damage. In other countries, there are regular accounts of fatalities in animals due to the use of Groundsel. This herb is strongly contraindicated, both externally and internally, for children and during pregnancy and breast-feeding.

Hawkweed

Hieracium spp.
Asteraceae—Undafífill

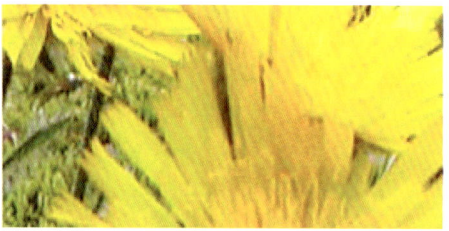

Action

Expectorant, antitussive, antispasmodic, diuretic, antibacterial, and vulnerary.

Uses

Hawkweeds are rarely used in Western herbal medicine nowadays. In the past, they were traditionally used for respiratory diseases, such as asthma, tuberculosis, whooping cough, and bronchitis. They were also thought effective for reducing heavy menstrual bleeding, for edema, for healing wounds and hernias, and for stopping nosebleeds. References suggest that *H. pilosella* is good for brucellosis, which is a bacterial infection caused by unpasteurized dairy products.

Research

In vivo and *in vitro* tests on *H. pilosella* show it to have mild antifungal action as well as diuretic and anti-inflammatory properties.[1]

Dosage

The fresh herb is said to be much more effective than the dried herb.

Tincture: 2–4 ml three times a day (1:5, 40%).

Syrup: 1–2 teaspoons three times a day.

Infusion: 1–2 teaspoons in a cup three times a day.

Infusions, tinctures, compresses, and ointments for external use.

Habitat

All species of Hawkweed are quite common all over Iceland, but the most common is Icelandic Hawkweed, *Pilosella islandica.*

Parts Used

The entire plant is used, except for the roots.

Harvesting

Hawkweed is collected in bloom from June–August.

Constituents

Coumarin, flavonoids, and phenolic acids.

History

Hawkweed is the common name for the following closely related Asteraceae: *H. aquiliforme, H. stictophyllum, H. alpinum, H. elegantiforme, H. thaectolepium, H. holopleurum,* and *P. islandica.* In other countries, *H. pilosella* has been used for medicinal purposes and references to its healing powers date back to the Middle Ages. Hawkweeds do not have the same properties as Dandelion, apart from their both being diuretic. The Icelandic word "und" from the name of the herb means wound and Hawkweed has been used for healing wounds.

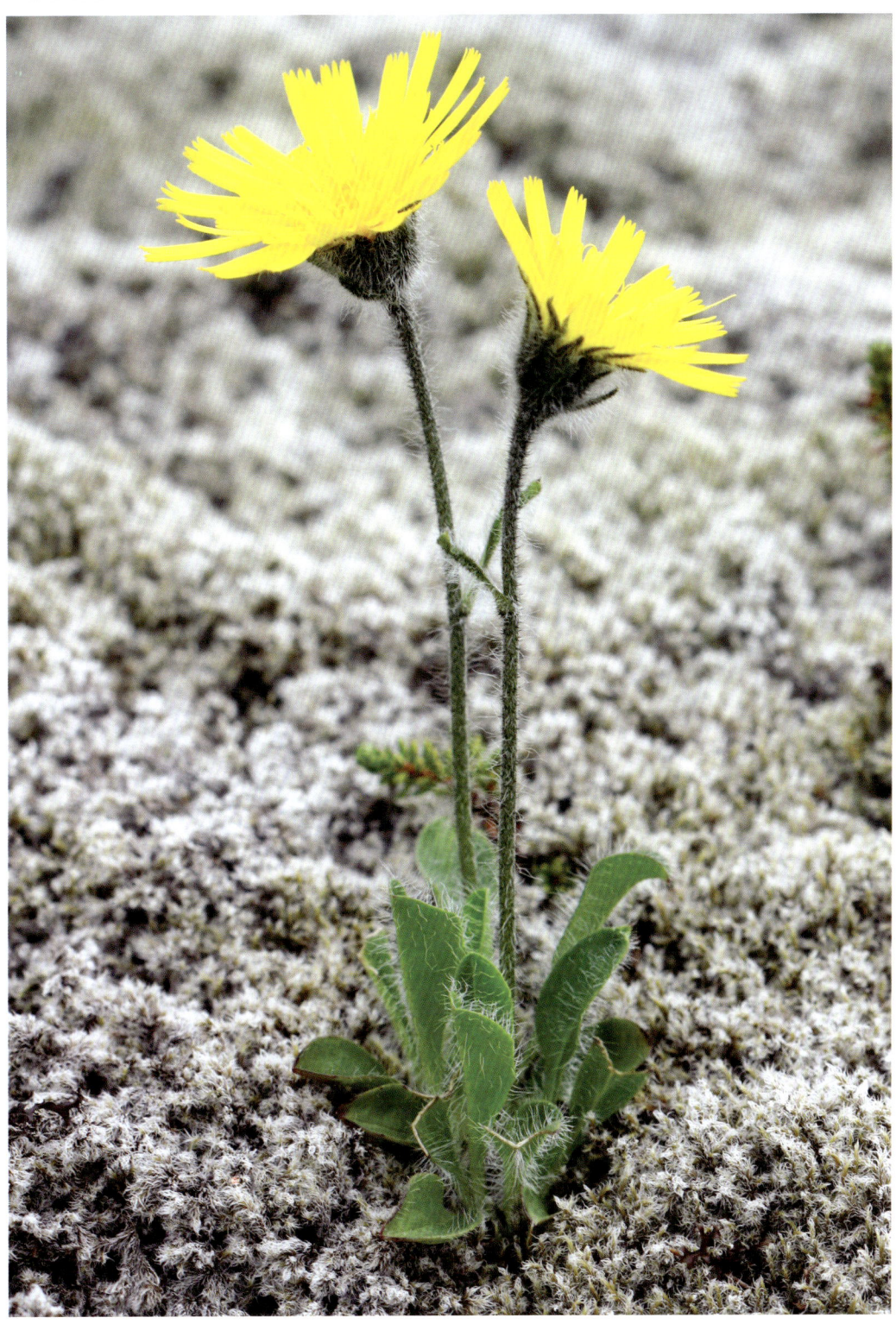

Heartsease

Viola tricolor
Violaceae—Þrenningarfjóla

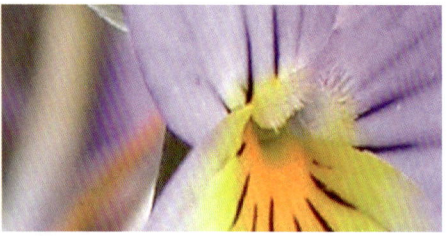

Habitat

Heartsease is common in some places in North and West Iceland, but in other areas it is rare. It grows mainly in stony ground or in sandy soil.

Parts Used

The entire plant is used, except for the root.

Harvesting

It is collected in bloom from May to June.

Constituents

Flavonoids (rutin) and phenolic acids (salicylic acid and methyl salicylate).

History

Heartsease was much used in the old days for love spells and indeed plays a role in the love spells in the Shakespeare play *A Midsummer Night's Dream*. As well as being promising for love spells, in the past Heartsease was also thought beneficial for disorders that plagued the heart, thus explaining its English name. In Icelandic, it is also called "Þrenningargras" (Tri-herb); the Latin name *tricolor* means three colors, because the flower is made up of three colors. Both the leaves and the flowers of Heartsease are traditionally used for cooking, and the flowers are especially beautiful in salads. The flowers of Heartsease have also been used to dye yarn and the leaves were formerly used as a dye for acid paper.

Action

Expectorant, diuretic, diaphoretic, anti-inflammatory, mild laxative, vulnerary, and reduces itching.

Uses

Heartsease has long been considered good, both internally and externally, for skin disorders such as eczema, psoriasis, impetigo, and acne. It has also been used for cradle cap, where the scalp is washed with an infusion of the herb. Heartsease contains both rutin and salicylic acid, which are anti-inflammatory and could explain its popularity for use with rheumatism over time. Rutin, which is mostly found in the flowers of Heartsease, is also thought to be very good for capillary veins and thus the plant is used for bruises, broken veins, and water retention. Rutin is also said to protect against atherosclerosis and to lower blood pressure. Heartsease has traditionally been used for lung diseases such as tuberculosis, bronchitis, and whooping cough. It is a mild laxative and is also considered to be good for cystitis. Traditionally, rashes are washed with an infusion of Heartsease as it has anti-itching properties, and likewise it is often used in ointments for skin disorders.

Research

In vitro and *in vivo* tests on Heartsease have shown that it has anti-inflammatory properties,[1,2] antioxidant action,[3,4] and inhibits growth of cancer cells.[5] In old research where animals with eczema were given Heartsease in their food for two months,[2] their eczema improved markedly.

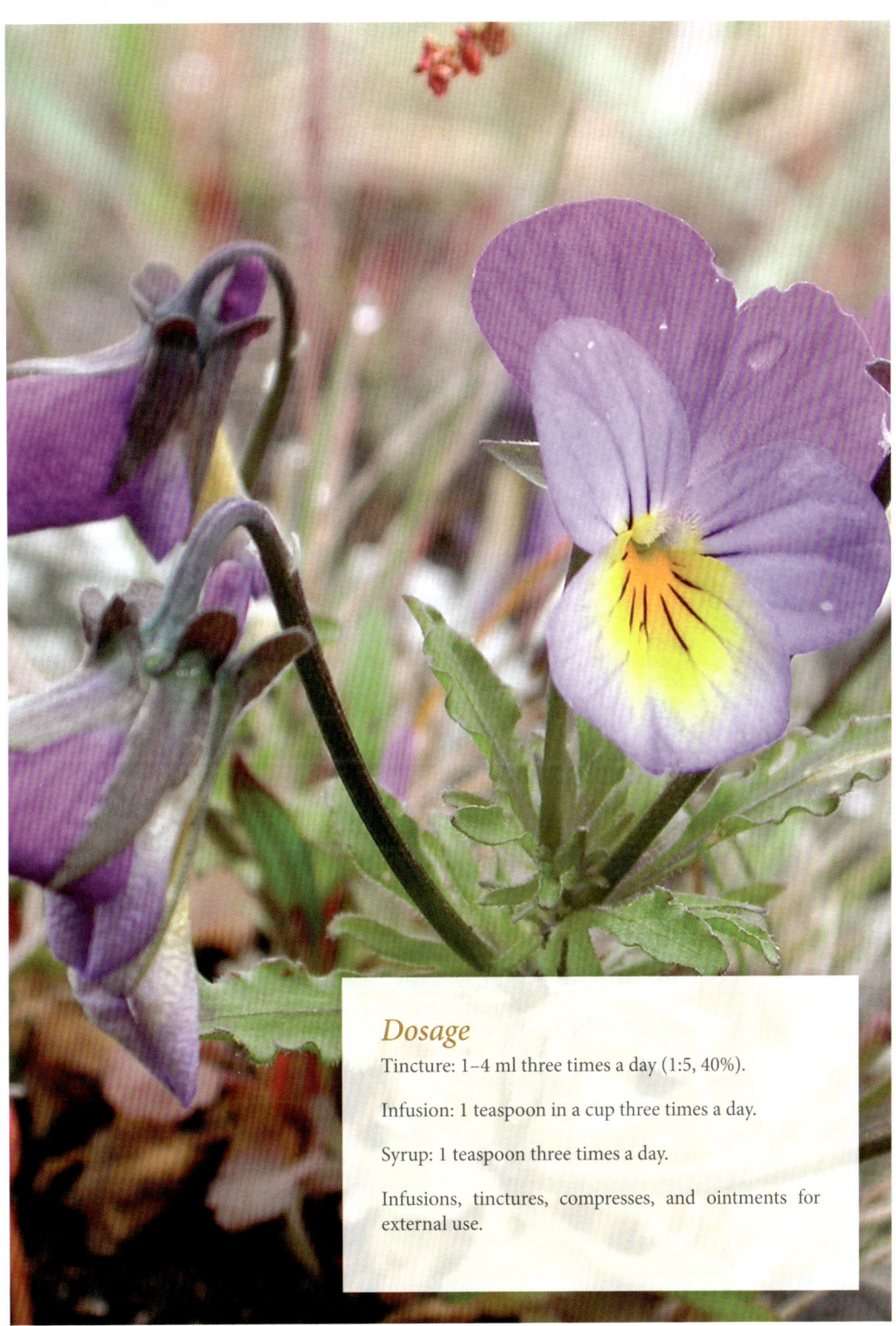

Dosage

Tincture: 1–4 ml three times a day (1:5, 40%).

Infusion: 1 teaspoon in a cup three times a day.

Syrup: 1 teaspoon three times a day.

Infusions, tinctures, compresses, and ointments for external use.

Heather

Calluna vulgaris
Ericaceae—Beitilyng

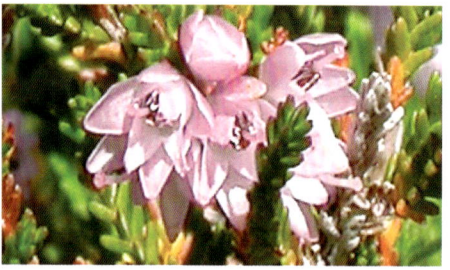

Habitat

Heather is common on moors and hillsides all over Iceland.

Parts Used

The entire plant is used, except for the root.

Harvesting

It is collected during bloom in August and September.

Constituents

Hydroquinones (arbutin), flavonoids (quercitrin), triterpenes (ursolic acid, uvaol), and coumarins.

History

The Latin genus name *Calluna* comes from the Greek verb "kallynein," meaning cleanse, beautify ,or sweep, and Heather was indeed used to make brooms in old times. There have been many uses for Heather over time (e.g., it was used to make mattresses, rope, straw bags, and beer, as well as dye). Gypsies in Europe today still sell heather on the streets as it is supposed to bring good luck, while honey from Heather is said to be delicious. Heather has a great, long history as a healing herb and is still used today in the same way as described by ancient sources.

Action

Antibacterial, diuretic, anti-inflammatory, mildly sedative, vulnerary, and strengthens the urinary system and kidneys.

Uses

Heather has long been used for infections in the urinary system and is excellent for cystitis. It has also been used for kidney stones and other kidney diseases. Heather is well known for arthritic problems such as arthritis and gout. It is thought to have diuretic properties and is used for inflammation of the prostate gland and incontinence. It is also known for treatment of stomach cramps, gastritis, and diarrhea. It has been used for insomnia and restlessness because of its slightly sedative effect. It is also reputed to be good for coughs, fevers, and colds. It is used externally as a compress on joints to relieve pain and also as an ointment to heal sores. It is traditionally used as a rinse to relieve swollen eyes and for vaginal discharges.

Research

In vitro testing shows that Heather kills bacteria and fungi and is anti-inflammatory as well as inhibitory for the growth of certain cancer cells.[1–7] It has also shown antioxidant properties.[8] The presence of quercitrin is the reason why Heather is used to strengthen and calm nerves.[9]

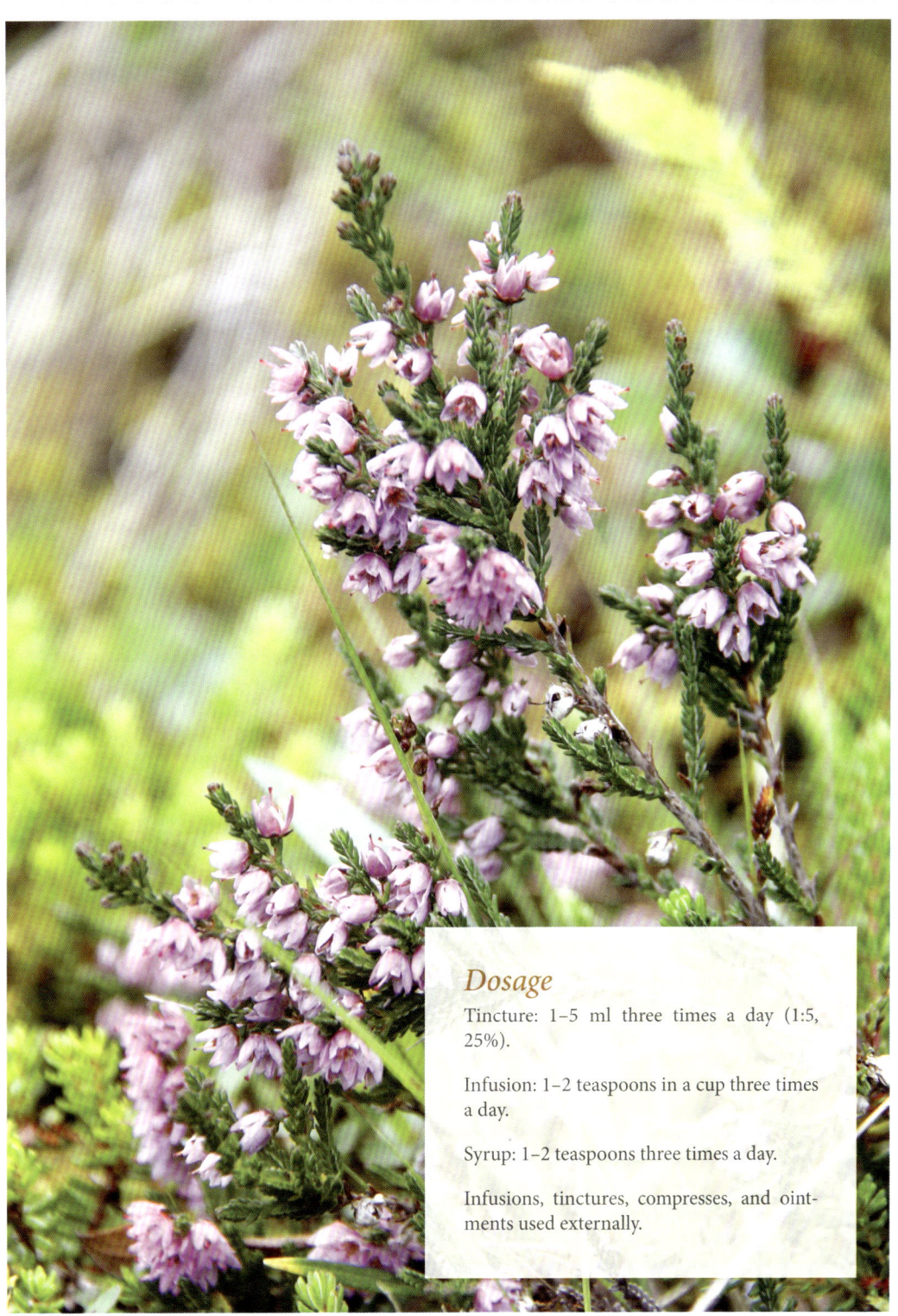

Dosage

Tincture: 1–5 ml three times a day (1:5, 25%).

Infusion: 1–2 teaspoons in a cup three times a day.

Syrup: 1–2 teaspoons three times a day.

Infusions, tinctures, compresses, and ointments used externally.

Hemp-nettle

Galeopsis tetrahit
Labiatae—*Garðahjálmgras*

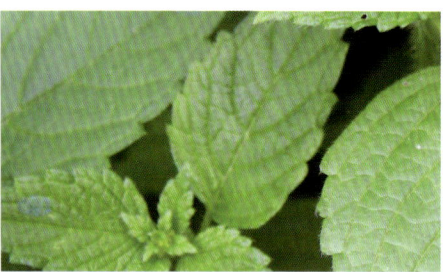

Habitat

Hemp-nettle is rather rare in Iceland but is found close to farmsteads and urban areas, mainly in Southwest Iceland.

Parts Used

Leaves and flowers.

Harvesting

Hemp-nettle is picked while in bloom in July.

Constituents

Phenylpropanoids, iridoids, flavonoids, tannins, silicic acid, and saponin.

History

Native Americans have used Hemp-nettle for lung diseases as well as drinking a decoction of the root to induce vomiting and to protect against evil spells. Oil produced from Hemp-nettle has been used on leather, and the stem fiber have been used to make rope. Hemp-nettle has also been used in cooking, with the young leaves being boiled in soups.

Action

Astringent, expectorant, antitussive, and anti-inflammatory.

Uses

Hemp-nettle is not used much in Western herbal medicine nowadays. It is known to be an expectorant and is used for coughs and chronic lung diseases such as bronchitis. It is also thought to be rich in minerals and therefore good for anemia.

Research

In vitro tests have shown that Hemp-nettle and other herbs of the same family have antioxidant properties.[1]

Dosage

Tincture: 2–5 ml three times a day (1:5, 25%).

Infusion: 1–2 teaspoons in a cup three times a day.

Warning

There are references to the toxic effect of other plants from the same family on livestock. These refer specifically to the active substances in the seeds, so care should be taken to not use the seeds.

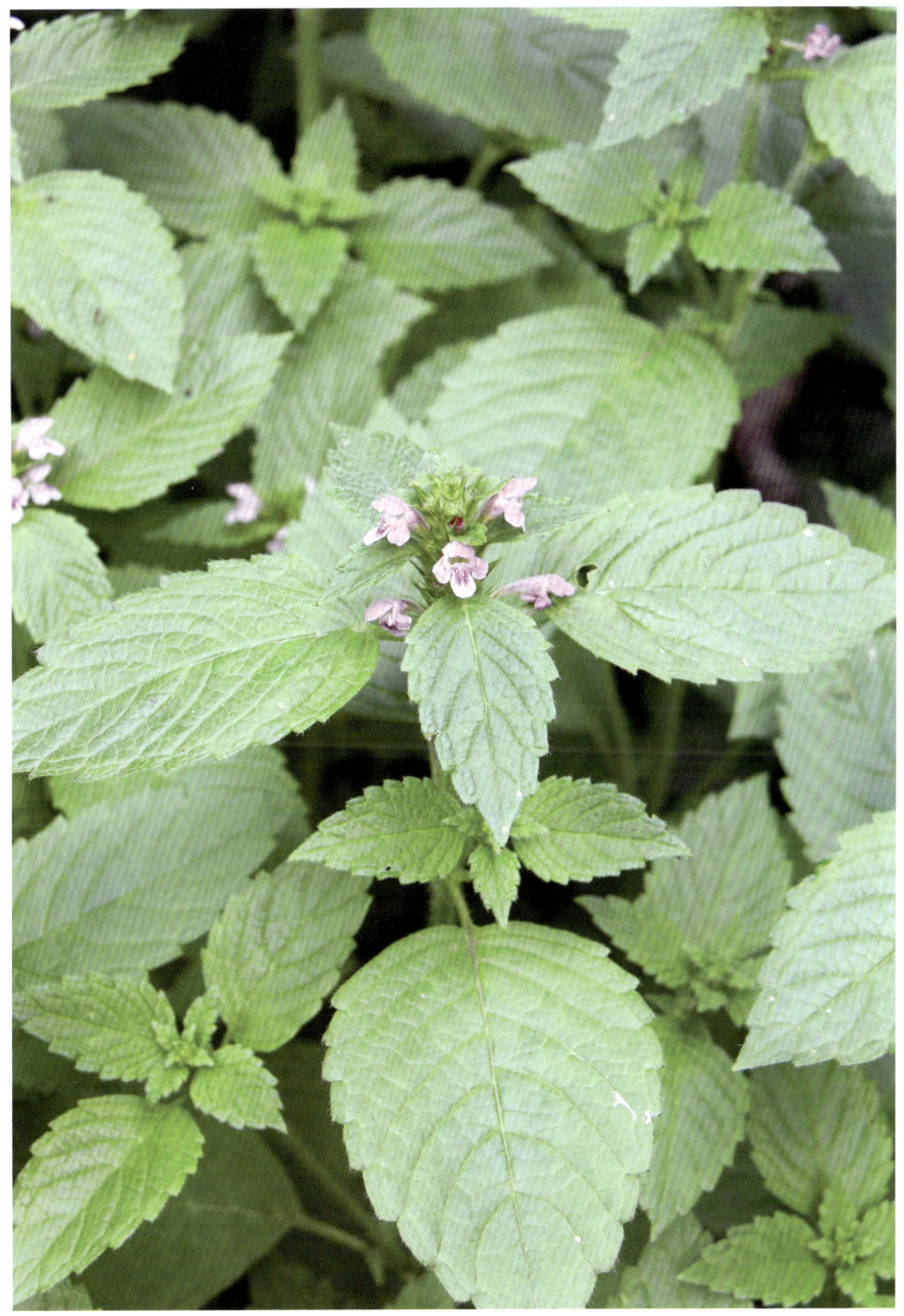

Horsetail

Equisetum arvense
Equisetaceae—*Klóelfting*

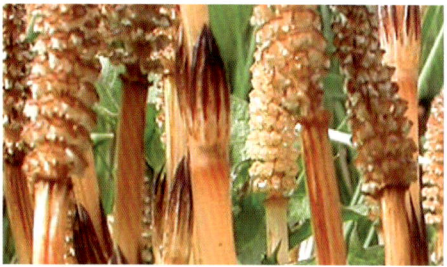

Habitat

Horsetail grows all over Iceland, in cultivated fields, pastures, and wetlands. It is easy to confuse Horsetail with Meadow Horsetail (*E. pratense*), which is not used for medicinal purposes.

Parts Used

Only the green stems are used. Early in spring, before the green stems are formed, fertile, spore-bearing stems are seen that are light brown. These are not used for medicinal purposes.

Harvesting

Horsetail is picked in early summer. When drying, Horsetail should be well spread out in order to avoid any danger of it going moldy.

Constituents

Silicic acid, alkaloids, flavonoids (quercitrin), sterols, phenolic acids, and saponins.

History

Horsetail is a fern and forms spores rather than the seeds or flowers of flowering plants. Horsetail is actually descended from giant tree plants that thrived about 600 million years ago. References to the medicinal use of Horsetail date back to the Roman and Greek eras, 130–200 BC. The genus name *Equisetum* is derived from the Latin words *equus* (horse) and *setum* (bristle), hence the English name Horsetail. Another name, Bottlebrush, refers to its use as a bottle cleaner. It was also used to polish pots, pans, and wooden furniture, as the high silica content made this task much easier.

There are many references to the medicinal properties of Horsetail (e.g., Culpepper, a 17th century British herbalist), used Horsetail for urinary retention and to stop bleeding, reduce inflammation, and heal wounds. Indian herbalists recommended Horsetail for benign enlargement of the prostate gland and the Native Americans used Horsetail for coughs, colds, urine retention, edema, kidney problems, urinary tract infections, headaches, arthritis, backache, diarrhea, constipation, and stimulating placental birth. Externally, Horsetail was thought to work well for skin rashes, wounds, and itchiness.

The Old Icelandic name for Horsetail was "kveisugras" (gripe grass) or "draumagras" (dream grass) as it was said to provide knowledge, through dreams, of whatever the dreamer

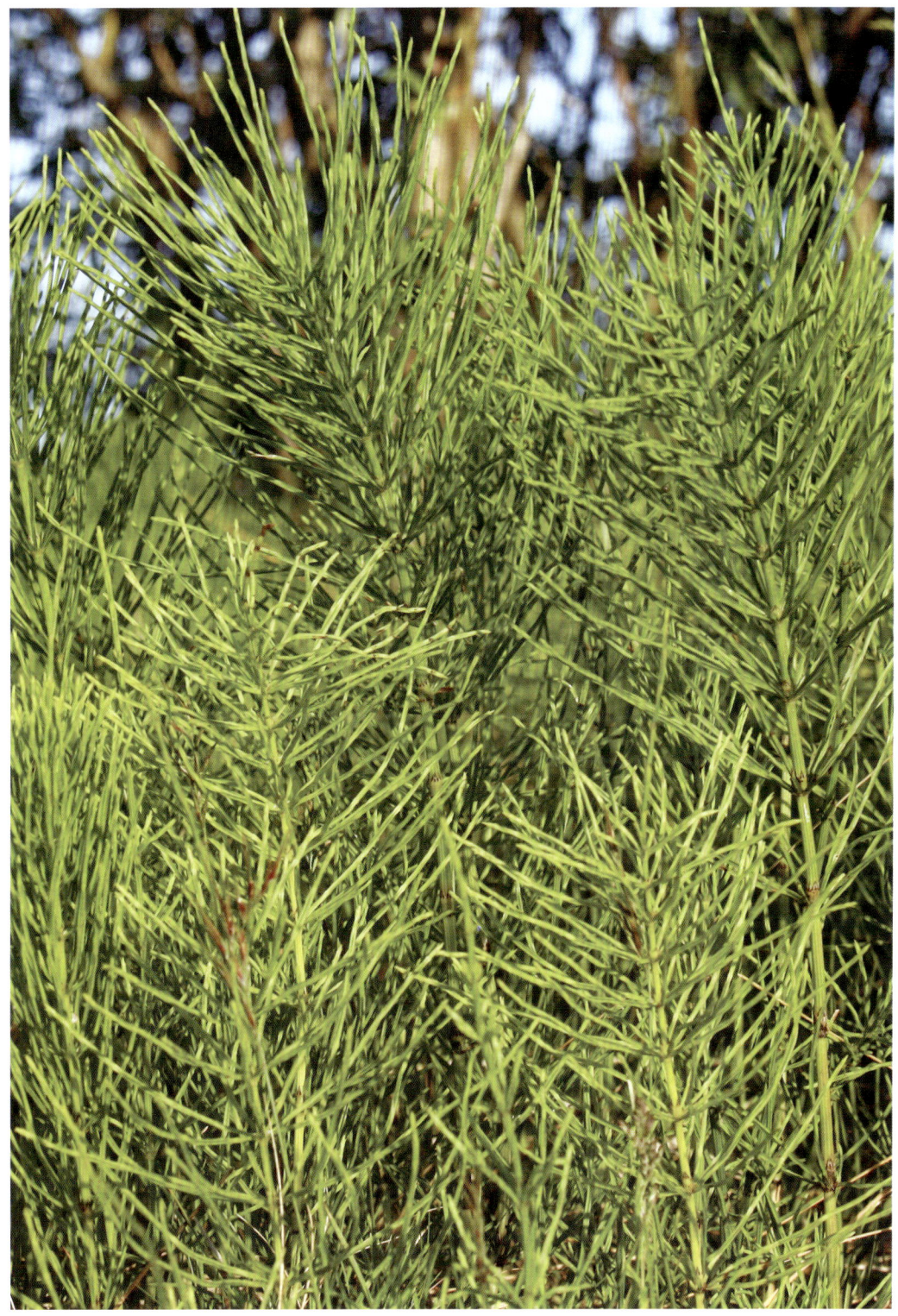

desired to know. The brown, spore-bearing stems are edible and were fried in butter or eaten in porridge.

Action

Astringent, diuretic, vulnerary, hemostatic, and strengthens connective tissue.

. . . .

Uses

Horsetail has been used for a long time to stop bleeding and to heal wounds and skin rashes. It was traditionally used to stop nosebleeds and internal bleeding. It is diuretic and is deemed good for cystitis, urinary tract infections, frequent urination, and incontinence. It is also thought to be powerful against benign enlargement of the prostate gland. Horsetail contains high amounts of silica and is therefore considered to strengthen connective tissue, hair, nails, bones, and ligaments as well as guarding against osteoporosis and accelerating the healing of broken bones. Its strengthening effect on connective tissue is said to be another reason why Horsetail is good for arthritis, osteoarthritis, and lung diseases (e.g., emphysema). A decoction of Horsetail in the bath will speed up the healing of skin disorders, pulled muscles, and broken bones. It is also thought to be good for healing wounds and any kind of rash. In Asia, the traditional use of Horsetail is similar to that in Western herbal medicine, but there it is also thought to be a febrifuge, diaphoretic, and carminative, as well as being used for venereal diseases and hepatitis.

Research

Research was done on 122 post-menopausal women with osteoporosis, who were given a supplement containing Horsetail and calcium for two years. The results showed that their bone density increased.[1] *In vitro* tests on Horsetail have shown its antioxidant[2-9] and antibacterial effects.[2,6,10] *In vivo* tests have shown that it is sedative and antispasmodic[11] as well as having analgesic and anti-inflammatory effects.[12] Horsetail is also part of an herbal compound used in clinical and *in vivo* testing that is thought to be beneficial for treatment of inflammation of the prostate gland.[13,14] *In vivo* testing has also shown that Horsetail can lower blood sugar and therefore could possibly be useful in the treatment of diabetes mellitus type 2.[15,16] Open clinical trials on patients with heart failure and edema show the diuretic effects of Horsetail,[2] while *in vivo* tests have also indicated similar effects[17] and the possible prevention of kidney stones.[18] Research also shows that Horsetail has no damaging effects on liver function;[19] on the contrary, it has a protective effect on the liver[20] and possibly protects against blood clots.[2] *In vitro* tests on Horsetail show its inhibiting effect on cancer cell growth[3] and research on a blend of Horsetail and other herbs shows similar action.[21-23] *In vitro* tests show a slight stimulating effect of Horsetail on uterine muscles.[2]

Dosage

Tincture: 2–6 ml three times a day (1:5, 25%).

Infusion: 1–2 teaspoons in a cup three times a day.

Infusions, tinctures, compresses, and ointments for external use.

Warning

It is not recommended to take Horsetail internally in large doses for longer than six weeks unless under the supervision of a professional, as it can cause irritation in the digestive tract. Be careful not to confuse Marsh Horsetail (*E. palustre*) with Horsetail, as the former contains toxic alkaloids and is not used for medicinal purposes.

Tea for Hair and Nails

2 parts Horsetail

1 part Stinging Nettle leaves

1 part Downy Birch

Put 3–4 tablespoons of the blend into a 750 ml vacuum flask and add boiling water. Sieve the infusion into a cup and then place the herbs back into the flask. Allow to stand all day. Drink one flask during the day.

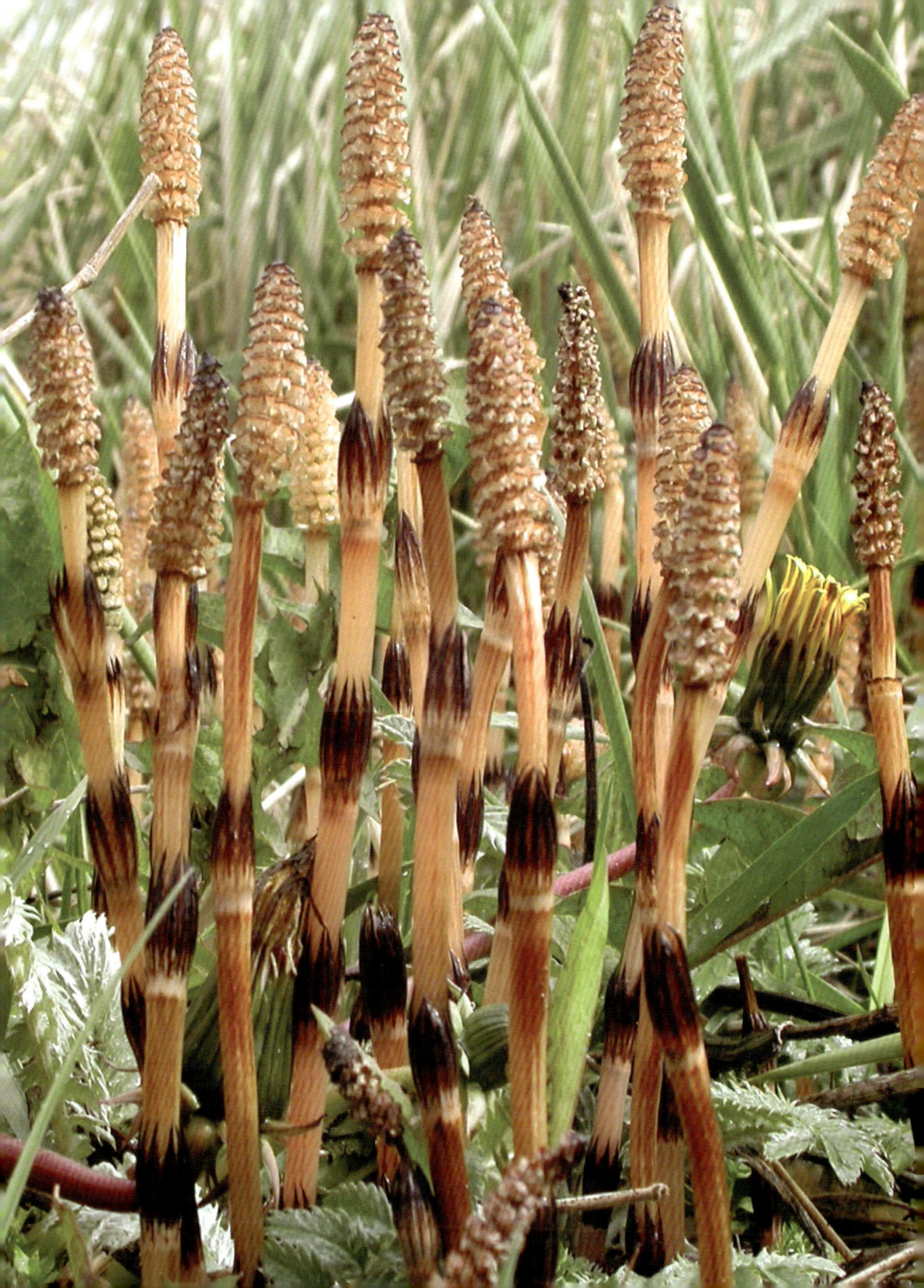

Iceland Moss

Cetraria islandica
Parmeliaceae—*Fjallagrös*

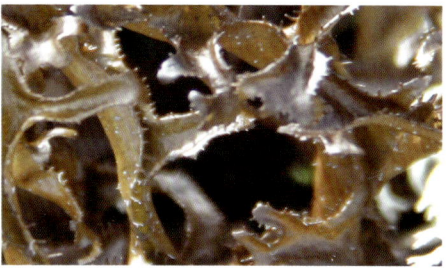

Habitat

Common all over Iceland.

Parts Used

The entire lichen.

Harvesting

Iceland Moss can be collected from the time the snow thaws in spring until the first snowfall in autumn. It is easier to collect it while wet than dry. Caution should be taken not to take too much at once as Iceland Moss takes about 5–10 years to reach maximum size. The plants accumulate lead so it is very important to collect in unpolluted areas.

Constituents

Lichen acids (protolichesteric acid), poly-saccharides, minerals (iron, calcium), and fiber.

History

Iceland Moss is not actually an herb but a lichen which lives symbiotically with fungi and algae. It grows in many parts of Europe but is associated with Iceland, in both the Latin and English

This grass, or rightly said, moss, is best for healing tuberculosis as well as all bloating, all crudities and other ailments of the stomach. It has often been confirmed that half a meal of this moss with milk, well-prepared, has kept the health, strength and stamina of men longer than most other food. The bitters, which are on the leaves of the moss, soften faeces or cause diarrhea, and thus foreigners have called this moss Catharticus. But the bitterness goes if it is soaked in water for a while before eating. Drinking a decoction of this moss like tea is good for bloating and worms in the stomach or intestines of man. Moss porridge, boiled thoroughly into a mash, with milk, is a very nourishing and strengthening food and cures diarrhea.

Björn Halldórsson, Uses of Herbs, *1783*

names as well as in other languages such as Danish, French, and German.

It has been used for centuries in cooking and as a medicinal herb and the first reference to Iceland Moss in Iceland can be found in the second law code for Iceland called "Jónsbók." Iceland Moss was very valuable and used as currency, and the law code stated that the collection of Iceland Moss on another's land was prohibited. In fact, going up in the mountains to collect Iceland Moss before winter set in was a deep-rooted custom in Iceland. Iceland Moss was a real asset and was used in breads, blood pudding, cough syrups, soups, porridges, and drinks, as well as for dyeing yarn.

Action

Anti-inflammatory, demulcent, vulnerary, expect-orant, nourishing, anti-emetic, antitussive, anthelmintic, laxative, and antibacterial.

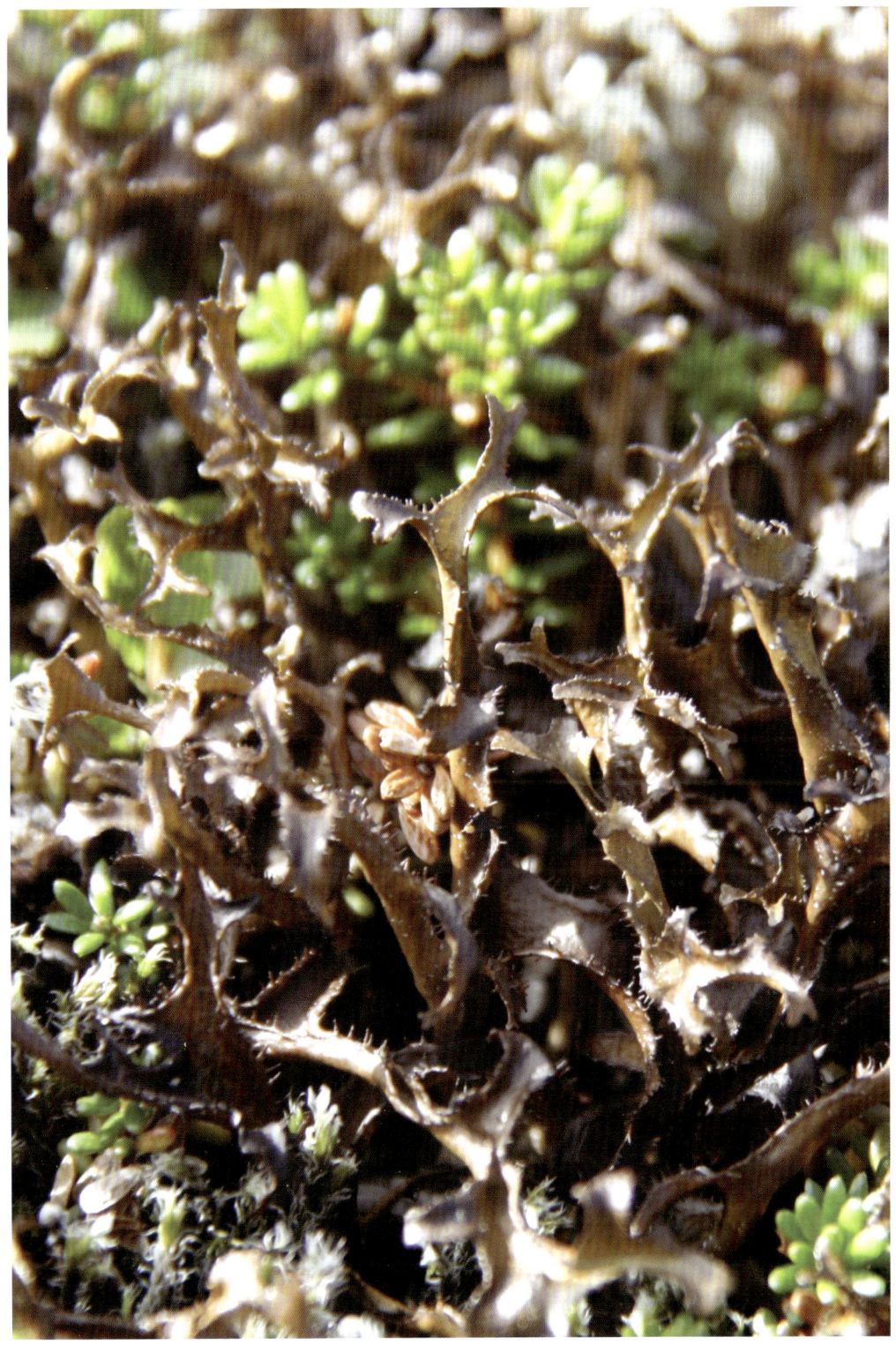

Uses

Iceland Moss contains mucilage, which is especially good for irritated and sore throats, as well as for stimulating digestion. There is a long tradition of using it for coughs, throat infections, asthma, and bronchitis. Iceland Moss is unique in that it contains both mucilage and bitters, which is a rare combination in herbs. It is considered good for all sorts of digestive problems where the mucilage soothes and protects the mucous membrane of the stomach and the bitters strengthen and stimulate digestion. It works well for indigestion, gastritis, stomach and duodenal ulcers, irritable bowel syndrome, and constipation, and is also considered good for eliminating worms. Iceland Moss is known to be good for nausea and to stimulate digestion after chronic illness. Topically, Iceland Moss compresses are used to heal wounds and rashes.

Research

Clinical research was done involving 61 patients, shortly after nose surgery that caused dryness and inflammation in the mouth. They were given Iceland Moss lozenges and after five days they showed significant improvement.[1] In another trial involving 100 patients with sore throats and bronchitis who were given Iceland Moss lozenges, positive effects were found by 86 of them.[2] *In vitro* and *in vivo* tests on Iceland Moss have indicated its anti-inflammatory[3,4] and antioxidant properties.[5] The antibacterial properties of Iceland Moss have also been demonstrated during *in vitro* and *in vivo* tests[6] against *Helicobacter pylori*, which can cause gastritis and stomach ulcers,[7] and *Mycobacterium aurum*.[8] *In vitro* testing has also revealed that Iceland Moss has an inhibiting effect on the HIV-1 RT virus,[9] a stimulating effect on the immune system,[8, 10-12] and an inhibiting effect on the growth of cancer cells.[4,13-15]

Dosage

Tincture: 1–4 ml three times a day (1:5, 25%).

Infusion: 1 teaspoon in a cup three times a day.

Decoction: 1 teaspoon in a cup, boiled for 3 minutes and allowed to stand for 10 minutes. 1 cup, three times a day.

Syrup: 1–2 teaspoons, three times a day.

Infusions, decoctions, tinctures, compresses, and ointments for external use.

Warning

Iceland Moss has been known to cause allergic reaction, such as nausea and stomach pain, but this is rare.

Iceland Moss Soup

25 g Iceland Moss

1 liter milk

1 tablespoon brown or white sugar

Salt

Clean the lichen thoroughly, squeeze the water out of it, and chop it, finely. Put milk in a pot and bring to a boil. Add the lichen and sugar. Simmer for 5–10 minutes. Add salt. (Nanna Rögnvaldardóttir, *Matarást*, 1998.)

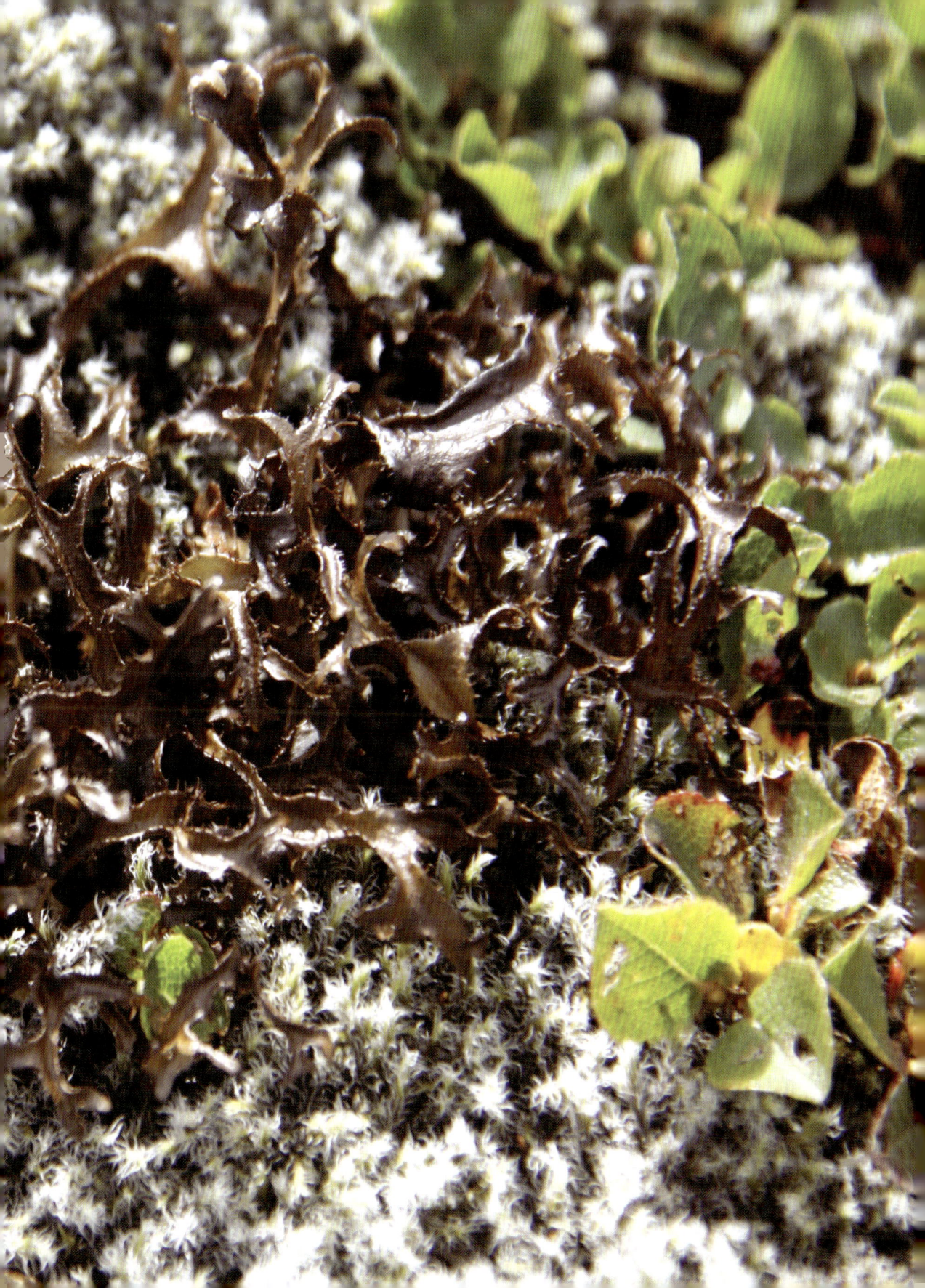

Irish Moss

Chondrus crispus

Gigartinaceae—*Fjörugrös*

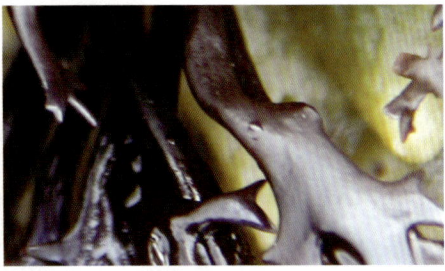

Habitat

Irish Moss is found on beaches (as indicated by the Icelandic name, Fjörugrös, meaning Beach Weed) and is most common in Southwest Iceland.

Parts Used

The entire seaweed.

Harvesting

Irish Moss is collected in early summer.

Constituents

Mucilage (carrageen), protein, amino acids, iodine, bromine, and various minerals.

History

Irish Moss is used as a jelly or binder in the food and cosmetics industry throughout the world. A jelly-like substance called carrageen is formed when Irish Moss is boiled, thus another English name for this plant is Carrageen Moss. This plant has a high content of mucilage, which forms a gel similar to that of Iceland Moss. As the name indicates, Irish Moss is traditionally used in Ireland. *Mastocarpus stellatus* (Cat's Puff) looks very similar to Irish Moss and they often grow close to each other and have the same

> This Irish Moss is soaked, then chopped well and boiled in milk; an edible porridge is made which causes loose bowel movements for those who eat too much. For bloating and problems in the stomach, this porridge is good, as it is easily digested and supports the digestion of hard foods.
>
> *Björn Halldórsson,* Uses of Herbs, *1783*

properties. In Ireland no differentiation is made between the two when picking. It was common in Ireland to use Irish Moss for colds, coughs, tuberculosis, and other lung diseases and documentation also exists for its use in kidney problems and burns. A non-alcoholic drink called Sobriety was made from Irish Moss and enjoyed great popularity. In Iceland, Irish Moss was also used for cooking, in porridge or mixed with skyr (an Icelandic dairy product, similar to yogurt). It was considered to be the food of the poor and not as good as Dulse.

Action

Demulcent, nourishing, expectorant, antitussive, and anti-inflammatory.

Uses

Irish Moss is hardly used in Western herbal medicine today, but it has traditionally been used for coughs, bronchitis, and tuberculosis. It is also thought to protect the mucous membrane of the stomach and works well for indigestion, gastritis, stomach and duodenal ulcers, and cystitis. It is also considered a good source of nourishment for those who are thin and need to put on weight. It helps to ease inflammations of the skin when applied topically.

Research

In vitro tests on carrageen have shown that it inhibits the herpes simplex virus 1 and 2 and HIV as well as having a healing effect on wounds.[1]

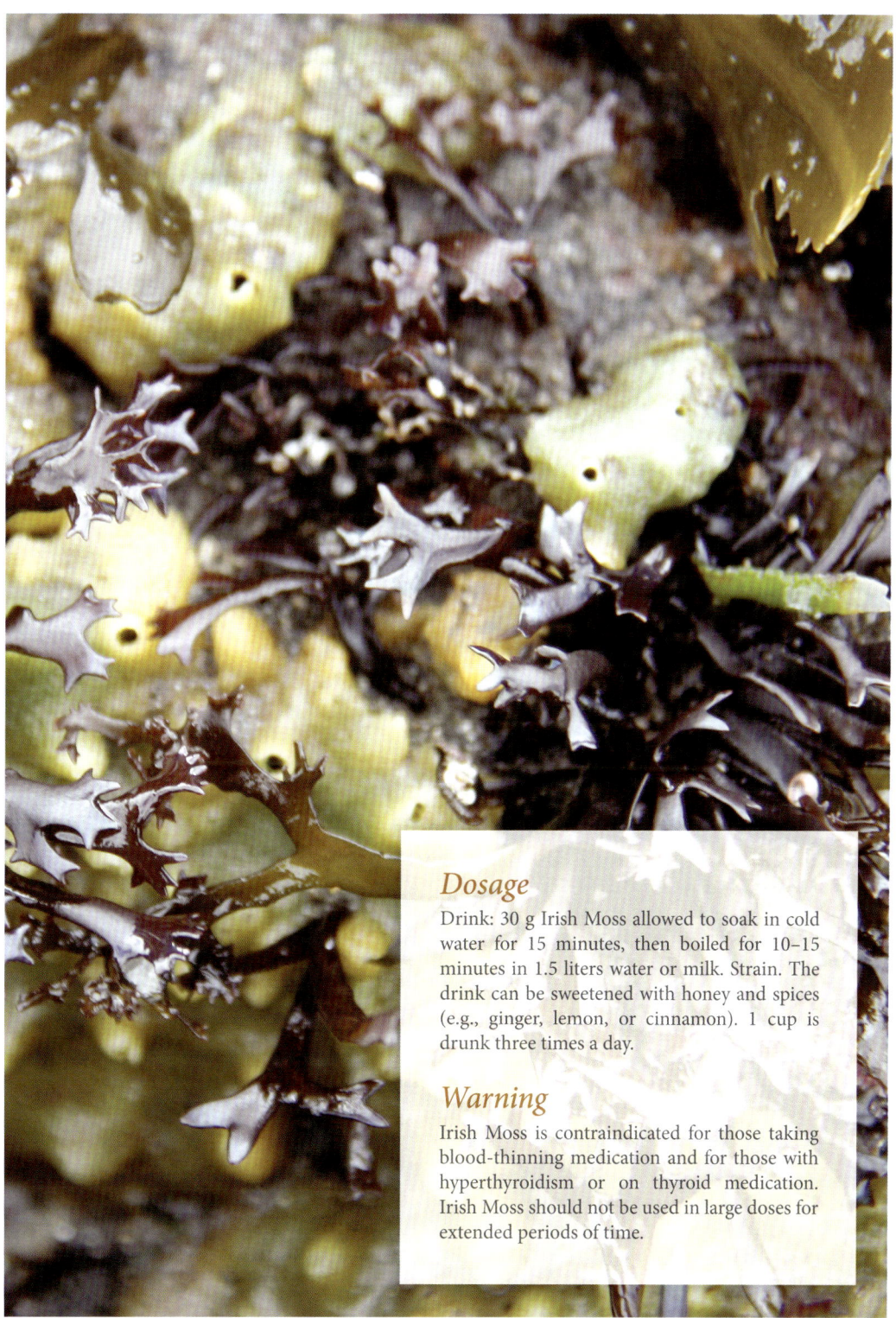

Dosage

Drink: 30 g Irish Moss allowed to soak in cold water for 15 minutes, then boiled for 10–15 minutes in 1.5 liters water or milk. Strain. The drink can be sweetened with honey and spices (e.g., ginger, lemon, or cinnamon). 1 cup is drunk three times a day.

Warning

Irish Moss is contraindicated for those taking blood-thinning medication and for those with hyperthyroidism or on thyroid medication. Irish Moss should not be used in large doses for extended periods of time.

Juniper

Juniperus communis
Cupressaceae—*Einir*

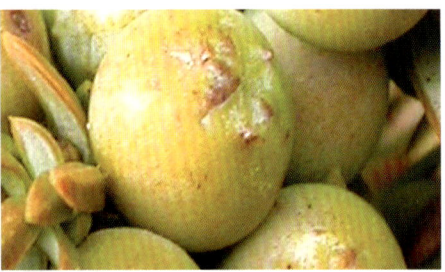

Habitat

Juniper is the only wild conifer found in Iceland. It is a low bush with sharp needles and is fairly common all over the country.

Parts Used

Berries and branches.

Harvesting

Mature berries are collected in the autumn. They are green the first year and mature in the second or third year when they become a blue-black color. There are often both green and black berries on the same branch. The branches are collected all summer and into autumn.

Constituents

Essential oils, tannins, diterpenes, flavonoids, sugars, resins, and vitamin C.

History

Juniper has long been used as a medicinal herb (e.g., Romans used a Juniper berry decoction as a hair wash to prevent hair loss). In the past, branches of Juniper were burned in Europe as protection from evil spirits and Black Death, while burning Juniper branches over pregnant women was supposed to keep the devil at a reasonable distance. Juniper berry is the main flavoring in gin and it is commonly used as a cooking spice (e.g., in jam-making or in meat marinades). The essential oil is distilled from the berry.

In the old days, a traditional custom in Iceland, particularly in the Southeast, was to eat dried fish with butter and juniper berries, which were sold by weight. The Native Americans used both the berries and the branches of Juniper for medicinal purposes. It was highly honored for use in various respiratory problems such as colds, flu, fever, coughs, throat infections, asthma, and tuberculosis. It was also used for stomach pains, heartburn, sores, and diarrhea. Juniper was used to speed up birth and to protect against infection after birth. Juniper branches were used as an incense to purify houses and to disinfect and heal wounds. They were also used for kidney pain, urinary infections, and venereal diseases. Juniper was reported to be good for muscle pain, lumbago, and arthritis, as well as for lowering blood pressure and calming nerves. It was also used in good luck rituals and to

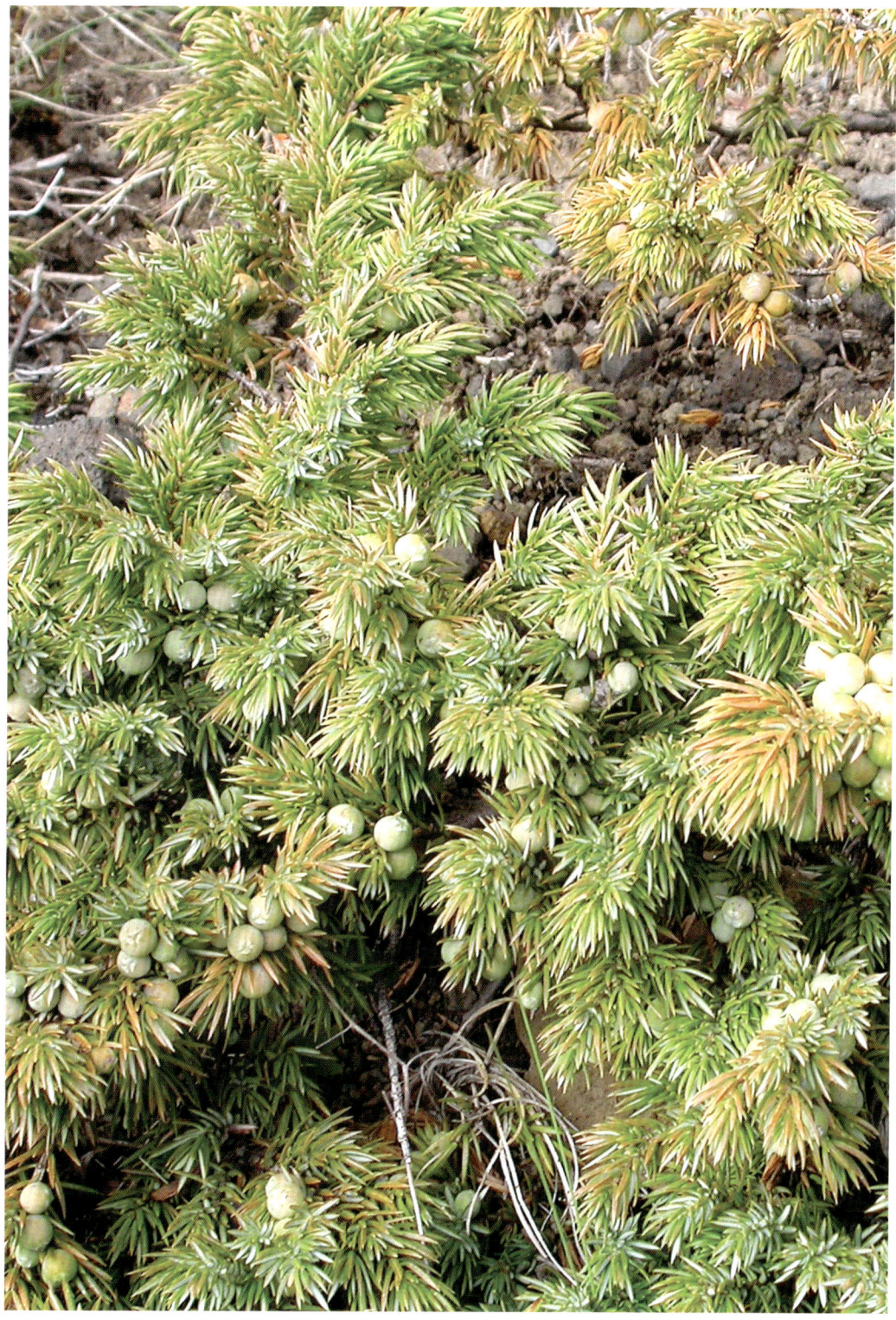

protect against evil spirits. Juniper berries were sewn on clothes as decoration and also used to make necklaces.

Action

Diuretic, antibacterial, cholagogue, anti-inflammatory, analgesic, carminative, and emmenagogue.

. . . .

Uses

Juniper berries are excellent for cystitis and edema and are considered more effective than the branches. The berries are also good for stomach cramps, bloating, and flatulence, and for stimulating menstruation. Juniper berry is traditionally used, both internally and externally, for muscle and joint pain and is considered to be good for arthritis, gout, and other arthritic diseases. In mainland Europe, juniper berry syrup is traditionally used for colds, throat infections, and bronchitis.

Research

In vitro tests on the essential oil of both the berry and the branches have shown Juniper's antibacterial and antifungal properties.[1–4] Tinctures and decoctions of the berries and the branches have shown antibacterial properties.[5–7] *In vitro* studies on the roots, berries, and branches of Juniper have also shown an inhibiting effect on the tuberculosis bacteria *Mycobacterium tuberculosis* and *M. aurum*.[8–10] In other *in vitro* studies on both the berries and the branches, antioxidant properties[11,12] were shown as well as an inhibiting effect on the growth of breast cancer cells.[13] *In vivo* tests using a decoction of Juniper berries showed a lowering of blood-sugar levels.[14,15]

Dosage

Tincture: 0.5–2 ml three times a day (1:5, 40%).

Infusion: ½-1 teaspoon in a cup three times a day.

Syrup: 1 teaspoon three times a day.

Infusions, tinctures, compresses, and ointments for external use.

Warning

Large doses or prolonged use of Juniper berries may cause kidney damage, so those with a kidney infection or kidney weakness should not use Juniper berries. Juniper is also contraindicated for pregnant women and for heavy menstruation.

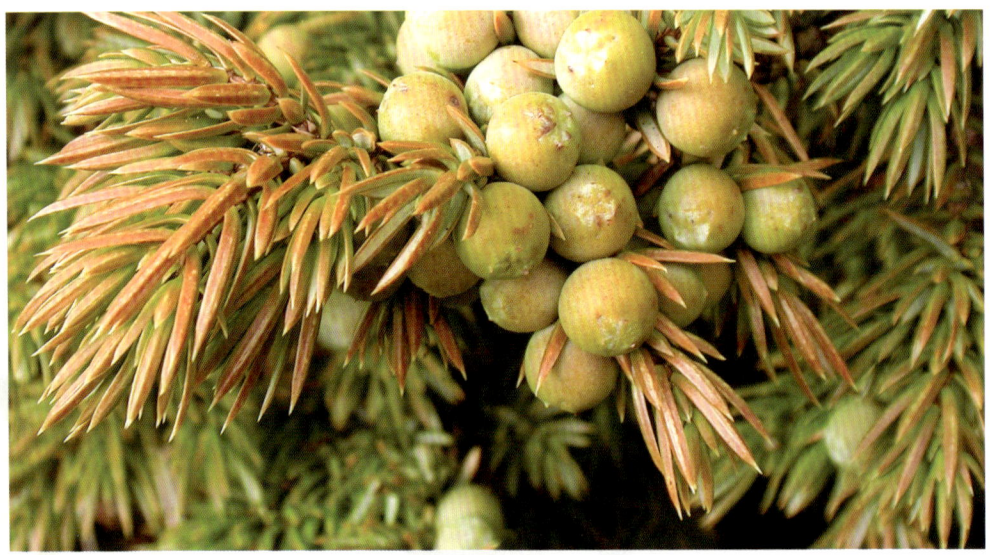

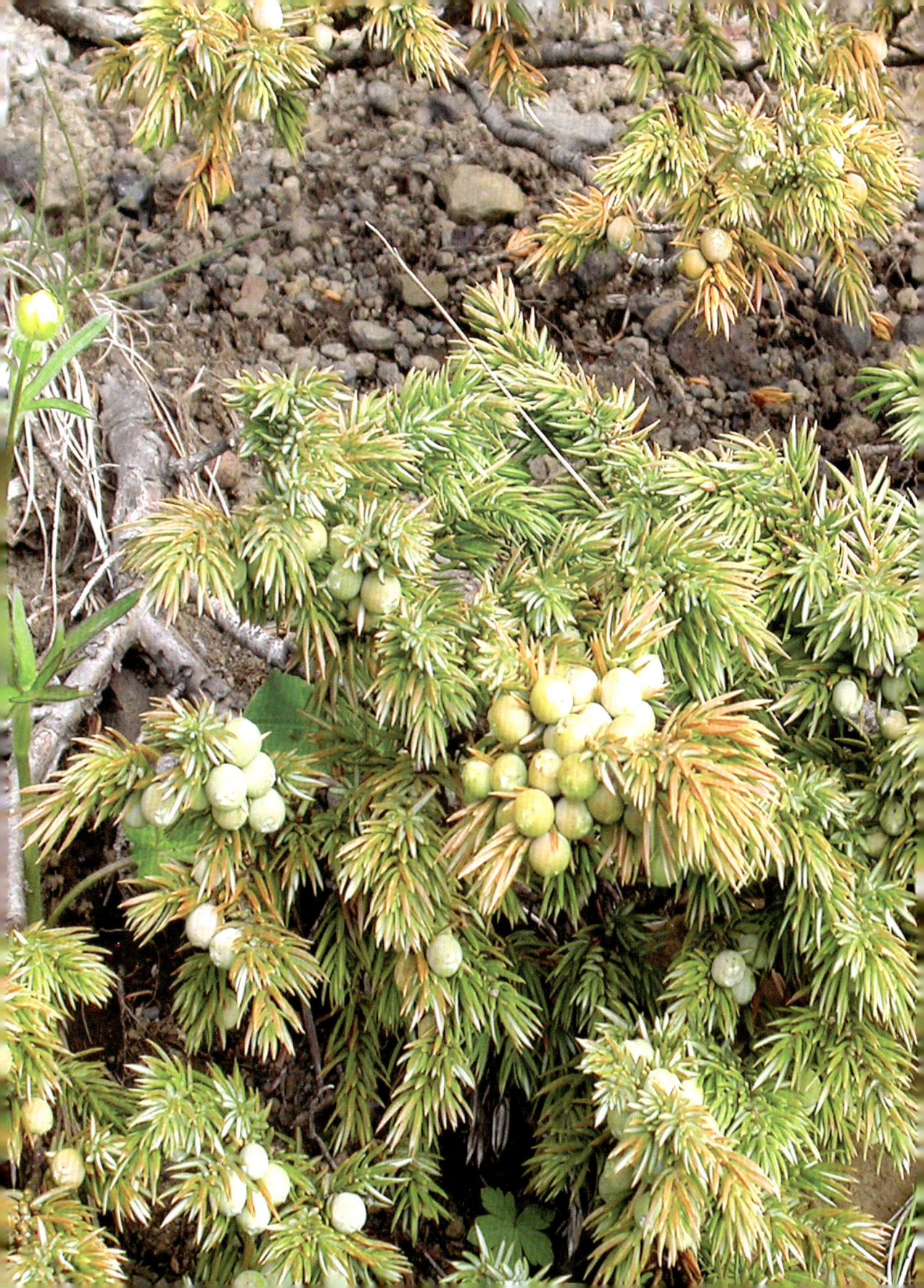

Kidney Vetch

Anthyllis vulneraria
Fabaceae—*Gullkollur*

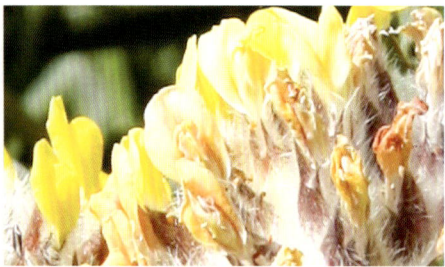

Habitat

Kidney Vetch grows in sandy soil, dry grasslands, and on roadsides. It is rare in Iceland but grows on the Reykjanes Peninsula and in Mosfellssveit.

Parts Used

The entire plant is used, except for the root.

Harvesting

Harvesting Kidney Vetch is not recommended as it is a rare plant in Iceland.

Constituents

Tannins, mucilage, saponins, and flavonoids.

History

The Latin name *vulneraria* is derived from the word "vulnus", which is the Latin for wound. This name indicates that Kidney Vetch was used to heal sores and wounds.

Action

Vulnerary, astringent, expectorant, mild laxative, and antitussive.

Uses

Kidney Vetch is not used much in Western herbal medicine today. It is thought to be good for skin rashes, sores, burns, and bruises, but is also used for constipation. Kidney Vetch can safely be given to children. It is also thought to work well against coughs, while in some cases it can ease vomiting in children.

Research

In vitro testing on Kidney Vetch has shown antiviral properties (i.e., against herpes simplex virus 1 and 2 and poliovirus type 2),[1] as well as antioxidant properties.[2]

Dosage

Tincture: 1–5 ml three times a day (1:5, 25%).

Infusion: 1–2 teaspoons in a cup three times a day.

Infusions, tinctures, compresses, and ointments for external use.

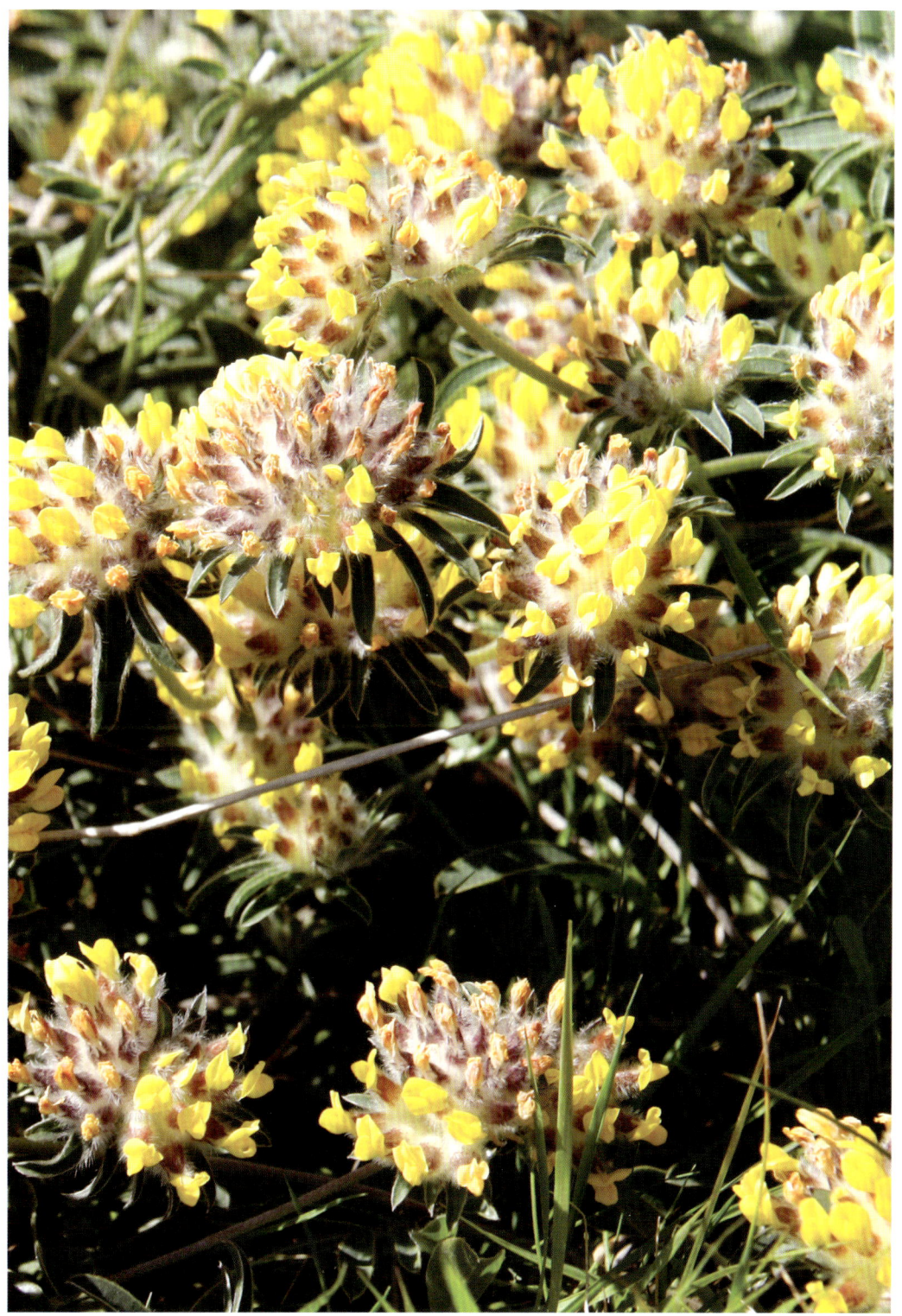

Knotgrass

Polygonum aviculare
Polygonaceae—*Blóðarfi*

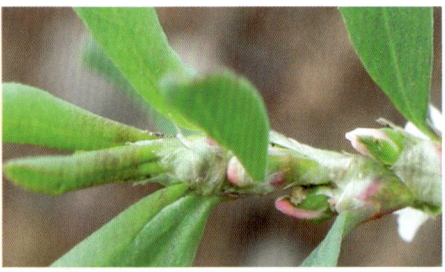

Habitat

Knotgrass grows all over Iceland. It thrives on farms and in areas with a lot of manure.

Parts Used

The entire plant is used, including the root.

Harvesting

It is collected all summer.

Constituents

Polyphenols (gallic and caffeic acid), flavonoids, silicic acids, and mucilage.

History

The species name *aviculare* is taken from the Latin word "aviculus," a diminutive of "avis," meaning bird. The seeds of Knotgrass are eaten by many small birds, thus the connection to the name. The word Knotgrass refers to the swollen jointed stems of the plant. Other names, such as Hogweed or Cowgrass in Britain, indicate that it was eaten by livestock as fodder. In the Shakespeare play *A Midsummer Night's Dream*, mention is made of "the hindering Knotgrass," referring to the belief that a decoction of Knotgrass could hinder the growth of children and young pets. This belief also existed in Iceland. The Icelandic name for Knotgrass is Blóðarfi (Blood Weed), referring to its small red flowers and also to its use in stopping bleeding. Knotgrass has a long, well-documented history as a medicinal herb all over the world. The Chinese have believed for two thousand years that Knotgrass is a diuretic and it is traditionally used in India today as well. The Native Americans use it for cases of painful urination, blood in the urine, and diarrhea, and to prevent miscarriage. It is used externally both as a vulnerary and as an analgesic.

Action

Astringent, hemostatic, diuretic, anthelmintic, anti-inflammatory, antibacterial, and antifungal.

Uses

Knotgrass is not used as much today in Western herbal medicine as it was in the past. Traditionally it has been used to ease diarrhea, menstrual bleeding, nosebleeds, and bleeding wounds. It is also considered good for hemorrhoids and gingivitis, and to eliminate worms. Knotgrass is used traditionally for respiratory diseases: it contains silicic acid, which strengthens the connective tissue of the lungs, and is thought to be good for colds, sore throats, coughs, and bronchitis.

In China, Knotgrass is considered to be diuretic and very effective against urinary infections,

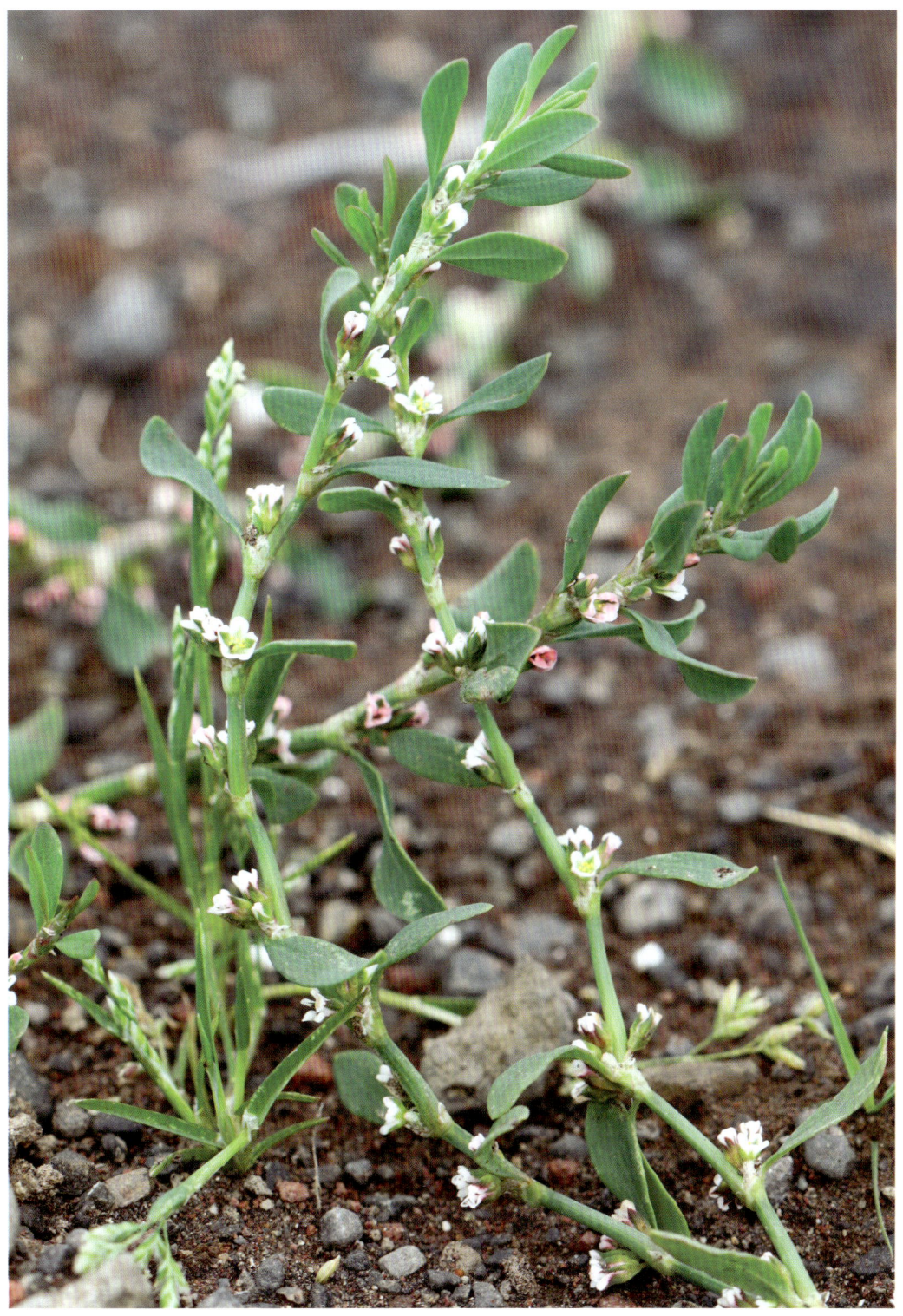

painful urination, and blood in the urine. It is also considered to relieve itching and is used to ease vaginal itching, skin fungus, and eczema. Knotgrass is known to kill parasites in the digestive tract, such as tapeworms, hookworms, and pinworms. Knotgrass has been used in China in cases of diarrhea, dysentery, cholera, hemorrhoids, kidney stones, gout, venereal diseases, and jaundice. In India, there is a long tradition of using Knotgrass as a medicinal herb in a similar way to that in China, but in India it has also been used for diabetes and malaria and is considered especially good for bleeding of any kind, as in Western herbal medicine.

Research

Clinical research was done to find out the effects of Knotgrass on gingivitis. Sixty dentistry students used only a mouthwash from Knotgrass twice a day for two weeks. They were not allowed to brush their teeth while the research was ongoing. After two weeks, Knotgrass was shown to have a positive effect on gingivitis and bacterial formation in the mouth.[1] Clinical research was also done on the efficacy of Knotgrass on dysentery; of 108 subjects, 104 were symptom-free after five days.[2] *In vitro* testing on Knotgrass has revealed its antibacterial and antifungal properties,[3,4] and its antioxidant[5] and anti-inflammatory effects.[6,7] *In vivo* testing showed that Knotgrass decreased abnormal connective tissue growth in the liver,[8] while both *in vivo* and *in vitro* tests show that Knotgrass can lower blood pressure and thin the blood.[4]

Dosage

Tincture: 1–3 ml three times a day (1:5, 25%).

Infusion: 1–2 teaspoons in a cup three times a day.

Decoction: 1–2 teaspoons in a cup three times a day.

Infusions, decoctions, tinctures, compresses, and ointments used externally.

Tea for Diarrhea

1 part Knotgrass

1 part Meadowsweet

1 part Silverweed

Put 3–4 tablespoons of the blend into a 750 ml vacuum flask and pour boiling water into it. Strain the tea into cups and then return the herbs to the flask and allow to stand the whole day. Drink from the flask throughout the day.

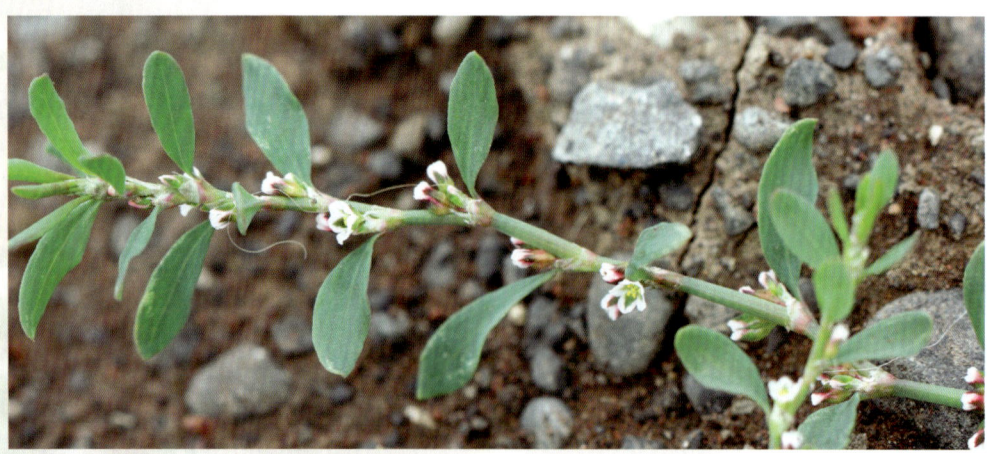

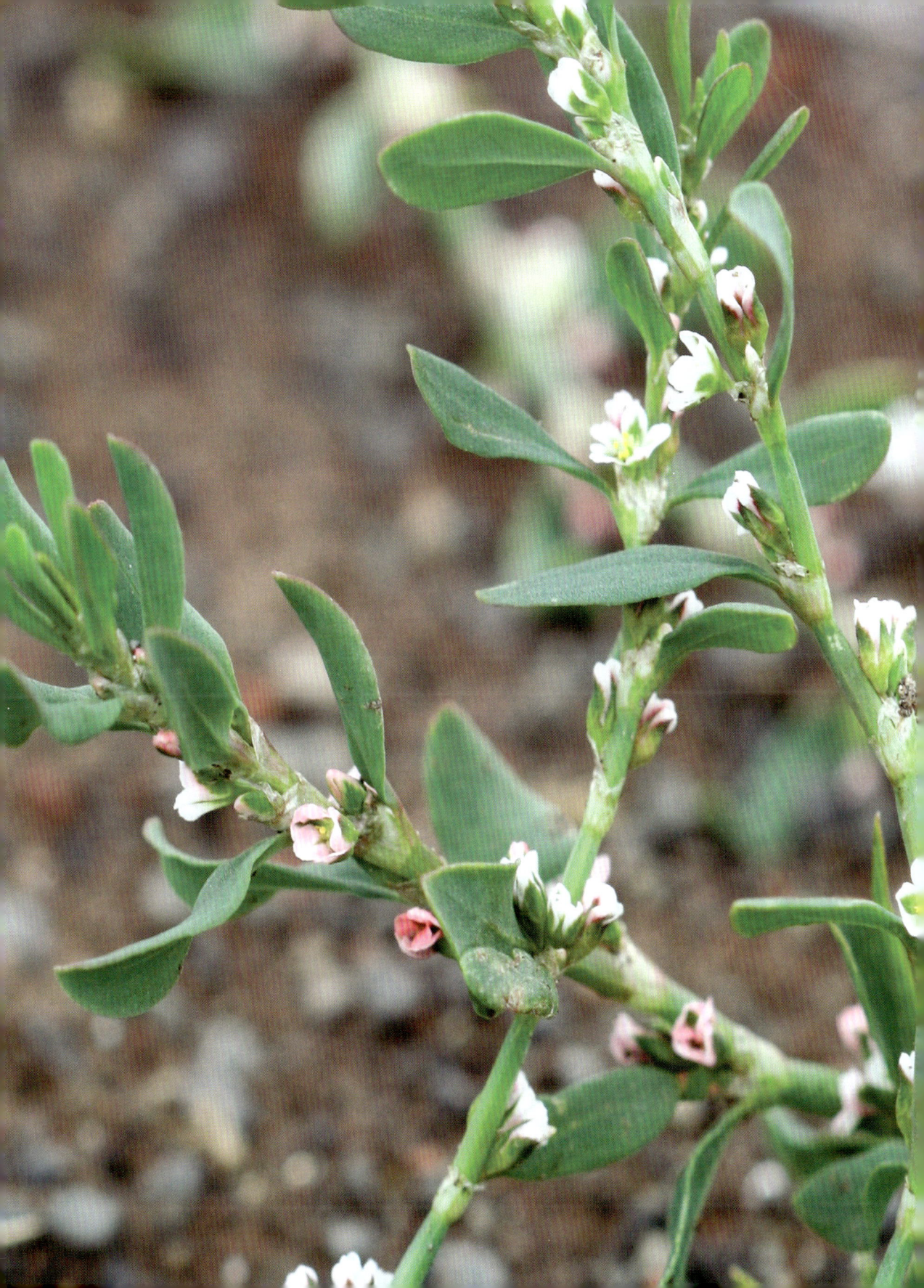

Lady's Bedstraw

Galium verum
Rubiceae—*Gulmaðra*

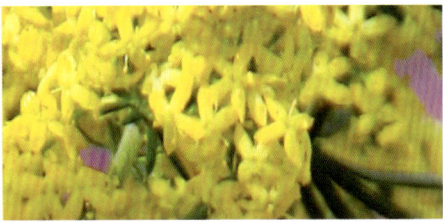

Habitat

Lady's Bedstraw is common all over Iceland and grows on heaths.

Parts Used

The entire plant is used, except for the root.

Harvesting

Picked just before bloom in June–July. If Lady's Bedstraw is used as a tea, it needs to be dried rapidly and used within a few weeks, as it loses its quality very quickly.

Constituents

Iridoids, flavonoids (quercitrin), anthraquinones, and alkanes.

History

The Latin genus name *Galium* is drawn from the Greek word "gala," which means milk. The name came about because Lady's Bedstraw was used to curdle milk in cheese processing. Up until the 19th century, Lady's Bedstraw was frequently used as a rennet, but it was withdrawn when other rennet agents came into use.

In old times, Lady's Bedstraw was often used to fill mattresses, as the name implies. In German folklore

This herb reduces bleeding if it is dried and ground and the powder allowed to enter the wound. It is also good for burns. If the blossoms are boiled in milk, cheese can be made from them which will be soft and a beautiful yellow. Men say that the milk curdles better and the cheese will be bigger. [...] Where Bedstraw grows in fields, women complain that their milk curdles immediately, and that is exactly the action of Bedstraw.

Björn Halldórsson, Uses of Herbs, 1783

it is mentioned that Virgin Mary laid her son Jesus in a cradle filled with Lady's Bedstraw.

It has also been used to dye yarn, and in Ireland the herb was traditionally put in cupboards to protect against moths and produce a nice smell. The Old Icelandic name for it is "ólúagras" (Not Worn Out), as it was thought to work against fatigue, but it was also considered a diaphoretic and good for epilepsy. There is documentation about Northern Bedstraw (*G. boreale*) having similar properties to Lady's Bedstraw.

Action

Diuretic, astringent, vulnerary, antispasmodic, and sedative.

Uses

It is diuretic and is used for edema, especially in connection with the lymphatic system and the kidneys. Lady's Bedstraw is used for kidney and bladder stones, urinary tract infections, and cystitis. It is also taken for skin problems (e.g., eczema and psoriasis), and topically for wounds and rashes. In France it is traditionally used for epilepsy. It is considered to be a sedative and is used for nervousness, headaches, and arrhythmia. It is also used for arthritis; its diuretic properties are probably responsible for this action.

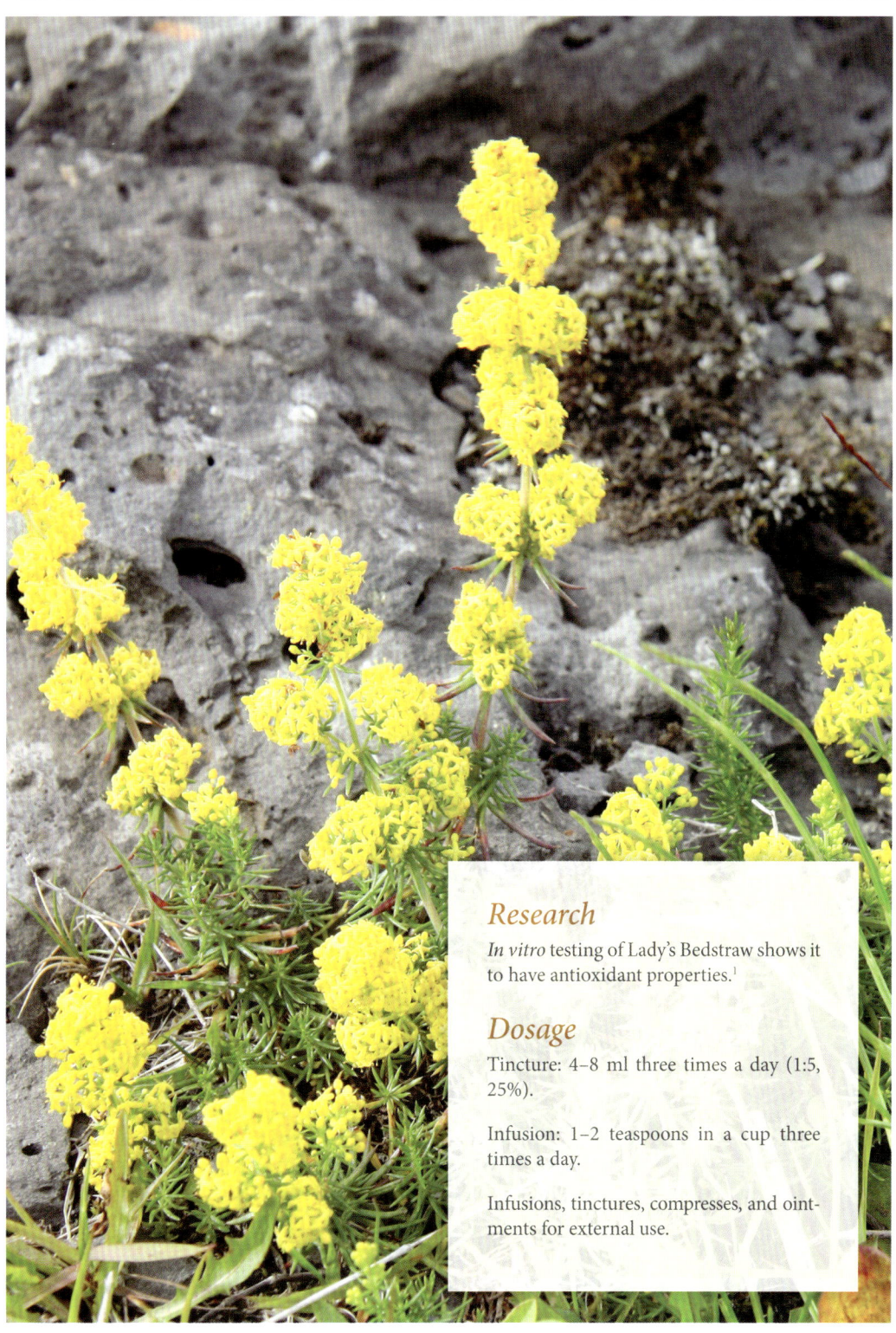

Research

In vitro testing of Lady's Bedstraw shows it to have antioxidant properties.[1]

Dosage

Tincture: 4–8 ml three times a day (1:5, 25%).

Infusion: 1–2 teaspoons in a cup three times a day.

Infusions, tinctures, compresses, and ointments for external use.

Lady's Mantle

Alchemilla vulgaris
Rosaceae—Maríustakkur

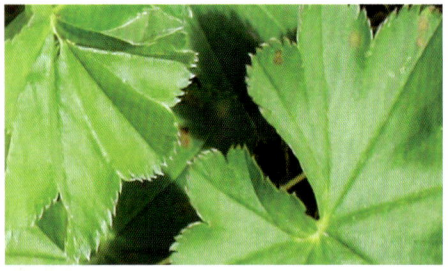

Habitat

Lady's Mantle is common all over Iceland and grows mainly in ravines and alongside streams.

Parts Used

The entire plant, except for the root.

Harvesting

Lady's Mantle is collected in bloom in June.

Constituents

Tannins, flavonoids (quercitrin), and phyto-sterols.

History

There are many kinds of Lady's Mantle, but in most sources on medicinal herbs the generic name *Alchemilla vulgaris* is used, which includes about 30 different varieties. In Iceland, there are four varieites of Lady's Mantle: Hairy Lady's Mantle (*A. filicaulis*), Clustered Lady's Mantle (*A. glomerulans*), Rock Lady's Mantle (*A. wichurae*) and Smooth Lady's Mantle (*A. glabra*). They are all used for medicinal purposes and there is no differentiation of their properties. Garden Lady's Mantle (*A. mollis*), which grows mainly in gardens, is also found close to towns, but it is much larger and is not used for medicinal purposes.

The genus name *Alchemilla* is said to be derived from the Arabic "alkemelych," which refers to alchemists of the Middle Ages who believed in the magical powers of Lady's Mantle. It is also believed that the name refers to the transpiration drops on the leaves, which resemble dewdrops and were coveted by alchemists at this time. The English name is thought to have arisen in the Middle Ages and refers to the Virgin Mary, like the names of many herbs during this period. The lobes of the leaves were said to resemble a Virgin's cloak. In Italian references from the 16th century it is recommended to blend the dried root of Lady's Mantle with red wine to heal internal and external wounds, while an infusion made with the fresh leaves was said to work well on the broken bones of infants. The references also state that if Lady's Mantle were to be drunk regularly for 15 days, it would hinder female infertility caused by the uterus being "slippery."

The contracting and astringent effects of Lady's Mantle were also supposed to tighten the female genitalia so much that women became virgins again. In other references, it is recommended to place the herb under the pillow in the evenings to get the best sleep. Culpepper, a 17th-century British herbalist, recommended Lady's Mantle for all wounds and female troubles as well as for women with big, drooping breasts, as both ingestion and washing with Lady's Mantle would help the breasts to become firm again. Old Icelandic references allege that Alpine Lady's Mantle (*A. alpina*) can be used in a similar way

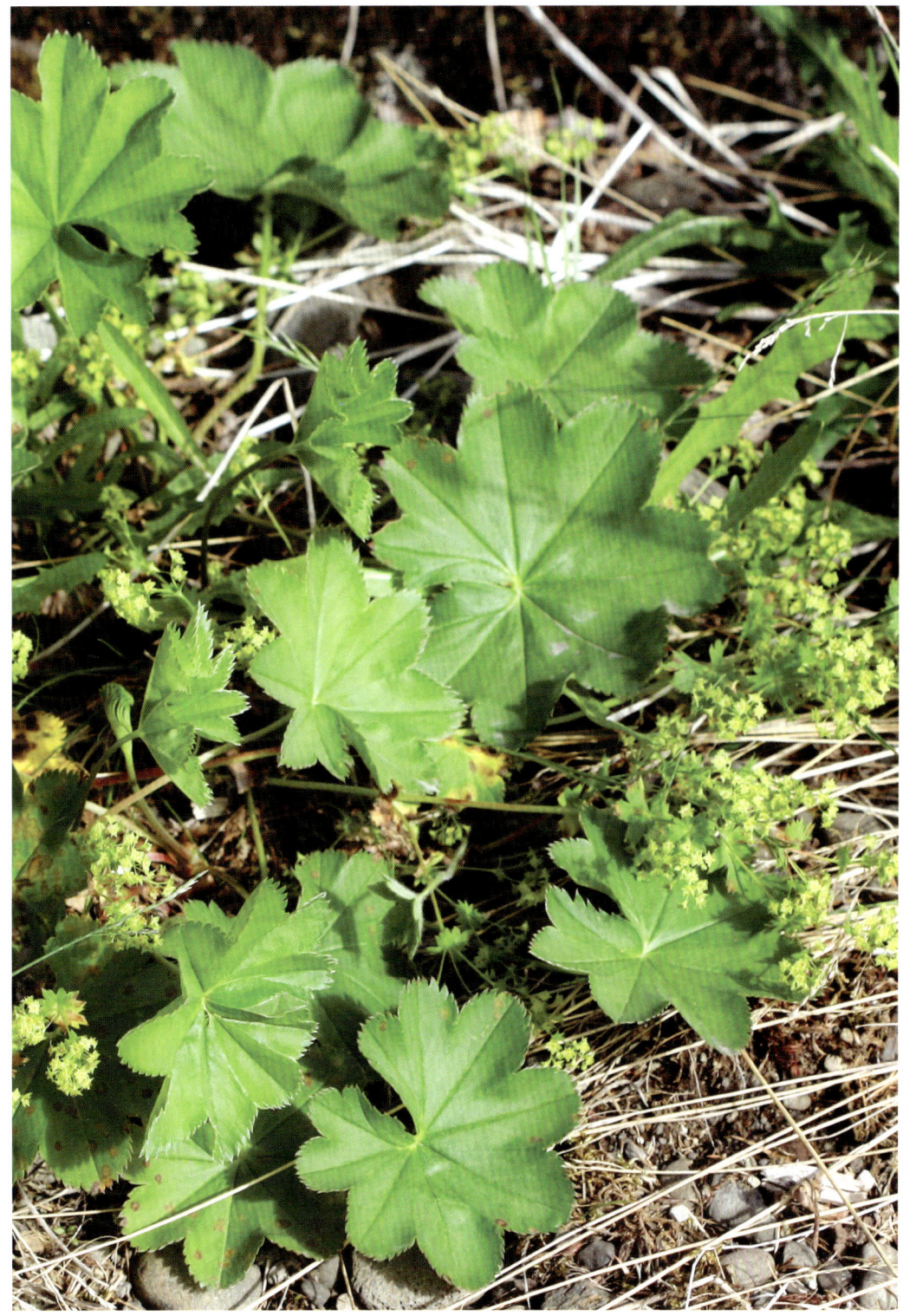

to Lady's Mantle, but there is little reference to its use and it is not used in Western herbal medicine today.

Action

Regulates the menstrual cycle, hemostatic, astringent, anti-inflammatory and vulnerary.

. . . .

Uses

Lady's Mantle is the main Icelandic medicinal herb for gynecological diseases. It helps to regulate menstruation, to control excessive and intermenstrual bleeding, and to ease menstrual pain. As strange as it may sound, Lady's Mantle has also been used to stimulate menstruation and to regulate the menstrual cycle as well as relieving the symptoms of menopause. It is also thought to be good against benign uterine tumors and endometriosis and is used for infertility, premenstrual tension, menstrual-related acne, and migraines. Lady's Mantle is also used, either as a rinse or an ointment, for vaginal discharges and itching. It is also strengthening for the digestive system and is used for gastritis, colitis, and diarrhea. Traditionally, it is used to heal wounds, both internal and external. Lady's Mantle can also be used as a mouthwash for mouth ulcers, gingivitis, laryngitis, and throat infections. Lady's Mantle is thought to have a strengthening effect on the venous system and is effective for ailments such as hemorrhoids and varicose veins, as well as for discomfort and pain in the legs.

Research

A clinical trial involving 341 young women with excessive menstruation, often with short intervals between periods, showed that Lady's Mantle worked well to lessen the bleeding. It also showed good results as a preventive if given 10–15 days before menstruation.[1] In another clinical trial on 48 individuals with mouth ulcers, Lady's Mantle showed positive effects.[2] Lady's Mantle has also shown to be anti-inflammatory[1] and vulnerary,[3] and to have antioxidant properties.[1,4,5] Similarly, *in vitro* tests have shown the antibacterial effects of Lady's Mantle,[1] its tonic effect on veins,[6] and its protective effect on the heart.[7] *In vitro* and *in vivo* tests on a blend of

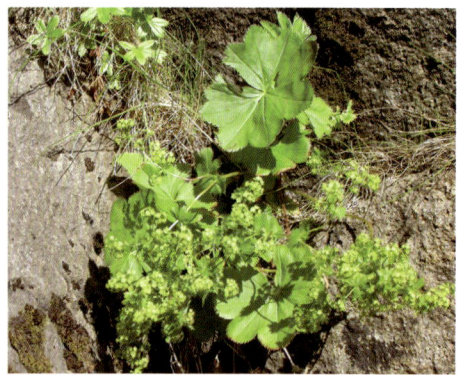

Lady's Mantle and three other medicinal herbs, *Olea europaea, Mentha longifolia,* and *Cuminum cyminum,* demonstrate its possible effect for weight loss in overweight individuals.[8]

Dosage

Tincture: 2–4 ml three times a day (1:5, 25%).

Infusion: 1–2 teaspoons in a cup three times a day.

Infusions, tinctures, compresses, and ointments for external use.

Warning

When abnormally excessive bleeding is present, it is essential to rule out malignant changes before treating with Lady's Mantle or other herbs. Internal use of Lady's Mantle during pregnancy is not recommended.

Tea for Menopause

2 parts Lady's Mantle

1 part Stinging Nettle leaves

1 part Yarrow

Put 3–4 tablespoons of the blend into a 750 ml vacuum flask and pour boiling water into it. Strain the tea into cups and then put the herbs back into the flask and allow to stand the whole day. Drink from the flask throughout the day.

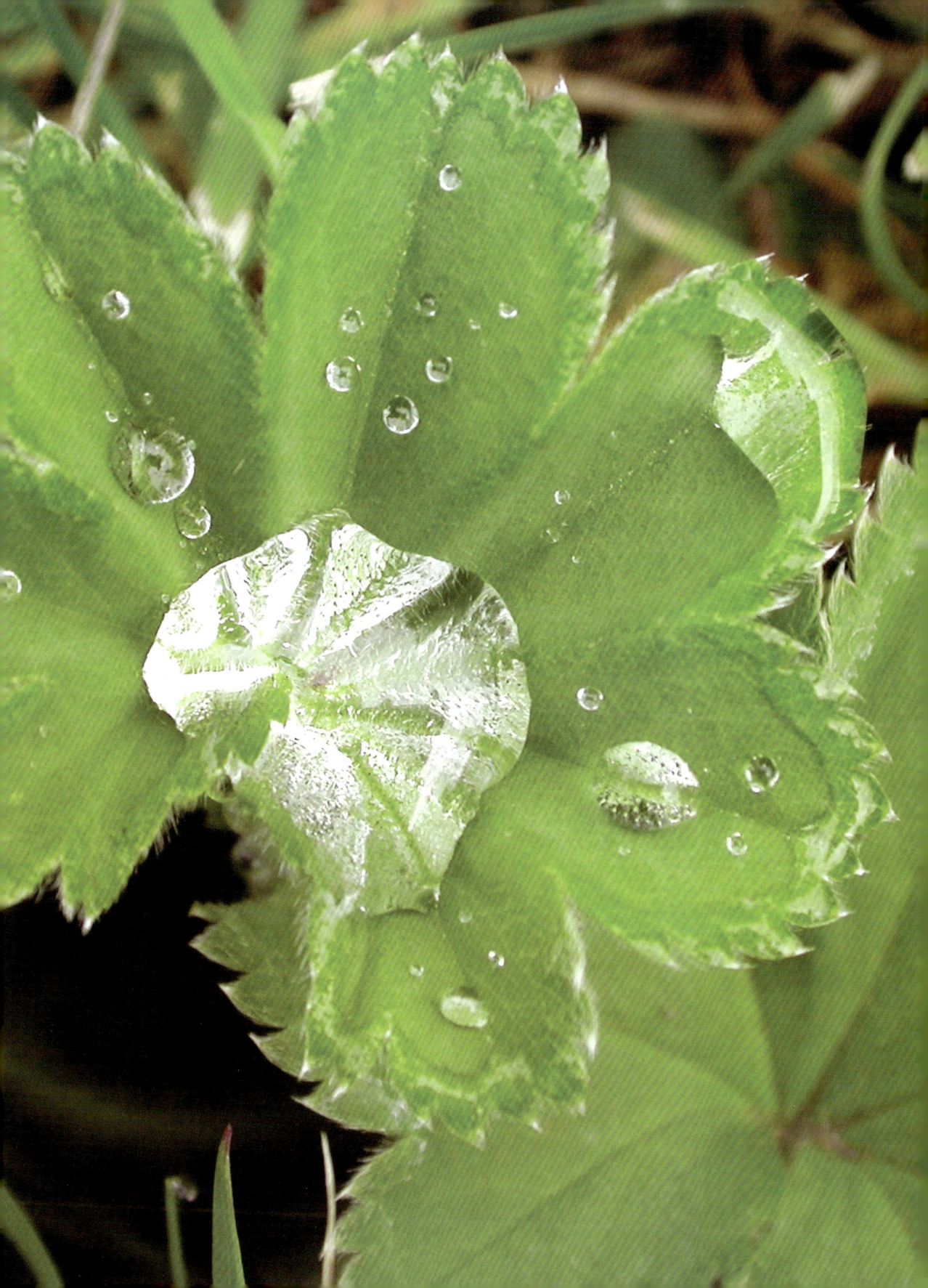

Large-flowered Wintergreen

Pyrola grandiflora
Pyrolaceae—Björlulilja

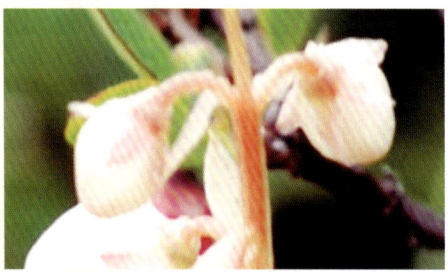

Habitat

It is rare and grows mainly in the moist ground of Northeast Iceland.

Parts Used

The entire plant is used, including roots.

Harvesting

Because it is so rare in Iceland, harvesting is not recommended.

Constituents

Phenols (arbutine), phenolic acid, essential oils, and flavonoids (quercetin).

History

The genus name *Pyrola* is drawn from the word "pyrus," meaning pear. The leaves of several Pyrolaceae resemble the leaves of the pear tree. The second name, *grandiflora*, refers to the size of the flowers, which are the biggest in this family. The name Large-flowered Wintergreen refers to how long the leaves remain green. It is not to be confused with the well-known American Wintergreen (*Gaultheria procumbens*) from which wintergreen essential oil is processed.

Canadian Inuits have used this herb and other types of wintergreen as a tea for children's coughs, earache, and eye problems and have put the chewed fresh roots over wounds. Both roots and leaves are used as diuretics and to ease childbirth. The leaves were considered laxative, the roots were chewed for sore throats, and root compresses were placed over swollen glands of the throat. Alaskan sources reveal that the herb was used in cooking, the seeds being used with fish roe, either baked whole, ground into powder, ,or raw. *Pyrola minor*, Common Wintergreen, is common all over Iceland and is said to have similar properties to the Large-flowered Wintergreen.

Action

Diuretic, antibacterial, astringent, and mildly antispasmodic.

Uses

This herb is not used much in Western herbal medicine nowadays, but sources reveal extensive use in the past. It is diuretic and considered effective for urinary infections (e.g., cystitis). It is also said to be mildly antispasmodic and is used in cases of painful urination due to urinary

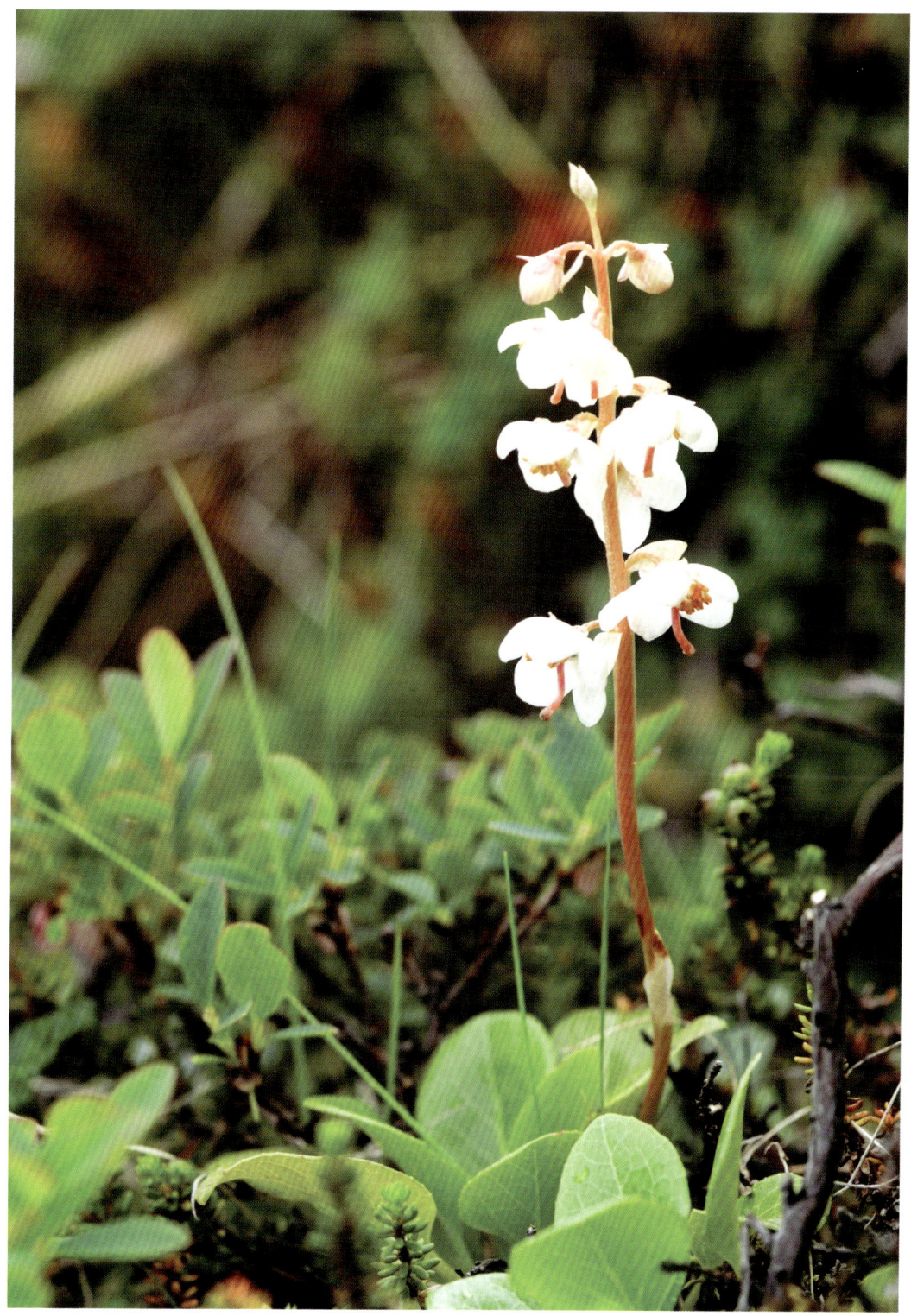

infections. It is used for swollen eyes and is good for skin diseases and healing wounds. It is also used as a mouthwash for swollen gums and sore throats. It is taken internally for epilepsy and to strengthen nerves. It is a popular herb in China, where it is used for tuberculosis sufferers, arthritic pain, as a calmative, and to strengthen bones and muscle attachments. The bruised fresh plant is used against insect, dog, and snake bites. It is also good for stopping bleeding (e.g., nosebleeds, menstrual bleeding, and bleeding from an injury).

Research

In a clinical trial, 18 lung disease patients were injected with methylhydroquinone, a compound isolated from Large-flowered Wintergreen; 16 got better, 2 did not. The same active constituent has been used with good results to treat infections in the digestive tract that cause diarrhea as well as for urinary infections.[1] Methylhydroquinone from *Pyrola grandiflora* also kills *Staphylococcus aureus*, *Micrococcus luteus*, *Salmonella typhi*, *Escherichia coli,* and other bacteria.[1,2] The decoction of the herb kills several species of bacteria.[1]

It is known that antibiotics can cause damage to the inner ear and kidneys and therefore lead to deafness. Protection against the toxic effect of antibiotics was shown by *in vivo* tests when *P. grandiflora* was used as an injectable, together with a Chinese medicinal herb (*Astragalus membranaceus*).[3] A number of trials have shown the effect that *P. grandiflora* has on the heart (i.e., it reputedly lowers blood pressure and increases blood flow to the heart).[1,4] *In vivo* tests have shown that Large-flowered Wintergreen may also have contraceptive properties.[1]

Dosage

Tincture: 1–4 ml three times a day (1:5, 25%).

Infusion: 1 teaspoon in a cup three times a day.

Decoction: 1 teaspoon in a cup three times a day.

Infusions, decoctions, tinctures, compresses, and ointments for external use.

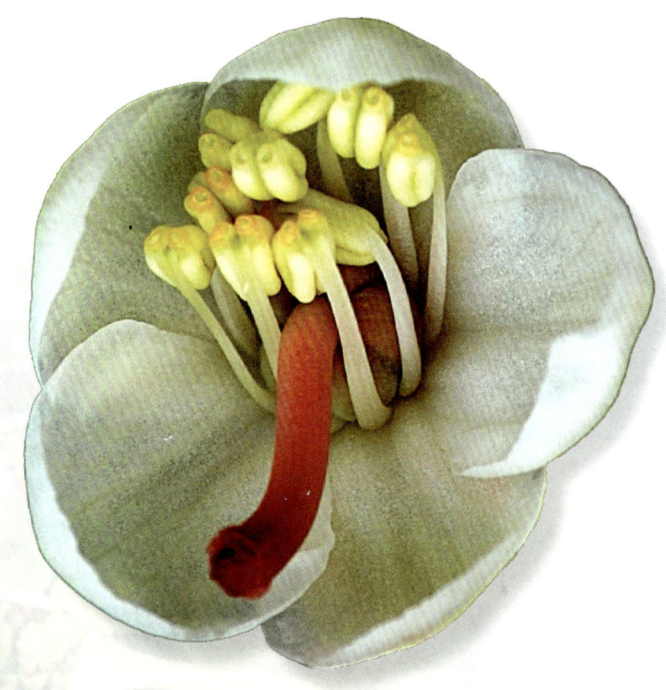

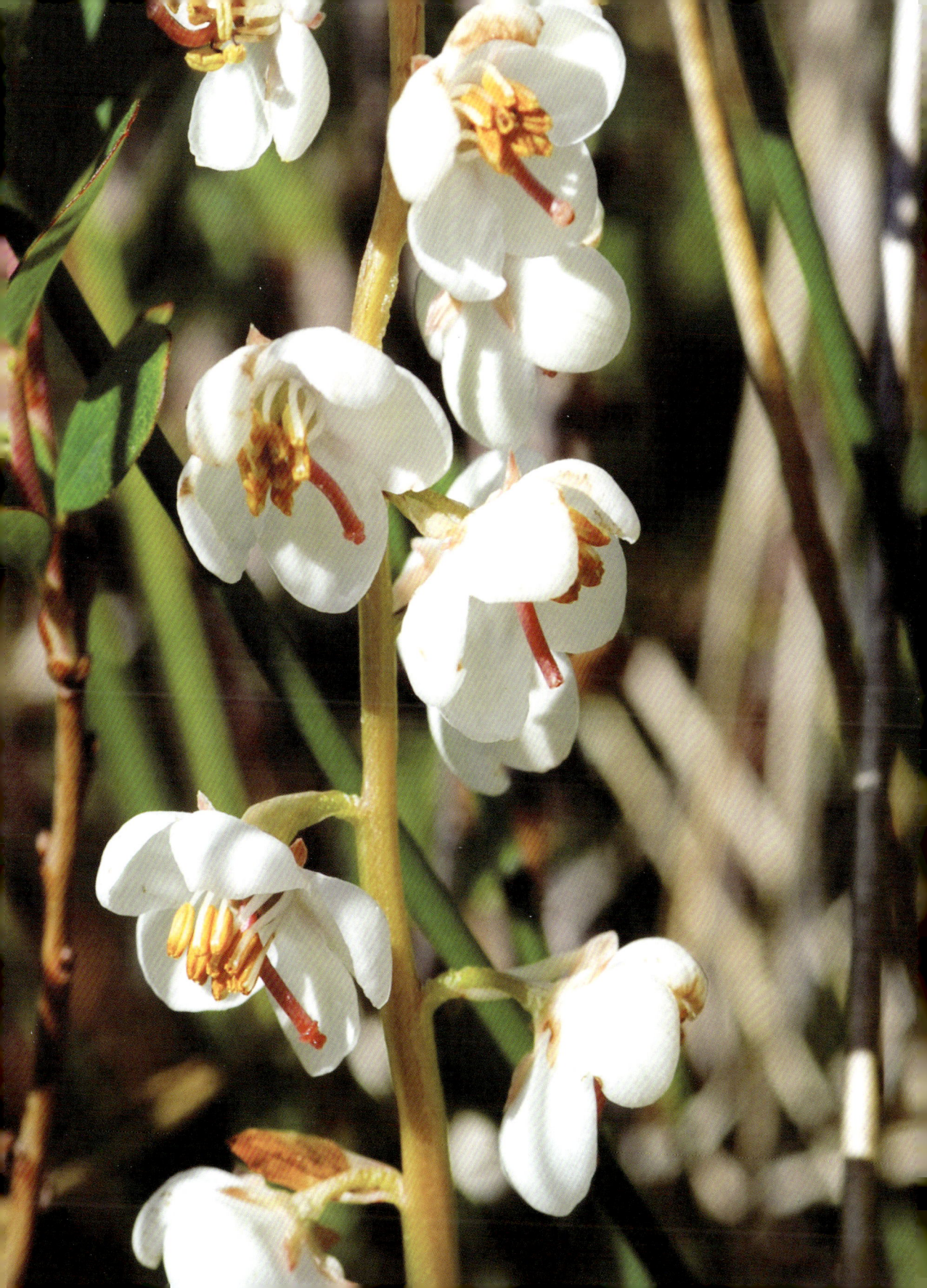

Male Fern

Dryopteris filix-mas
Dryopteridaceae—*Stóriburkni*

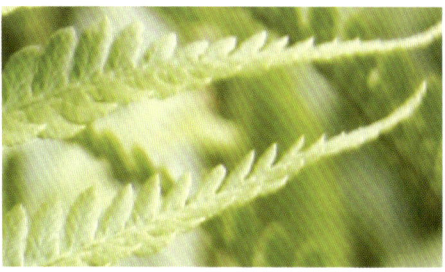

Habitat

Male Fern is rare and is found mainly in the West Fjords and on the Reykjanes Peninsula. It grows mostly in lava fissures and rocky clefts, although it is also found on grassy slopes.

Parts Used

The entire plant is used, including the root.

Harvesting

The leaves are picked all summer and the roots are harvested in autumn.

Constituents

Filicin, triterpenes, oils, resins, and essential oils.

History

There is a long tradition in Europe of using the root of Male Fern to expel intestinal worms, but soap was also made from the ashes of this herb.

Action

Anthelmintic.

Uses

Male Fern is rarely used in Western herbal medicine nowadays. It is considered to be one of the most effective herbs for eliminating worms, especially tapeworms. Fasting is necessary before the root is used for worms and a mild laxative must be used simultaneously, but the laxative must not contain oil as this could enhance the toxicity of Male Fern. Both the leaves and the roots have been used to make ointments for wounds and arthritis. Male Fern has also been used to ease bleeding, reduce inflammation, and lower fever.

Research

Research on isolated constituents of Male Fern in *in vitro* testing has revealed an inhibiting effect on the growth of cancer cells and the HIV virus 1.[1] *In vivo* tests have confirmed its anthelmintic properties.[2] Research on rats and mice with Male Fern revealed very strange side effects, as the penis of the males grew significantly when they were given Male Fern.[3]

Warning

Male Fern is poisonous and large doses can lead to nausea, vomiting, heart and lung failure, liver damage, and blindness. It should never be taken except under professional supervision. Male Fern should not be taken during pregnancy or if there is a history of heart or liver disease.

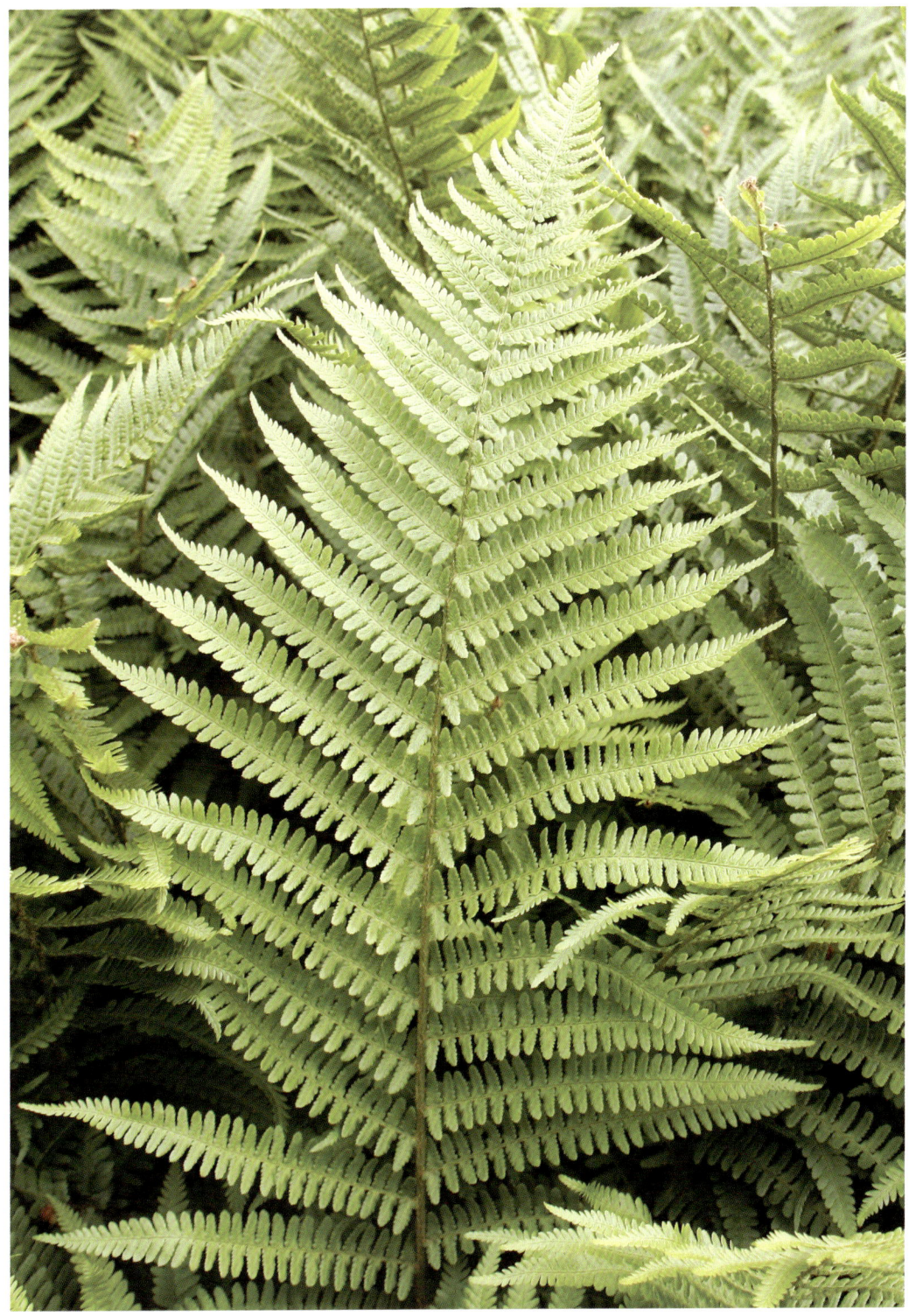

Mare's-tail

Hippuris vulgaris
Hippuridaceae—*Lófótur*

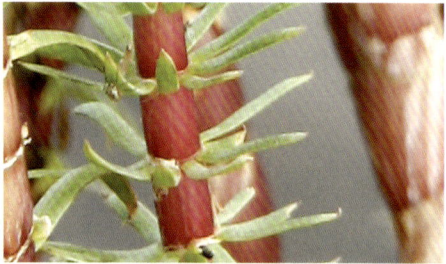

Habitat

Mare's-tail is a common aquatic plant and grows all over Iceland in large patches in shallow ponds.

Parts Used

The entire plant is used, except for the root.

Harvesting

All summer.

Constituents

Mucilage, phenolic acids, flavonoids, iridoids (aucubin), anthocyanins, and glycosides.

History

The genus name comes from the Greek "Hippuris," meaning mare's tail, thus the English name for this plant. The Inuits of Alaska have used Mare's-tail as a food for a long time, regarding it as a good vegetable, which is still the case today. It was mainly fried in seal fat and enjoyed all year round.

Action

Vulnerary, demulcent, and hemostatic.

Uses

Mare's-tail is rarely used in Western herbal medicine today, but in the past it was thought to help stop bleeding and heal wounds both externally and internally. In Tibet, Mare's-tail is thought to be good for the lungs, nerves, liver, and bones. It is also considered to be vulnerary, both internally and externally, and special mention is made of Mare's-tail being good internally for healing lung wounds caused by trauma.

Dosage

Tincture: 2–4 ml three times a day (1:5, 25%).

Infusion: 1–2 teaspoons in a cup three times a day.

Infusions, tinctures, compresses, and ointments for external use.

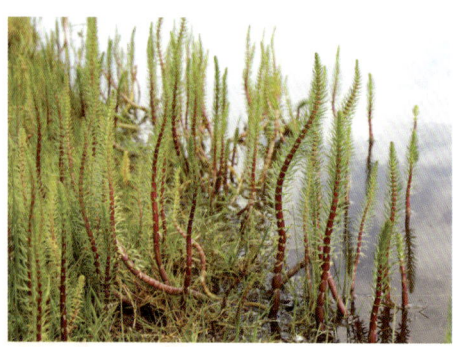

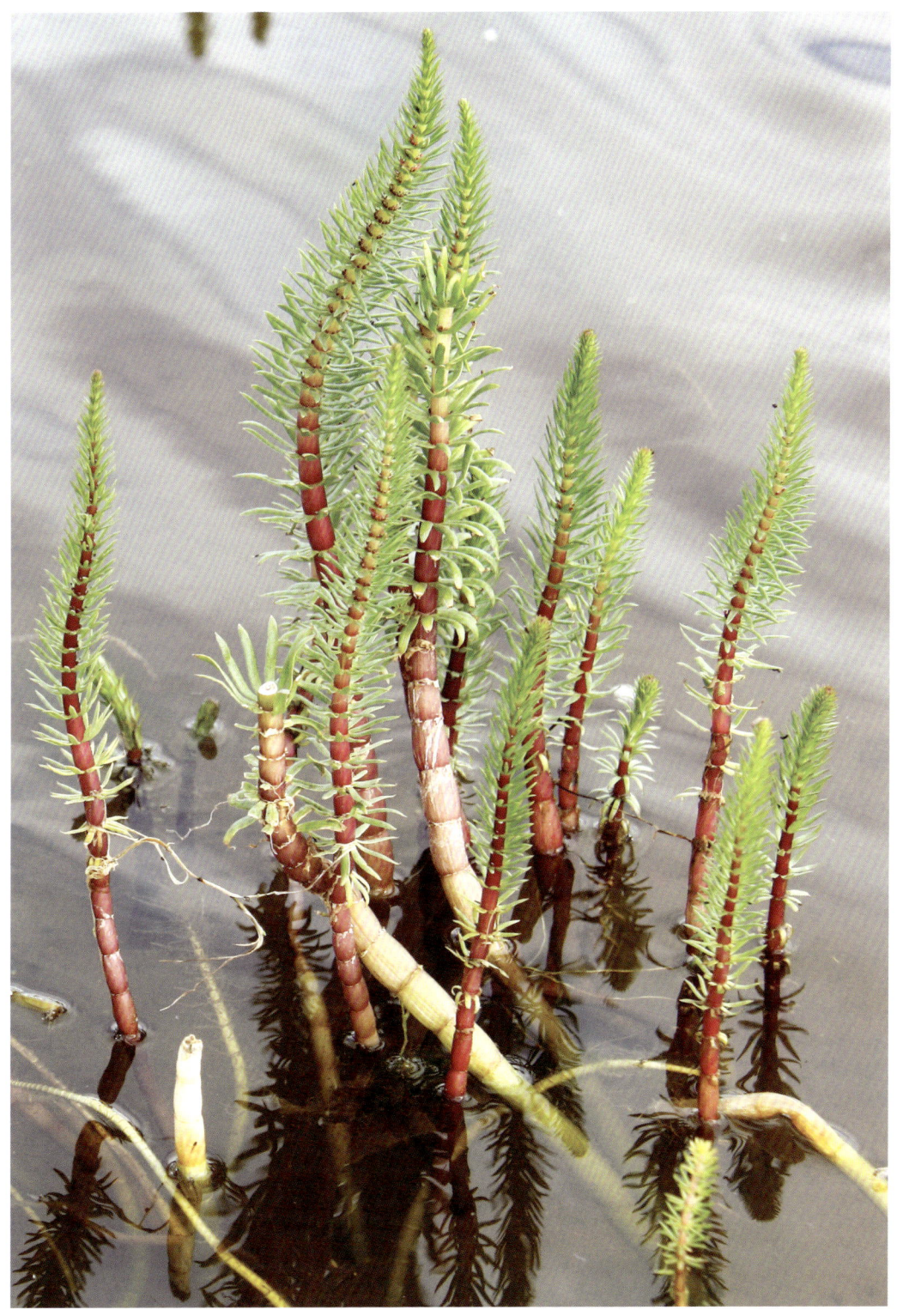

Marsh Marigold

Caltha palustris
Ranunculaceae—*Hófsóley*

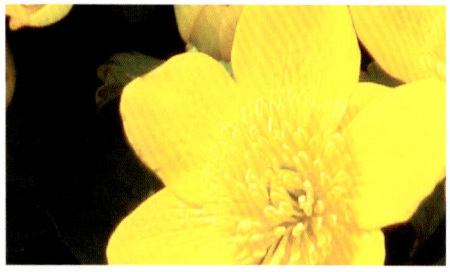

Habitat

Marsh Marigold is common all over Iceland. It grows mainly in marshes and alongside streams.

Parts Used

The entire plant is used, including the root.

Harvesting

Marsh Marigold is collected in May–June. Gloves should be worn while collecting as the juice from the plant can irritate the skin. Marsh Marigold contains a toxin, anemonin, which is destroyed by boiling and drying.

Constituents

Anemonin, alkaloids, choline, saponins, and coumarin.

History

The Latin genus name *Caltha* is derived from the Greek word "calathos", meaning cup or goblet, and refers to the shape of the flowers. The species name *palustris*, on the other hand, is drawn from the word "palus," meaning marsh, and refers to where Marsh Marigold grows. The English name Marigold refers to its use in church festivals in the Middle Ages, as it was one of the flowers dedicated to the Virgin Mary. Marigold has also been called Verrucaria, which is a direct indication that it was used to remove warts.

In past times, Marsh Marigold was used for epileptic seizures and a small amount of tincture was given for anemia. In Ireland, the flowers were boiled in soup and taken for a weak heart, while the leaves were boiled for a hot compress that was used on abesses. Native Americans have used the roots of Marsh Marigold as a diaphoretic and expectorant and to induce vomiting. The decoction of the herb was also mixed with maple syrup and was a popular cough syrup among settlers. A poultice of the boiled root was used on wounds and the decoction from the leaves was considered to be good for constipation. Many sources from the Native Americans warn of the toxicity of fresh Marsh Marigold and the need to boil it before use. There are also many references about Marsh Marigold being used in cooking and the young leaves, boiled as a vegetable, were considered a delicious meal. They are commonly eaten with butter and seasoned with salt and pepper. Similarly, the buds were often pickled like capers, although some references state that they are toxic as well if ingested. If Marsh Marigold leaves are eaten, they need to be boiled twice, with a change of water in between. It is also recommended to use only young leaves, because the older parts of the plant are more toxic than the younger parts.

The flowers of Marsh Marigold have been used to dye yarn yellow. They have also been used in hair rinses and as a beauty remedy for the skin.

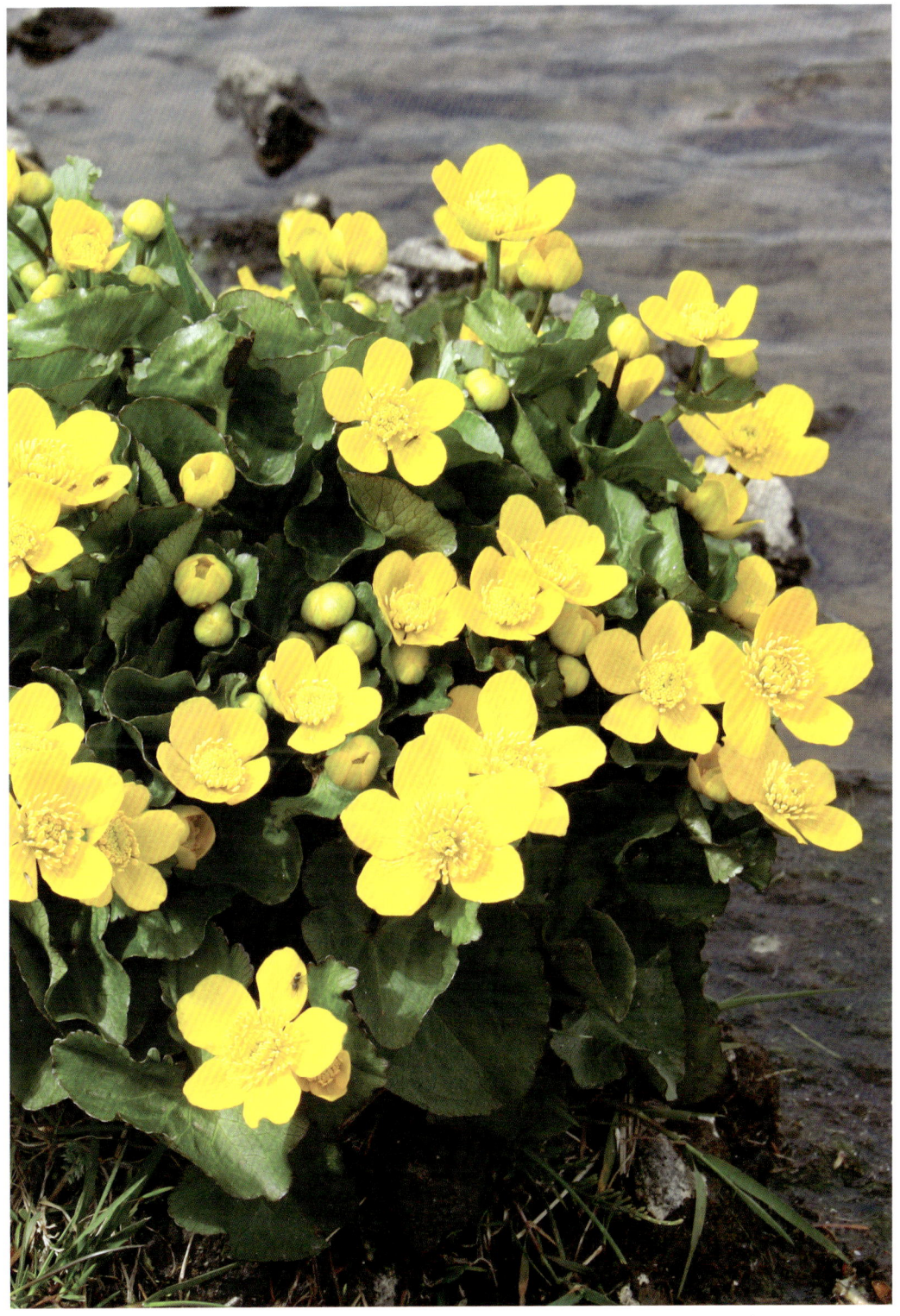

Action

Skin irritant, expectorant, antispasmodic, and removes warts.

Uses

It is not known if Marsh Marigold is still used in European herbal medicine. In the USA the dried leaves have been used internally in very small doses to release mucus from the lungs, digestive tract, and uterus. Infusions are made only from the dried herb, not the fresh herb. Externally, hot poultices of the leaves are used for lumbago, colon spasms, and Bell's Palsy. Marsh Marigold is also used to remove warts. Be aware that large doses of the infusion can cause nephritis and hepatitis. In China, the roots are used for arthritis.

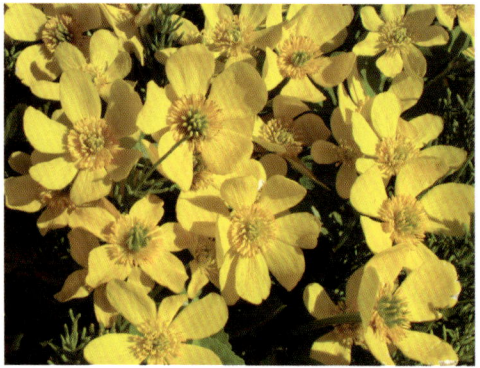

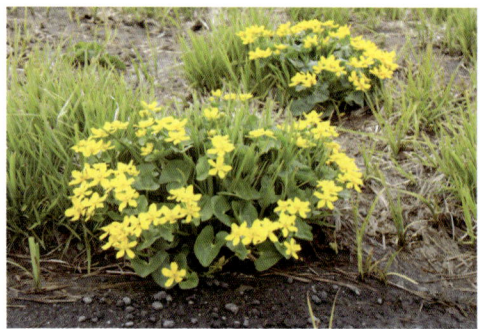

Research

The toxins anemonin in the ratio of 1:20 and proanemonin, in the ratio of 1:80 show inhibiting effects on cancer cells in *in vitro* tests. An infusion of Marsh Marigold showed mild inhibition of various cancer cells but also had toxic effects at the same time.[1]

Dosage

Infusion: ½ teaspoon in a cup once to twice a day.

N.B. The fresh herb must not be used, only the dried herb.

Poultices for external use.

Warning

The entire plant, especially the older parts, contains anemonin, which is toxic. Use of the fresh plant is not recommended, but anemonin is destroyed by boiling and drying the herb. The juice from the plant can irritate the skin. Internal use of Marsh Marigold is not recommended without consulting a professional.

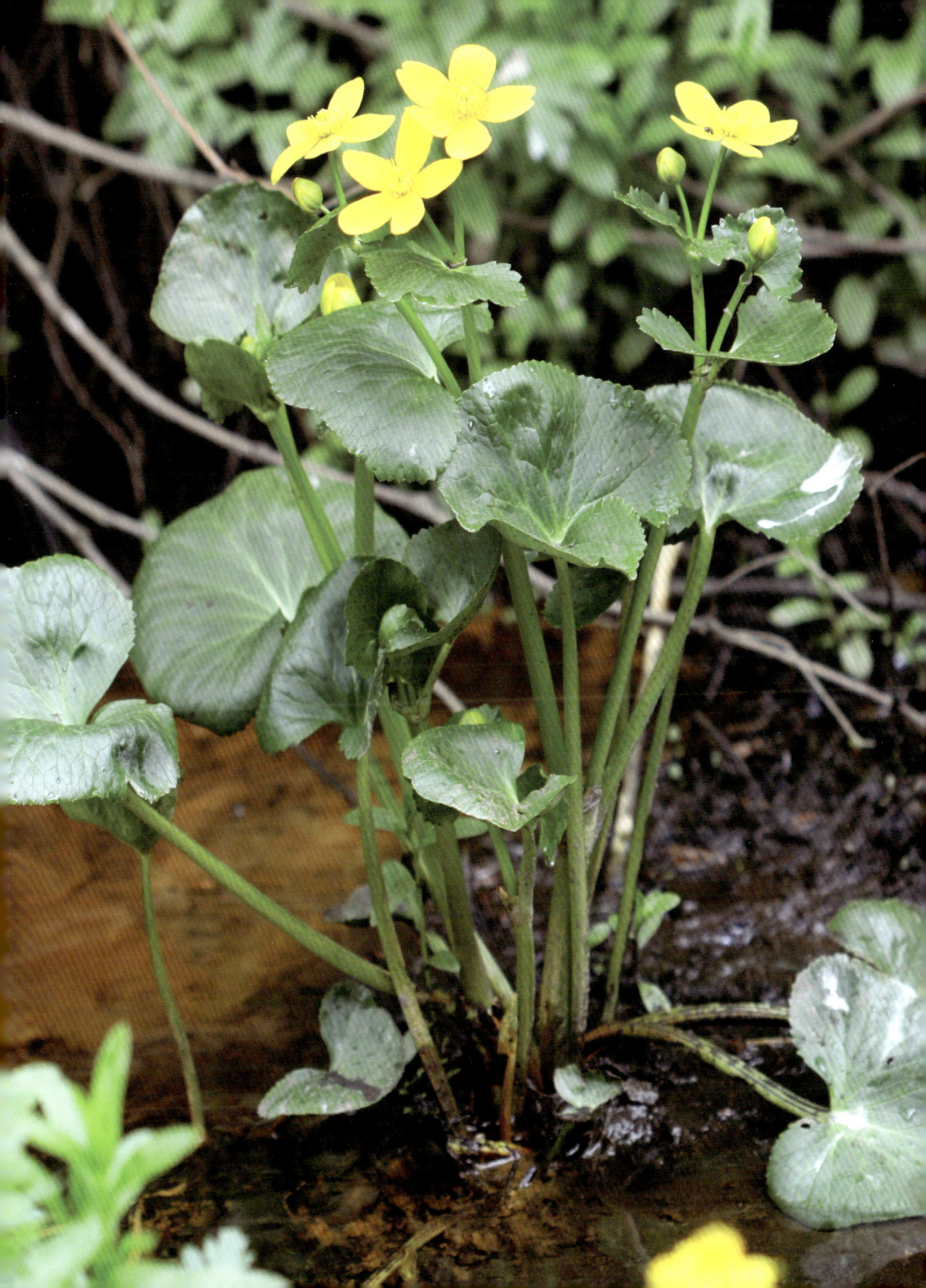

Meadow Buttercup

Ranunculus acris
Ranunculaceae—Brennisóley

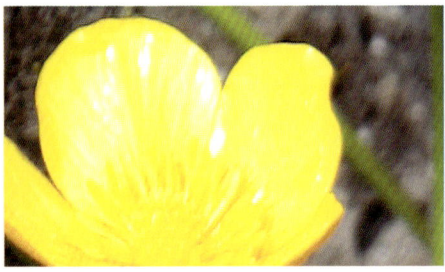

Habitat

Meadow Buttercup is prolific all over Iceland and grows well in old fields.

Parts Used

The entire plant, including the root.

Constituents

Aniemonole.

History

The Latin name *acris* means bitter or acrid, which is very apt because the herb is so bitter that it burns, just as the Icelandic name "Brennisóley" (Burning Buttercup) denotes. Sources from Britain report that Meadow Buttercup was used externally for gout, headaches, and removing warts. The Native Americans used the leaves of Meadow Buttercup externally for arthritis and nerve pains. Meadow Buttercup was used topically and was also sniffed for headaches. The roots were bruised and laid on abscesses, and a liquid was made that helped with diarrhea. Compresses of the fresh plant were laid on chests for colds and chest pains. The juice of the plant was considered to be soothing.

Action

Irritant, analgesic, causes redness and blisters on the skin.

Uses

There is no knowledge of Meadow Buttercup being used in Western herbal medicine today, but it is known in Tibet, where the flowers are used to heat, remove tumors, and draw out fluid.

Warning

Meadow Buttercup is toxic so its use as a medicinal herb is discouraged, both internally and externally. It causes burns and blisters on the skin and mucous membranes.

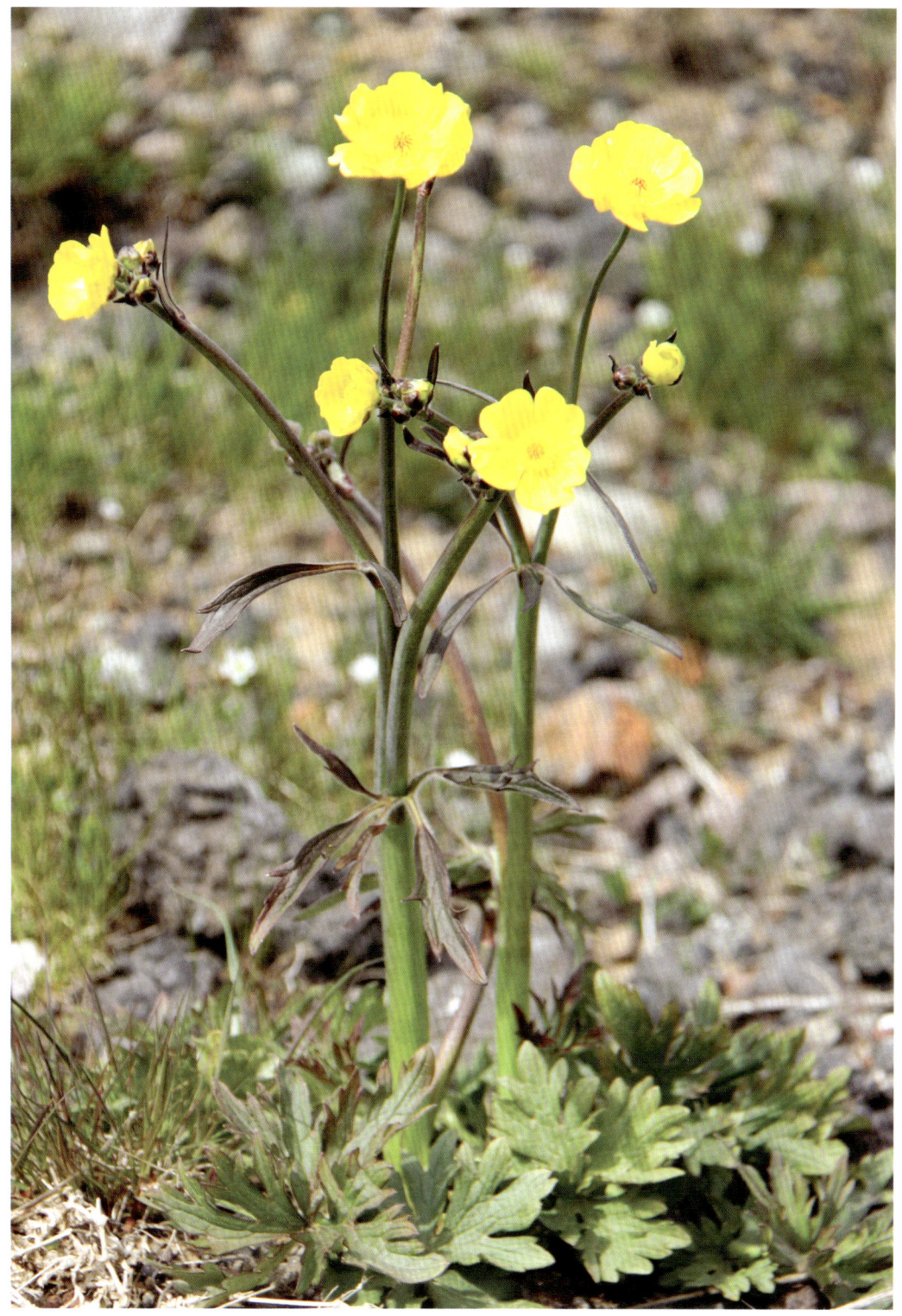

Meadowsweet

Filipendula ulmaria
Rosaceae—Mjaðjurt

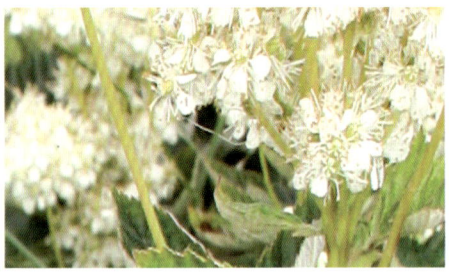

Habitat

Meadowsweet grows all over Iceland but mostly in the South in moist areas and in ditches.

Parts Used

The entire plant is used, except for the root.

Harvesting

Meadowsweet is collected just before bloom or when buds have newly opened in July.

Constituents

Essential oils (salicylaldehyde, methyl salicylate), phenolglycoside, flavonoids (rutin), and tannins.

History

The name Meadowsweet is derived from the word "mead," as Meadowsweet was used to make mead in the old days. It was one of the three sacred herbs of the Druids, who were seers, poets, and wizards of the ancient Celtic beliefs. Ever since then, the medicinal power of Meadowsweet has appeared in ancient scripts. The active ingredient salicin, which is analgesic and anti-inflammatory, was first isolated from the herb in 1827. Salicylic acid was later isolated in 1838. It was first made synthetically in 1859 and is the basis of aspirin, a painkiller first produced in 1899. The former Latin name for Meadowsweet was *Spiraea*, from which the word aspirin is derived. Aspirin in large doses can cause stomach ulcers, but Meadowsweet, on the contrary, heals stomach ulcers. Meadowsweet is a good example of how it is not always possible to understand the medicinal action of herbs from isolated constituents, and the entire herb should be considered holistically in this respect. According to ancient Icelandic folklore, Meadowsweet should be able to help one identify the person who has stolen one's belongings.

Action

Astringent, anti-inflammatory, febrifuge, analgesic, diaphoretic, antibacterial, diuretic, vulnerary, and reduces stomach acid.

Uses

Meadowsweet is one of the best Icelandic medicinal herbs for various digestive disturbances. It heals the mucous membrane of the stomach, balances gastric acid, and is used for indigestion, stomach pain, gastritis, stomach and duodenal ulcers, bloating, and flatulence. Meadowsweet is considered to be good for

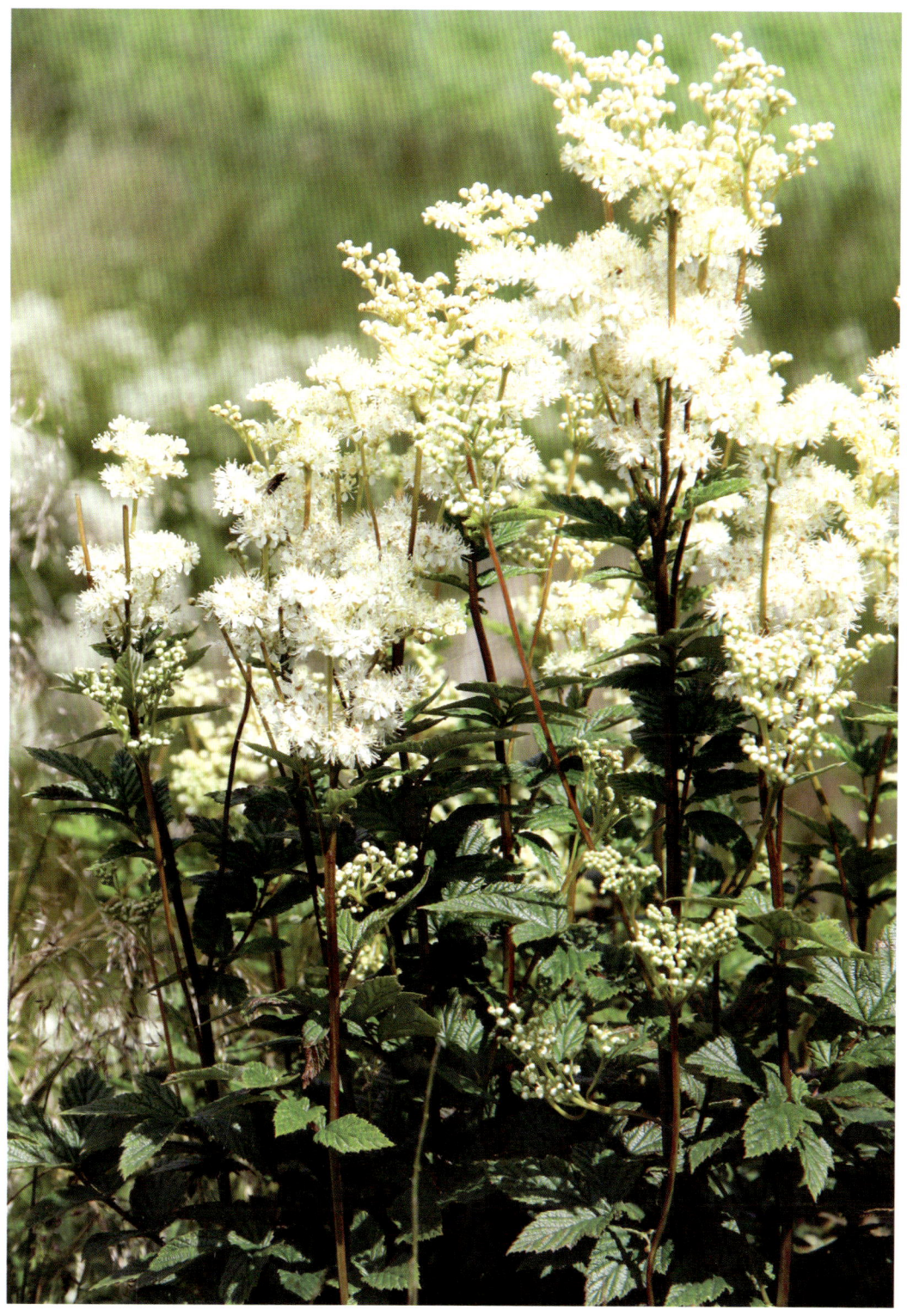

diarrhea, especially in children, as well as for sensitive colons. It is also traditionally used for colds, influenza, fevers, and various childhood diseases such as measles and chickenpox. In addition, Meadowsweet is used to treat arthritis and inflammation as well as being a diuretic and so is reputed to be good for cystitis. Externally it is considered beneficial for healing wounds, for arthritis and inflammation, and as a douche for vaginal discharges. In France, Meadowsweet is traditionally used as a painkiller for headache and toothache.

Research

Clinical research on 32 patients for the efficacy of Meadowsweet on cervical cancer showed positive results.[1] *In vitro* and *in vivo* tests revealed that the tincture of Meadowsweet had an inhibiting effect on the growth of cancer cells.[1,2] In research on 21 medicinal herbs, Meadowsweet was found to be one of the most effective against the *Helicobacter pylori* bacteria, which is thought to be a cause of stomach ulcers and stomach cancer.[3] Research on Meadowsweet showed that it has anti-inflammatory and cooling properties equal to conventional anti-inflammatory drugs,[4] while other research has also shown its anti-inflammatory action.[5] Meadowsweet has shown an inhibiting effect on bacteria,[6] antioxidant properties,[7,8] and a stimulating effect on the immune system.[5] Research on the leaves and seeds of Meadowsweet has revealed its blood-thinning properties.[9] It has also been shown that a decoction of Meadowsweet heals stomach ulcers.[10]

Dosage

Tincture: 2–4 ml three times a day (1:5, 25%).

Infusion: 1–2 teaspoons in a cup three times a day.

Infusions, tinctures, compresses, and ointments for external use.

Warning

Meadowsweet contains salicylic acid. Those allergic to aspirin or salicylic acid should not use Meadowsweet.

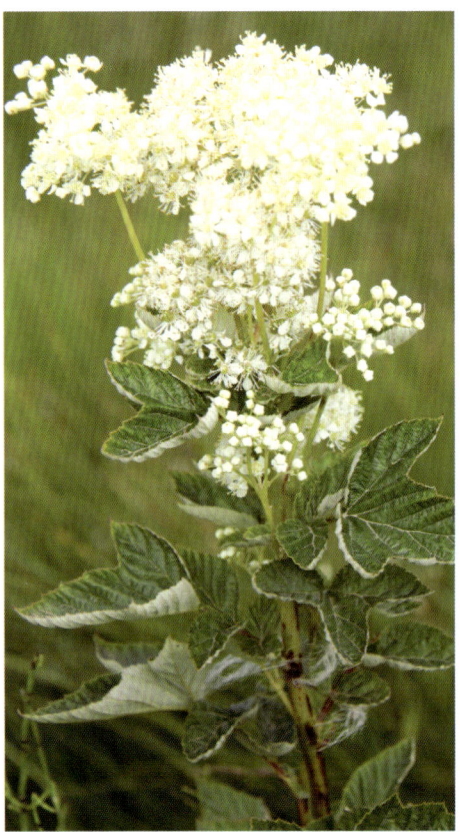

Tea for Gastritis

2 parts Meadowsweet

1 part Iceland Moss

1 part Lady's Mantle

Put 3–4 tablespoons of the blend into a 750 ml vacuum flask and pour boiling water into it. Sieve the tea into cups and then put the herbs back into the flask and allow to stand the whole day. Drink from the flask throughout the day.

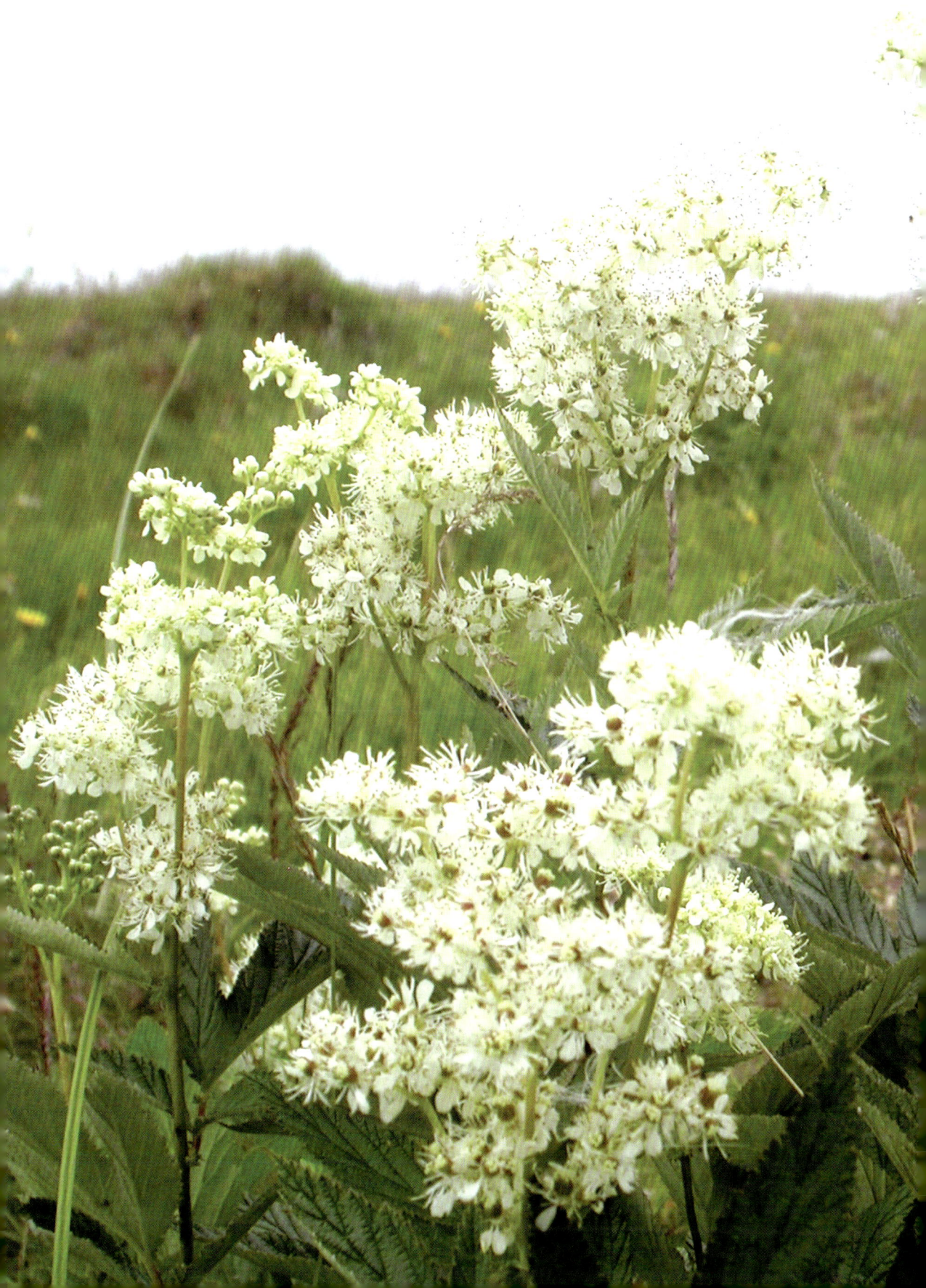

Mountain Avens

Dryas octopetala
Rosaceae—Holtasóley

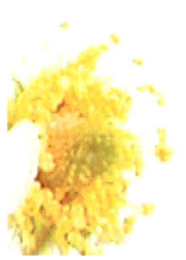 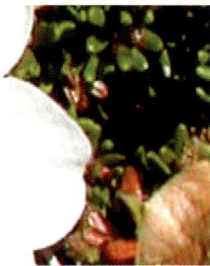

Habitat

Mountain Avens is common all over Iceland and grows in stony ground and on moors.

Parts Used

The entire plant is used, except for the root.

Harvesting

Mountain Avens is collected before bloom from May to June.

Constituents

Tannins, silicic acid, and minerals.

History

Mountain Avens was called Thief's Root because it was believed to grow best where thieves had been hanged. Thief's Root was also said to have the ability to attract money from the earth, but for this to happen one had to first steal money from a poor widow during Mass and place the money under Thief's Root. According to folklore, Thief's Root should have attracted as much money as was put under it so it was beneficial to steal money of significant value.

The leaves of Mountain Avens are also called "ptarmigan leaf" as they are an important food for ptarmigans. The leaves were also dried and crushed to spare tobacco, and tea was made from the leaves and drunk instead of black tea.

Action

Astringent and mild anti-inflammatory.

Uses

Mountain Avens is not much used in Western herbal medicine nowadays. It was formerly considered beneficial for stomach cramps and diarrhea as well as a mouthwash for gingivitis, mouth ulcers, and sore throats.

Dosage

Tincture: 1–5 ml three times a day (1:5, 25%).

Infusion: 1–2 teaspoons in a cup three times a day.

Infusions and tinctures as mouthwash.

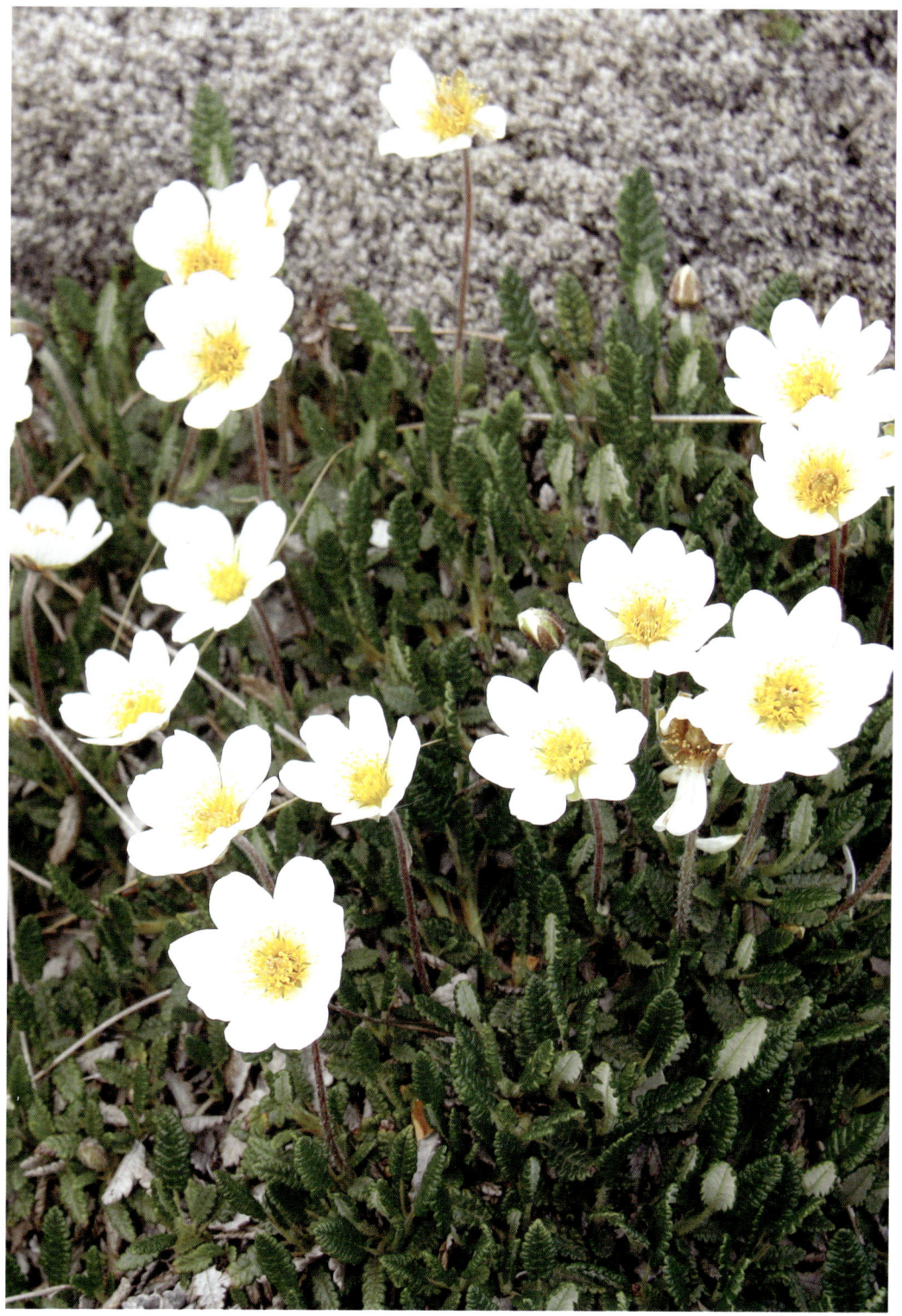

Nootka Lupine

Lupinus nootkatensis
Leguminosae—Alaskalúpína

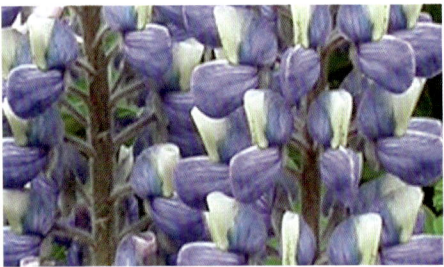

Habitat

An imported species introduced in the past decades, which has since spread all over Iceland.

Parts Used

Root.

Constituents

Alkaloids (lupinine, lupanine and sparteine).

History

Nootka Lupine originates from North America, where many different lupine species grow. *Lupinus alba* was used medicinally in Europe and the seeds were thought to lower blood sugar, heal wounds, eliminate worms, stimulate menstrual bleeding, and act as a diuretic. Lupine seeds contain alkaloids that can cause toxic reactions, though the amount of alkaloids differs between species. Warnings have been recorded that large amounts of *L. alba* root can cause serious inflammation of the digestive system. If seeds of any Lupine species are used, they should be soaked in water overnight and then rinsed thoroughly before boiling, similar to the cooking of beans.

References from North America report that the tea from the leaves of *L. caudatus* is used to clean sores on the faces of infants and then a compress from the powdered leaf is put on the area. Very little information is available from Native Americans about the use of Nootka Lupine although it is known that the root was both used as food and was toxic; there are no references to its medicinal use. They used many other species of the Lupine for food despite its reputation for being toxic. It was also used in net-making and in rituals. Most sources report its external use, (e.g., to heal wounds, earache, or nosebleeds, or for eye rinses).

In Iceland there was no evidence of the use of the Nootka Lupine for medicinal purposes until the 1990s, when Ævar Jóhannesson began producing a Lupine decoction and giving it to patients for health purposes. This decoction also contains Angelica (*Angelica archangelica* and *A. sylvestris*), Northern Dock (*Rumex longifolis*), and a lichen (*Parmelia omphalodes*).

Uses

Nootka Lupine is not known as a medicinal in modern Western herbalism, apart from the above-mentioned decoction of Ævar Jóhannesson.

Research

Three research studies have been done on Ævar's decoction. The first was in North America in 1994 where the effects of the decoction on cancer cells were studied, but showed no active results. In Iceland, clinical trials were done with a few individuals in 1995, studying its effects on high cholesterol. The research showed no active effects on cholesterol, but red blood cell count increased in those who were taking the decoction. In the same trial, evidence showed a stimulating effect on the immune system. A third research project shows that the decoction contains active immunostimulants, most likely polysaccharides in the root of Nootka Lupine and the lichen.[1]

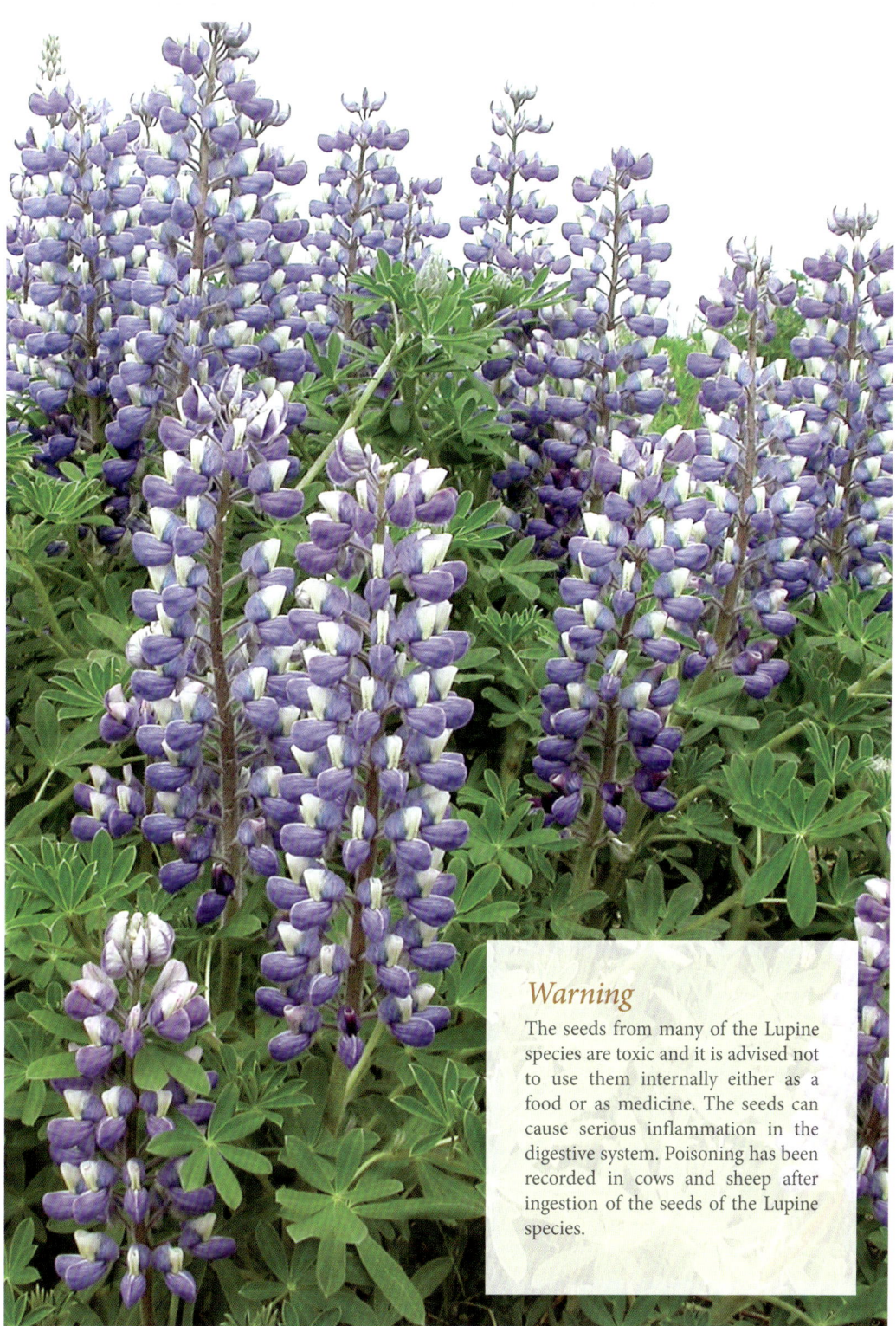

Warning

The seeds from many of the Lupine species are toxic and it is advised not to use them internally either as a food or as medicine. The seeds can cause serious inflammation in the digestive system. Poisoning has been recorded in cows and sheep after ingestion of the seeds of the Lupine species.

Northern Dock

Rumex longifolius
Polygonaceae—Njóli

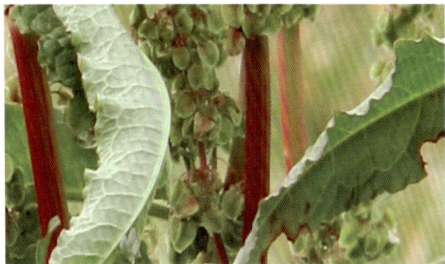

Habitat

Northern Dock grows all over Iceland and is commonly found close to towns and on uncultivated land.

Parts Used

Roots and seeds.

Harvesting

The seeds are collected in August and the roots are harvested in autumn.

Constituents

Anthraquinones, tannins, essential oils, and oxalic acid.

History

Many species from the genus *Rumex* are used for medicinal purposes. The best known in Western herbal medicine is Yellow Dock (*R. crispus*), but the Icelandic species *R. longifolius* is said to have very similar properties. In Europe it is well known that the rash and sting caused by touching Stinging Nettle can be relieved by placing the bruised leaves of Yellow Dock on the affected area. The leaves of Northern Dock were freq-

uently used as food in the past, and in Iceland its use in white sauce and soups is well known. Northern Dock has also been used to dye yarn.

Action

Root: Laxative, hepatic, cholagogue, vulnerary, and reduces itching.

Uses

Northern Dock is said to be good for constipation and jaundice and is also thought to be excellent for skin diseases, taken both externally and internally. The root is used internally for eczema, psoriasis, acne, boils, inflamed glands, and fungal infections. The root is also considered to be good for arthritis, especially osteoarthritis. Externally, Northern Dock root is thought to be

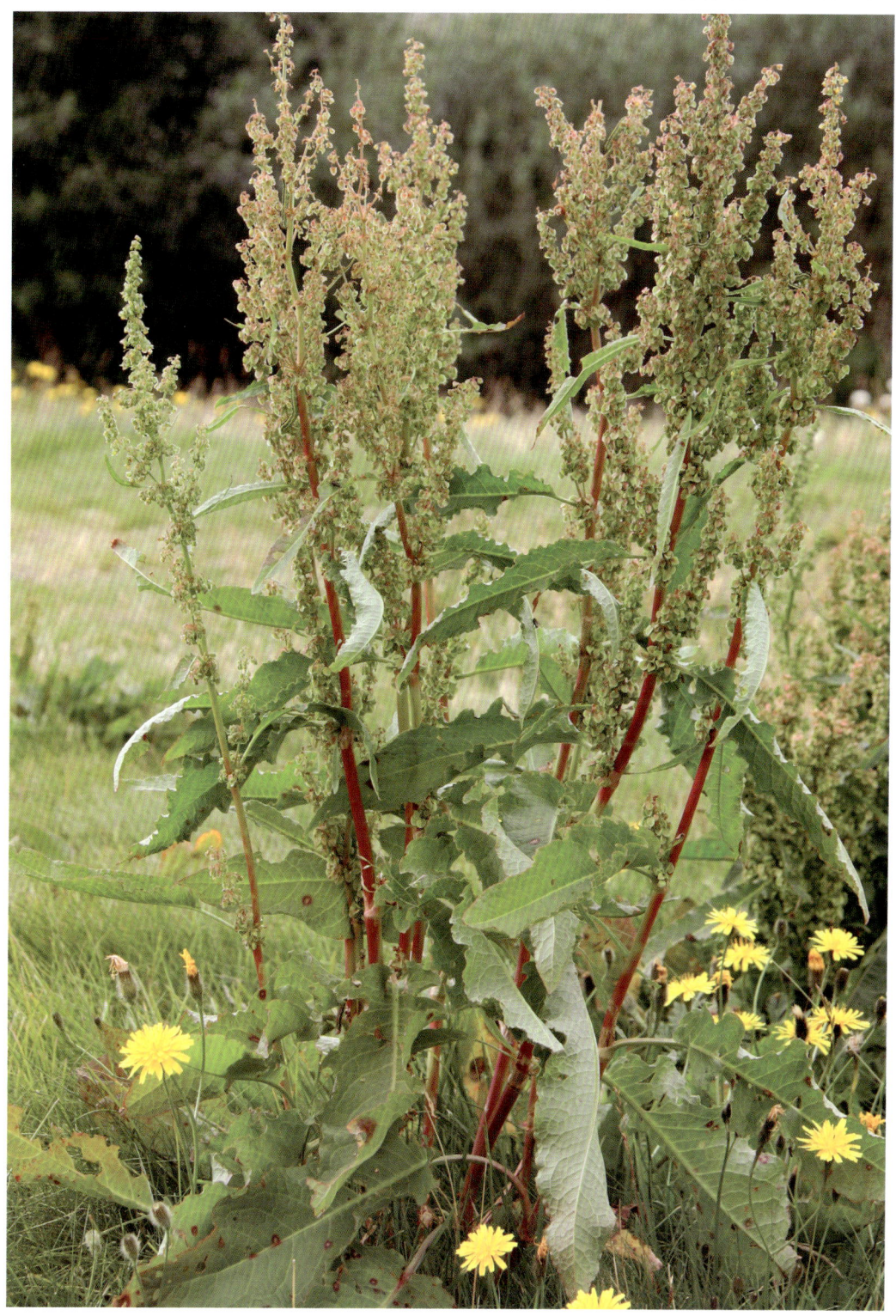

beneficial for itching, fungal infections, and gingivitis, and for healing wounds. The root is almost the only part of the plant used for medicinal purposes nowadays, but it is also known that the seeds are astringent and are considered good for diarrhea and for reducing bleeding. The leaves have been used externally for rashes.

Research

The following research has all been done on Yellow Dock, which does not grow in Iceland. However, this species is closely related to Northern Dock and references state that they have similar action. *In vitro* tests on Yellow Dock have shown it to be antioxidant[1-3] and anti-bacterial,[3] as well as having antifungal action on mold in barley.[4] There are known cases of death caused by eating Yellow Dock leaves and acute poisoning in sheep has been caused by oxalic acid in the leaves of Yellow Dock.[5]

Dosage

Tincture: 1–2 ml three times a day (1:5, 25%).

Decoction: 1 teaspoon in a cup three times a day.

Decoctions, tinctures, compresses, and ointments for external use.

Warning

Large doses of the leaves of Yellow Dock (*R. crispus*) have caused death in both humans and animals as the leaves have a high content of oxalic acid. Consumption of the leaves is therefore not recommended except in small amounts, and then boiled rather than fresh. It is recommended to use only the small fresh leaves in the spring as the oxalic acid content increases with the growth of the leaves. Those with kidney stones, arthritis, or high levels of gastric acid should not use Dock leaves. The root contains much less oxalic acid than the leaves but it should not be consumed in large doses as it can cause digestive disturbances, nausea, and diarrhea. Fresh Dock root can cause vomiting.

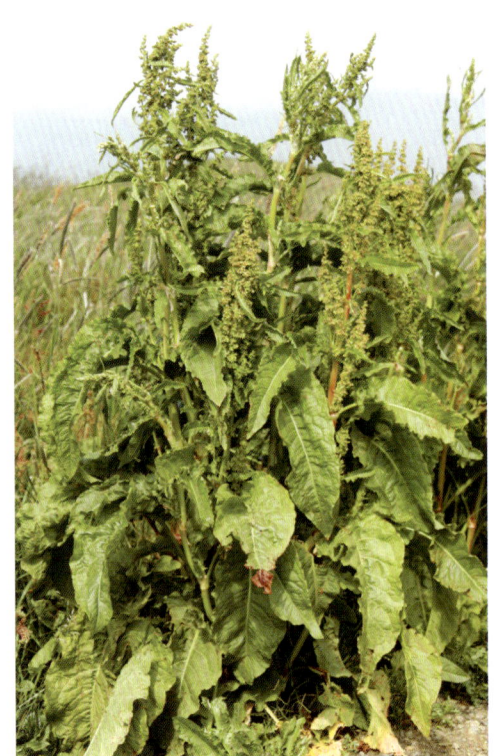

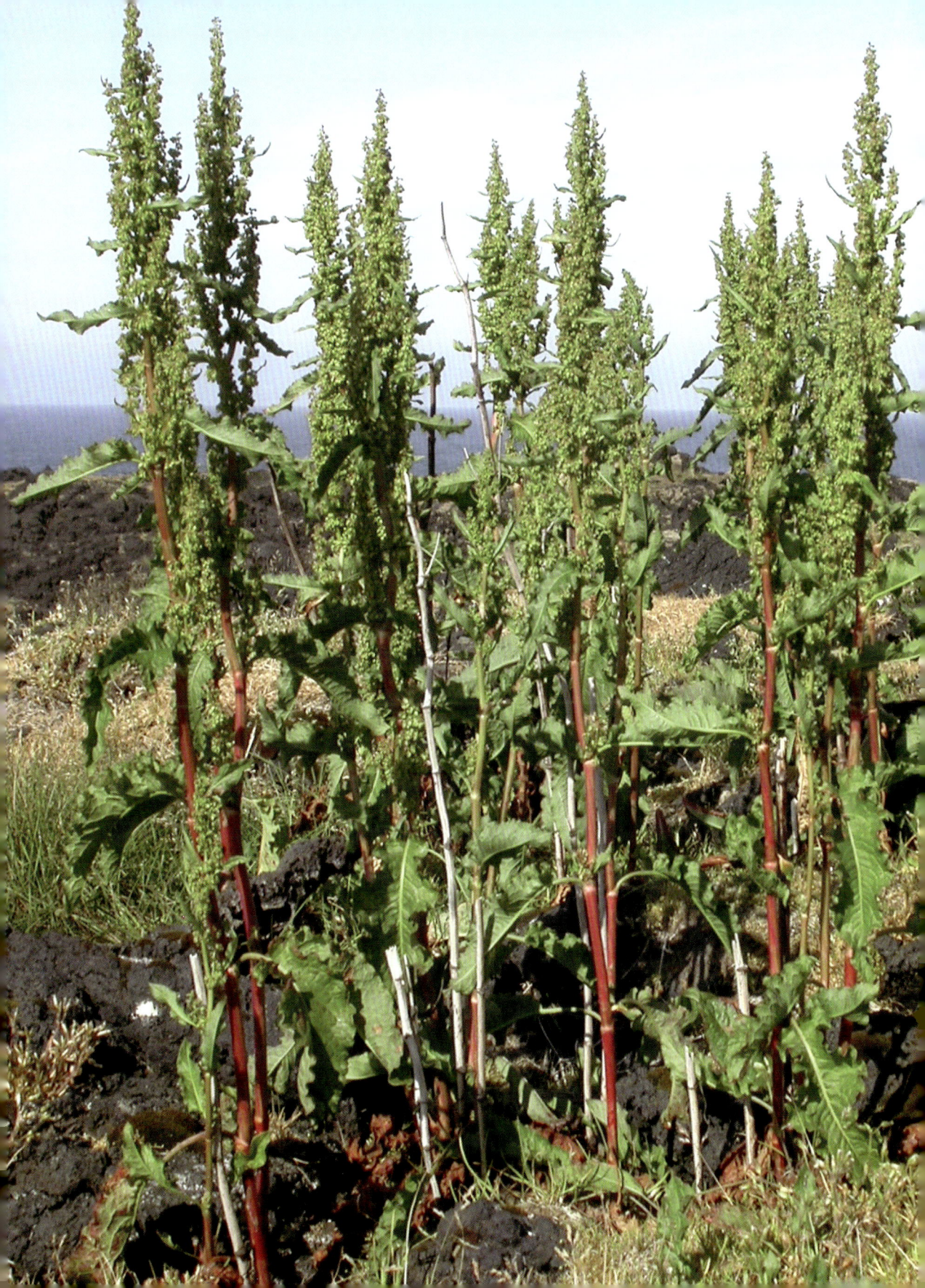

Pineappleweed

Lepidotheca suaveolens
Asteraceae—Hlaðkolla

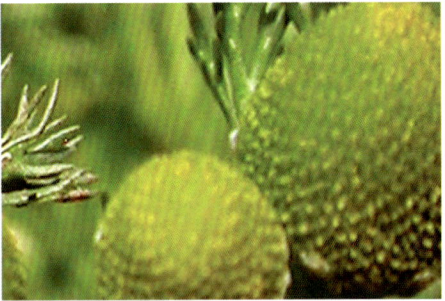

Habitat

Pineappleweed grows all over Iceland, especially in towns and industrial areas.

Parts Used

The entire plant is used, except for the root.

Harvesting

Pineappleweed is picked in bloom from July to September.

Constituents

Essential oils and terpenes.

History

Pineappleweed has sometimes been confused with Chamomile (*Chamomilla recutita*), which is a well-known medicinal herb that does not grow wild in Iceland. They are very closely related and dried Pineappleweed is similar to dried Chamomile in appearance. The old genus name for both Pineappleweed and Chamomile is *Matricaria*, meaning beloved mother. Chamomile is a well-known medicinal herb for various gynecological diseases and Pineappleweed has been used in a similar way.

The Native Americans used Pineappleweed for stomach pain, especially if there was excessive flatulence, diarrhea, sores, fever, and colds. They also used Pineappleweed for its pleasant smell, for cooking, and in rituals. The plant was considered good for regulating menstruation, for relieving menstrual pain, and for stimulating lactation. Pineappleweed is also used as an insect repellent.

Action

Sedative, carminative, antispasmodic, anthelmintic, vulnerary, and mild anti-inflammatory.

Uses

Pineappleweed is hardly used at all in Western herbal medicine these days. It is considered to be a sedative and is used for stomach pain and flatulence, colitis, and menstrual pain. It has also been used for colds and to eliminate worms. Topically it is good for reducing inflammation, healing wounds, and stopping itching.

Dosage

Tincture: 2–6 ml three times a day (1:5, 40%).

Infusion: 1–2 teaspoons in a cup three times a day.

Infusions, tinctures, compresses and ointments for external use.

Warning

Pineappleweed can cause allergies in those who are sensitive to plants belonging to the Asteraceae family. Large doses of the herb can cause nausea and vomiting.

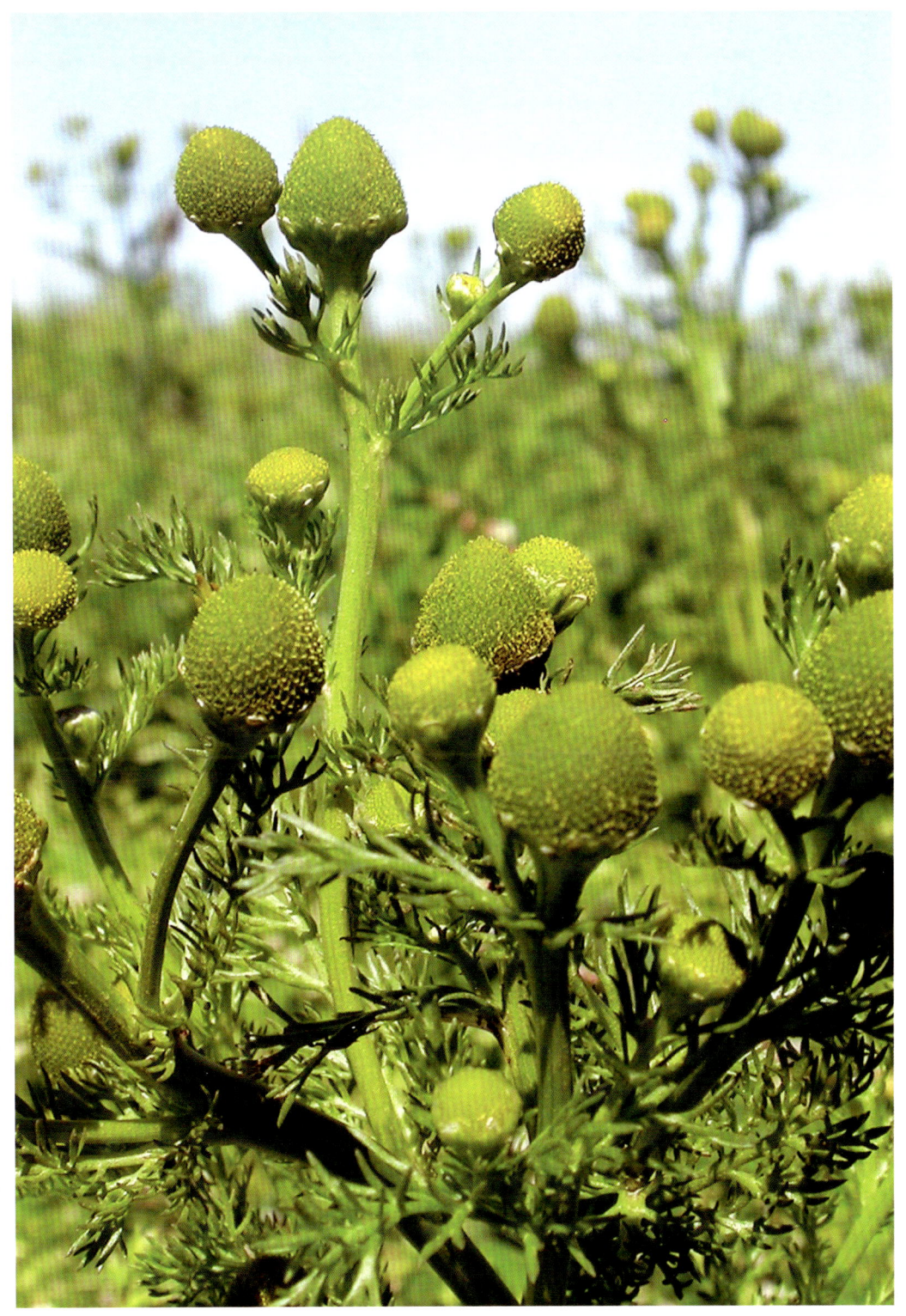

Polypody

Polypodium vulgare
Polypodiaceae—Köldugras

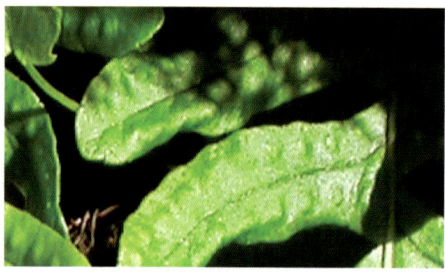

Habitat

Polypody is an evergreen fern that grows all over Iceland but is quite sparse in the North and Northeast. It grows mainly on sunny ridges.

Parts Used

The root is used.

Harvesting

The root is harvested in the autumn.

Constituents

Saponins, ecdysteroids, phloroglucin, essential oils, tannins, and oils.

History

The Icelandic name "Köldugras" (Arthritic Grass) indicates its efficacy for arthritic pain or for what Icelanders in the old days called cold diseases. In old references, Polypody is said to be good for gynecological problems as well as being diaphoretic and diuretic and good in cough syrup. Polypody root contains a sweetener that has been used in liqueurs and as a substitute for licorice root. Native Americans used the root for stomach pains and constipation. They chewed the root for sore throats and drank the decoction for colds, coughs, and lung diseases. They also used Polypody as a medicine for heart conditions and both internally and externally for rashes and skin inflammation. The root was also used fresh, baked or boiled in food, and as a sugar substitute.

Action

Cholagogue, laxative, and expectorant.

Uses

Polypody is rarely used today in Western herbal medicine but has traditionally been used for hepatitis and jaundice. The root was also thought to be good for stimulating appetite and bowel movements and it was safe to use as a laxative for children. Polypody root is considered to be good for mucus in the lungs, bronchitis, dry cough, pleurisy, and pneumonia, as well as for psoriasis and for eliminating worms. In China, the root is also thought to be good for urinary stones. Many closely related species of Polypody are used for medicinal purposes; one of the best known is *P. calaguala,* which is thought to be a good anti-inflammatory and analgesic, and effective for psoriasis and cancer.

Dosage

Tincture: 1–2 ml three times a day (1:5, 25%).

Decoction: ½-1 teaspoon in a cup three times a day.

Syrup: 1 teaspoon three times a day.

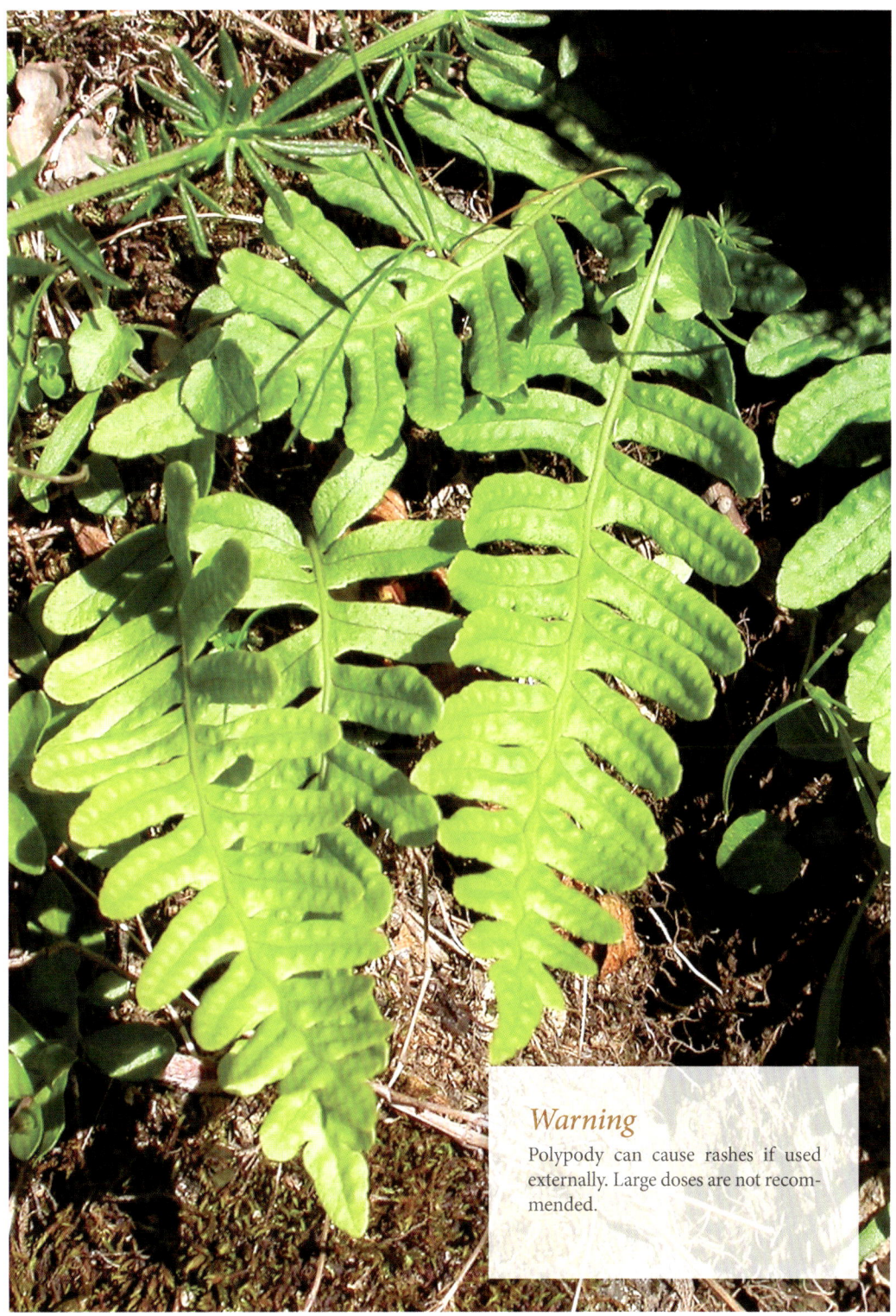

Warning

Polypody can cause rashes if used externally. Large doses are not recommended.

Purging Flax

Linum catharticum
Linaceae—Villilín

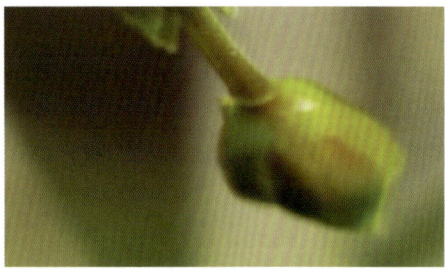

Action

Laxative and mild diuretic.

Uses

Purging Flax is no longer used in Western herbal medicine. In the past, it was thought to be good for constipation, edema, arthritis, and liver disease. When used for constipation, it is commonly blended with carminative herbs such as Caraway seeds.

Dosage

Tincture: 2–4 ml three times a day (1:5, 40%).

Infusion: 1–2 teaspoons in a cup three times a day.

Decoction: 1–2 teaspoons in a cup three times a day.

Habitat

Purging Flax grows on grassy slopes and ravines. It is not common, but is found in the North and parts of South Iceland.

Parts Used

The entire plant is used, including the root.

Harvesting

Purging Flax is collected in bloom in July and the root is harvested in autumn.

Constituents

Essential oils, polyphenols, and tannins.

History

Purging Flax was a popular medicinal herb in the past. It was thought to be a laxative, as indicated by the Latin name *catharticum*, which means cleansing. This can also be deduced from the Old Icelandic names, "laxerlín" (laxative flax) and "laxerurt" (laxative herb). Purging Flax is very closely related to flax and flaxseed is often used for constipation.

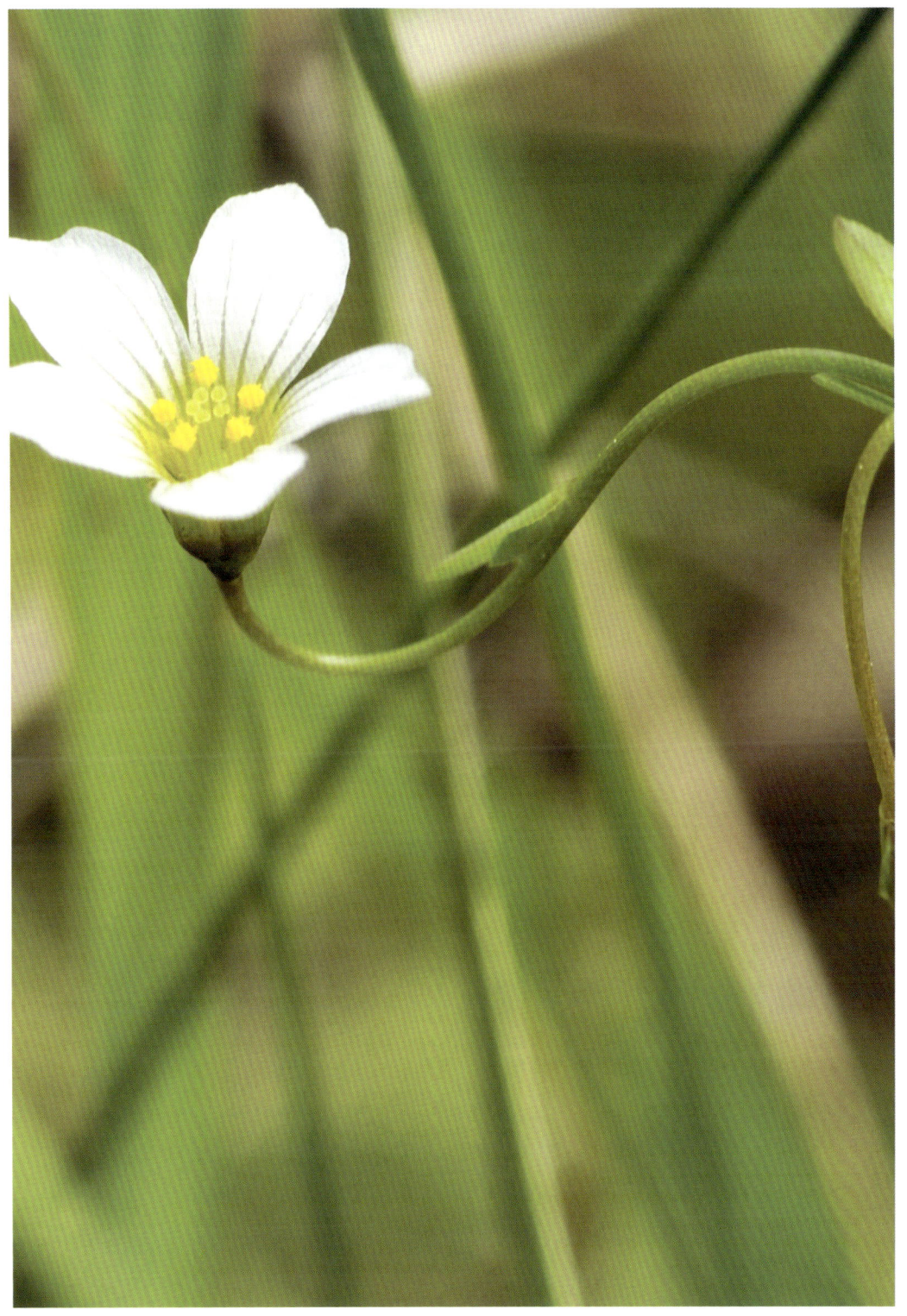

Purple Marshlocks

Comarum palustre
Rosaceae—Engjarós

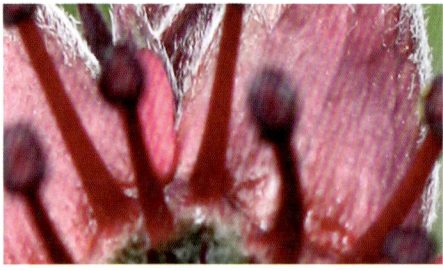

Habitat

Purple Marshlocks is found in marshy areas all over Iceland.

Parts Used

The entire plant, including the root.

Harvesting

The herb is collected before blossoming in June and the roots are harvested in autumn.

Constituents

Tannins, phenols, essential oils, resins, and saponins.

History

The old Latin name for Purple Marshlocks is *Potentilla palustris* and it is closely related to Silverweed, Tormentil, and other medicinal herbs from the Potentilla family. The Native Americans used both the leaves and roots for treatment of dysentery and stomach cramps. The leaves were also used as black tea before imported teas became popular. The flowers of the Purple Marshlocks have also been used to dye yarn.

Action

Astringent, anti-inflammatory, analgesic, and vulnerary.

Uses

Purple Marshlocks is not used much in Western herbalism except in Russia, where it is considered to be anti-inflammatory and analgesic and traditionally used for stomach pain, bronchitis, and tuberculosis. It is used especially for inflamed joints (e.g., rheumatism and osteoarthritis). Purple Marshlocks is also thought to be good for treating sores, both internally and externally.

Research

Russian research shows that Purple Marshlocks has anti-inflammatory properties[1-3] and positive effects on colitis,[4] nephritis,[5] and arthritis.[6]

Dosage

Tincture: 2–4 ml three times a day (1:5, 40%).

Infusion: 1–2 teaspoons in a cup three times a day.

Decoction: 1–2 teaspoons in a cup three times a day.

Infusions, decoctions, tinctures, compresses, and ointments for external use.

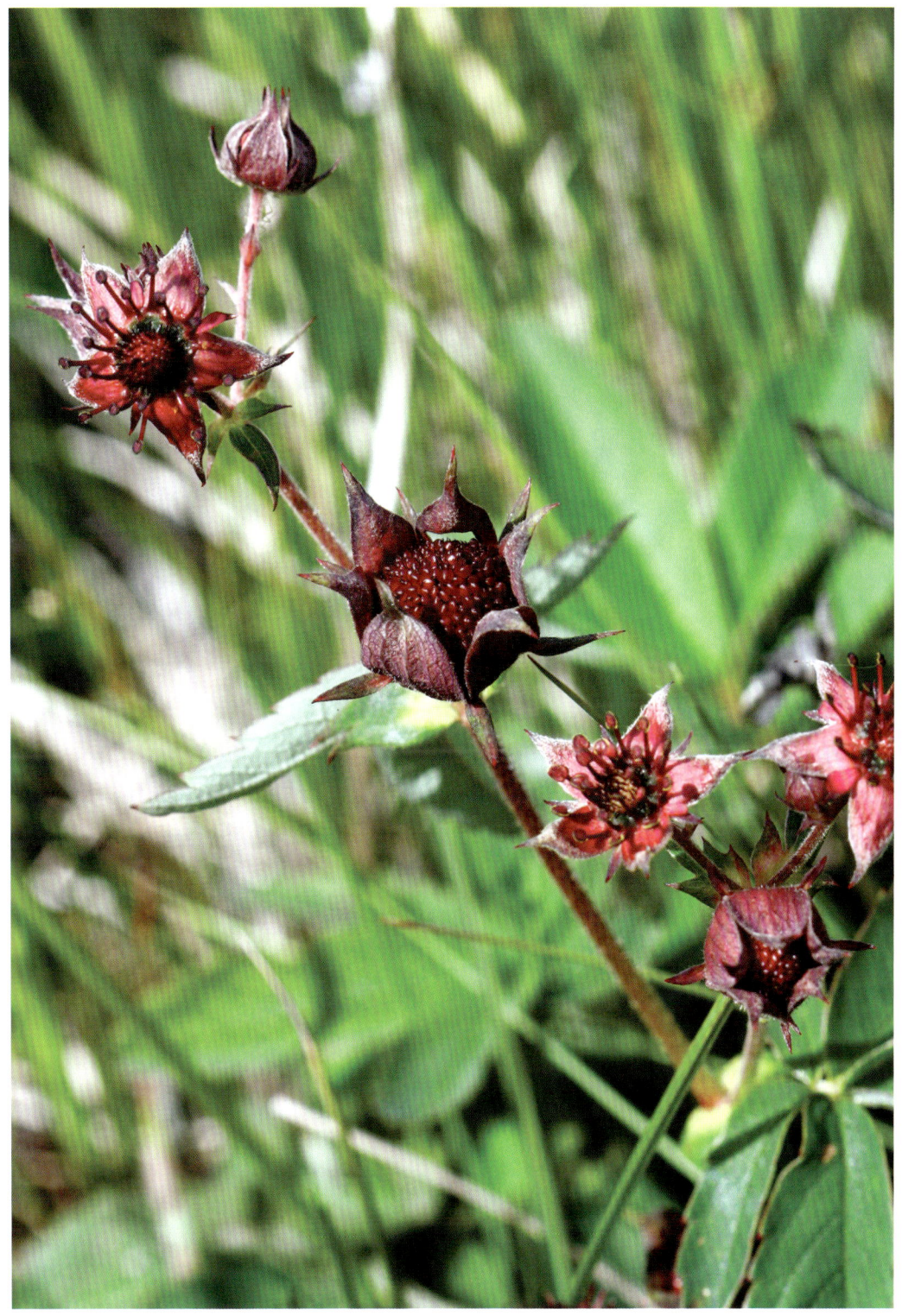

Red Clover

Trifolium pratense
Fabaceae—Rauðsmári

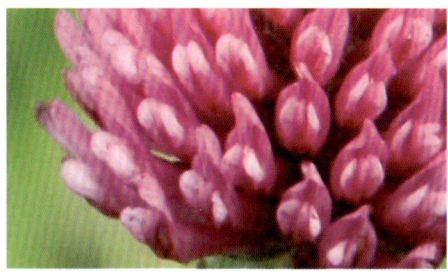

This herb is soothing, stimulating and analgesic. It is therefore good for inflammation, abscess, chest pain and jaundice. The infusion of the leaves is taken in cups 4 times daily. A soothing porridge is made from the buds and flowers of this herb, which is good for easing inflammation and for drawing out disease. The root, chopped and boiled in milk, is good healthy food.

Oddur Jónsson Hjaltalín,
Icelandic Botany, 1830

Habitat

Red Clover grows in the lowlands and is found scattered throughout Iceland.

Parts Used

The entire plant is used, except for the root.

Harvesting

Red Clover is collected in bloom in July–August.

Constituents

Flavonoids (isoflavonoids), essential oils, minerals, and vitamins.

History

Around 1930, Red Clover was a very popular medicinal herb for cancer, both for internal and external use. It was said to heal cancer of the breasts, ovaries, and lymph. Although Red Clover was used externally for cancers, bear in mind that cancer in those days did not necessarily have the same meaning as today and it could have meant bad wounds, not necessarily malignant. Older references state that the flowers of Red Clover were boiled into a thick porridge and then laid externally on cancerous breasts with the purpose of drawing the cancer out. Native Americans drank an infusion of Red Clover for fevers and kidney diseases, and as a blood cleanser. A cold infusion of the flowers was taken for menopause and was also used internally and externally for cancer. The leaves of Red Clover were also used as a vegetable.

Action

Expectorant, skin cleanser, mild antispasmodic, and vulnerary.

Uses

There is a long tradition of using Red Clover internally for skin diseases like eczema and psoriasis, and likewise it has seen long use externally for skin diseases and skin cancers. Red Clover has also traditionally been used for coughs, bronchitis, and asthma as well as a mouthwash for throat infections and mouth ulcers. Red Clover is said to have a cleansing effect on lymph nodes and the lymphatic system. Nowadays, Red Clover is also used for night sweats in menopause because of its effect on estrogen levels in the body. This particular use was first established in 1990, as a result of research, but there are differences of opinion about this effect among herbalists. Research has shown that Red Clover is thought to lower cholesterol and reduce the formation of wrinkles after menopause, and it is also said to be effective

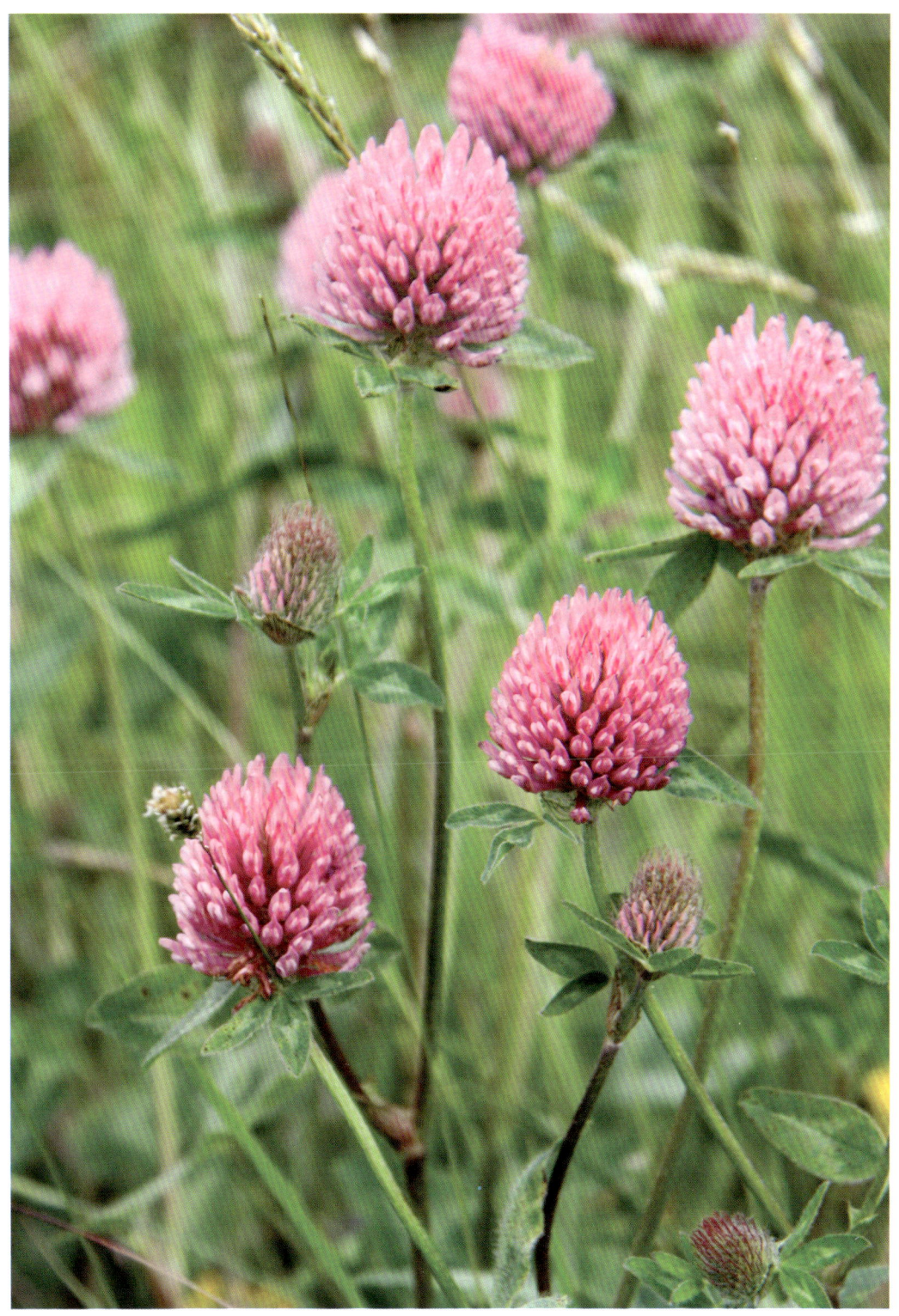

against osteoporosis. In addition, research indicates that Red Clover inhibits the growth of cancer cells. In China, Red Clover has been used for cancer, athlete's foot, burns, constipation, corns, gallbladder and liver problems, gout, rheumatism and osteoarthritis, skin problems and sensitive eyes.

Research

In many cases, the following research is directed at the isoflavonoids in Red Clover and not the plant as a whole.

Some clinical research has been done on the efficacy of Red Clover for night sweats and hot flashes in menopause, and some small clinical trials with less than 50 women have shown positive effects of Red Clover on hot flashes.[1,2] In one larger trial with 246 women wherein two types of supplements of Red Clover plus a placebo were tested, it was thought that Red Clover showed some effect on hot flashes but not enough to be able to assert that the results were significant.[3] Two other smaller clinical trials also did not show that Red Clover reduced meno-

pausal hot flashes and night sweats, or that it had a positive effect on memory.[4,5] A clinical trial on 107 post-menopausal women who had taken Red Clover for 3 months showed a positive effect on anxiety and depression.[6] Several in vitro and in vivo tests have shown that Red Clover increases estrogen levels, especially during menopause, which could have a positive effect on hot flashes and other symptoms.[1,7–15] Other research shows the opposite.[16] Estrogen levels drop during menopause, which negatively affects the skin and accelerates aging thereof. Research on Red Clover revealed that it reduces the negative effects on the skin caused by decreased estrogen levels.[17]

Two clinical trials on a small group of women have revealed that Red Clover lowers cholesterol,[18,19] but other research shows the opposite.[1,20–21] Further research studies involving in vitro and in vivo tests show a lowering of cholesterol,[8,22,23] but one test showed that cholesterol was not lowered.[24] In addition, other research indicates that Red Clover protects against heart and coronary disease.[25–27] Research

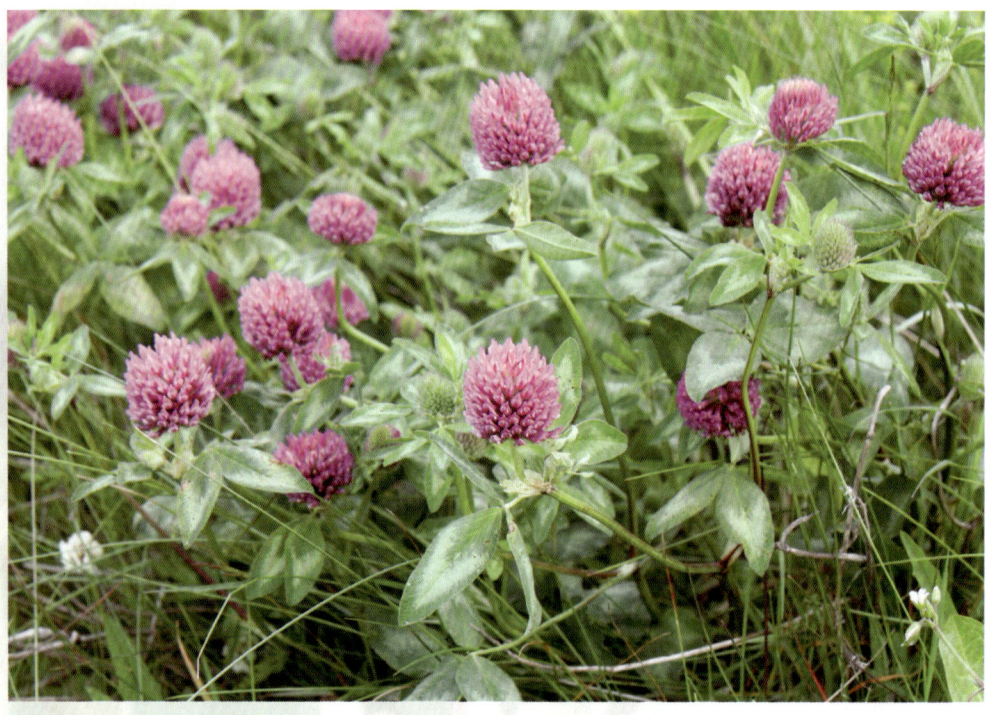

on 16 post-menopausal women with diabetes type 2 showed that Red Clover was hypotensive.[28]

Clinical research on a small group of women showed that bone density increased with the use of Red Clover for 6 months,[1] but other research shows the opposite.[29] In addition, several *in vitro* and *in vivo* tests indicate that Red Clover reduces the danger of osteoporosis in post-menopausal women.[10,30,31]

Several research trials on Red Clover show that it inhibits the growth of various cancer cells (e.g., in the prostate gland).[1,32–39] A small trial on men with prostate cancer who had undergone an operation showed that necrosis was more prevalent in those who received Red Clover than those who did not.[1] The effects of Red Clover were researched for 1 year on 20 men who had elevated PSA levels in the prostate gland but negative cancerous biopsies. No side effects were found, and after 1 year 30% experienced decreased PSA levels but elevated liver enzymes. It was also shown that Red Clover has no effect on sex hormones.[40]

In vitro tests on Red Clover reveal that it has anti-inflammatory[1,22,34,41,42] and antioxidant[8,11,12,43] properties and that it stimulates the immune system[44] and thyroid gland.[1] In Australia, large amounts of Red Clover found in sheep fodder have been linked to various side effects like sterility and abnormal lactation, the cause of which is attributed to the effects on estrogen from the isoflavonoids.[1] However, none of the research on women, who were given up to 160 mg of isoflavonoids a day, supports this speculation.[1] For three years, Red Clover was given to 401 women who were in a high-risk group for breast cancer due to family history. The research showed that Red Clover was a safe supplement and had no damaging effect on breast tissue, the circulatory system, or bone.[45] Further research indicates that Red Clover does not induce breast cancer or cellular proliferation of the endometrium.[46–48] It has also come to light that Red Clover does not contain coumarin and does not have blood-thinning properties as was previously believed.[1]

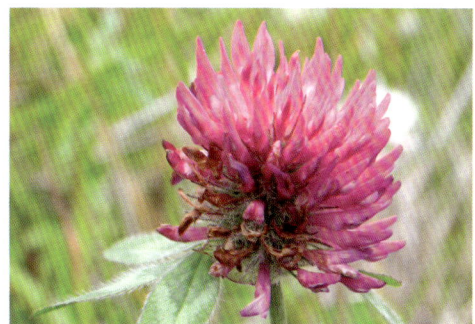

Dosage

Tincture: 2–4 ml three times a day (1:5, 40%).

Infusion: 1–2 teaspoons in a cup three times a day.

Infusions, tinctures, compresses, and ointments for external use.

Warning

Use of Red Clover internally is not recommended during pregnancy or while breastfeeding, or for children under 12 years of age.

Skin Cleansing Tea

1 part Red Clover

1 part Lady's Bedstraw

1 part Downy Birch

Put 3–4 tablespoons of the blend into a 750 ml vacuum flask and pour boiling water into it. Sieve the tea into cups and then return the herbs to the flask and allow to stand the whole day. Drink from the flask throughout the day.

Ribwort Plantain

Plantago lanceolata
Plantaginaceae—Selgresi

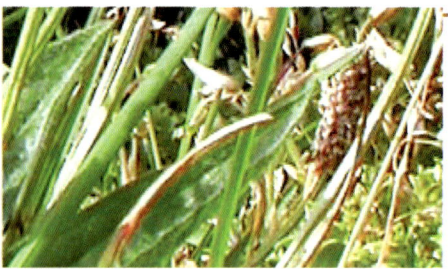

Habitat

Ribwort Plantain grows mainly at the foot of the Eyjafjall mountains and in Mýrdal in Southeast Iceland. In other places it only grows close to geothermal hot spots.

Parts Used

The entire plant is used, including the root.

Harvesting

Leaves and flowers are collected in bloom in July. Seeds are collected in late summer and roots are harvested in autumn.

Constituents

Mucilage, tannins, iridoid glycoside (aucubin), silicic acid, phenolic carboxylic acid, flavonoids, zinc, potassium, and saponins.

History

Ribwort Plantain has long been thought to have the same action as Greater Plantain (*P. major*) but is said to be more effective against lung diseases. There is also a long tradition of using Ribwort Plantain for skin cancer. The seeds of Ribwort Plantain are covered in mucilage, which is easy to remove if the seeds are soaked in hot water. This mucilage was used in the past to stiffen linen in France.

A decoction (of this herb) heals and dries. Taken in, it refreshes, and is good for colds, dysentery and diarrhea. It also kills worms in the digestive system. If this root be bruised together with Yarrow and then laid over a wound, it will heal even more. The root of this herb, boiled in wine, heals all the ailments of the bladder if it is then eaten. [...] Ribwort Plantain, cooked and eaten as cabbage, heals internal wounds, diarrhea and all blood-letting up and down. The liquid works the same way. It is good to soak a cloth in this juice and use for headaches. If it is used on the eyes and ears, it heals both sight and hearing. The same liquid heals mouth ulcers and inflammation in the mouth and throat if the mouth is rinsed often with it. The herb itself eliminates and reduces bacterial skin contagion and other hot inflammations.

Björn Halldórsson, Uses of Herbs, 1783

The Native Americans used Ribwort Plantain both externally and internally for snake bites and other poisonous stings. It was also thought to be good for digestive problems, vaginal discharges, blood in the urine, diarrhea, and dysentery, while a compress of the leaves was reported to work well for headaches, burns, blisters, wounds, and insect bites. The fresh juice of Ribwort Plantain was held to be good for conjunctivitis and an infusion of the leaves was placed in the ears for earache. Ribwort Plantain, together with other herbs, was also given to children to strengthen them while they were learning to walk.

Action

Anti-inflammatory, astringent, antitussive, hemostatic, antibacterial, vulnerary, demulcent, and mildly diuretic.

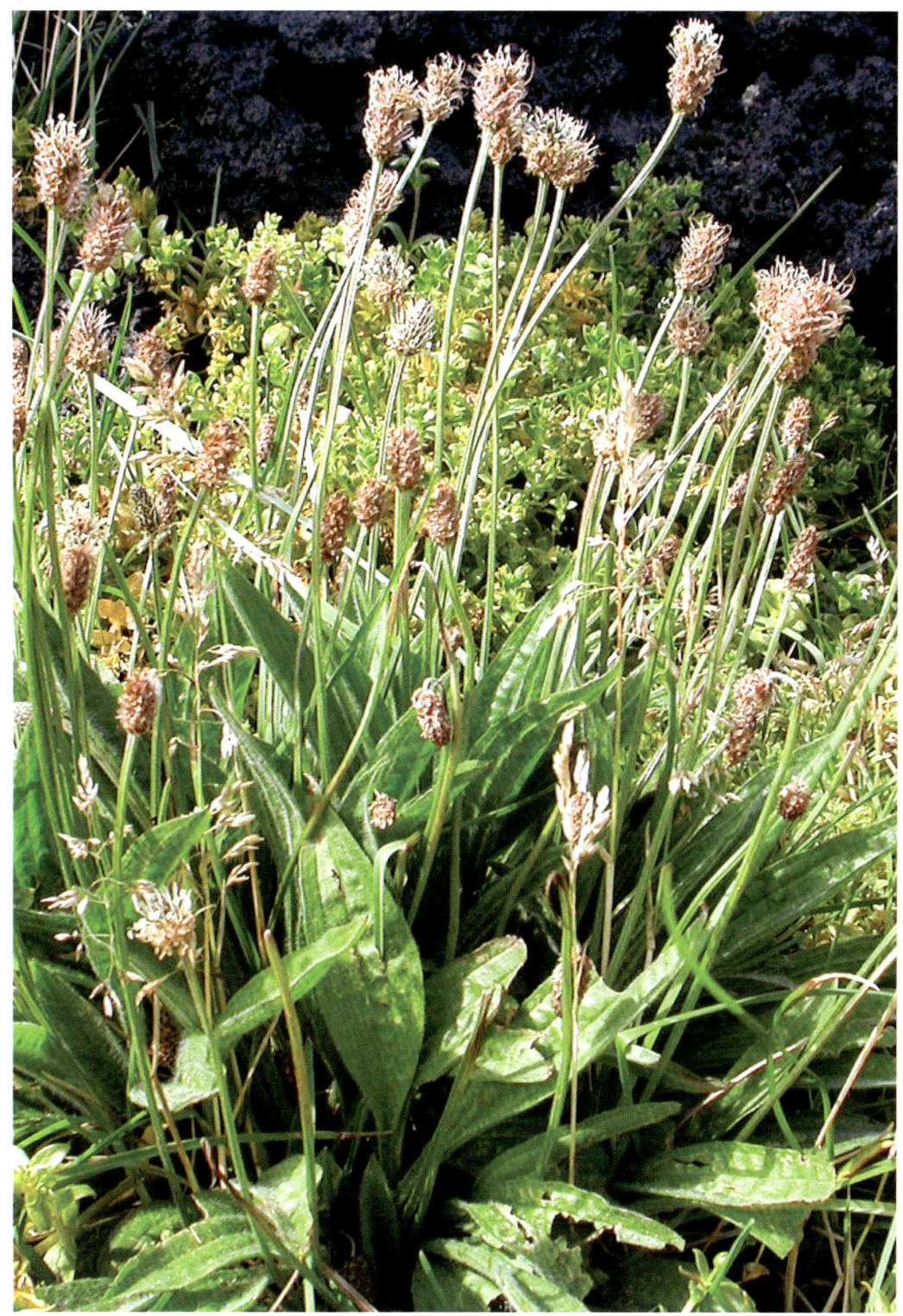

Uses

Ribwort Plantain strengthens the mucous membrane in the throat, ears, and sinuses and is thought to be very good for lung diseases, especially chronic bronchitis, tuberculosis, and persistent dry coughs. Ribwort Plantain is also said to be good for stomach ulcers, colon cramps, and colitis and the fresh juice is thought to be effective for earache. Externally, Ribwort Plantain works well for any wounds, inflammation, and insect bites and there is also a long tradition of using it for skin cancer. Cold infusions from Ribwort Plantain are made more often than hot ones as the antibacterial properties are believed to be destroyed by heat.

Research

Ribwort Plantain is anti-inflammatory according to *in vitro* and *in vivo* tests[1-7] and has a good effect on colitis.[8] It also has antioxidant properties[3,8–11] and an inhibiting effect on fungal infections[12] and worms.[13] Ribwort Plantain stimulates the immune system and is antitussive and antispasmodic, so it is recommended for persistent coughs, especially in children.[5,14] *In vitro* tests have also shown the strengthening effect of Ribwort Plantain on the digestive system[15] and the uterus.[16]

Dosage

Tincture: 2–5 ml three times a day (1:5, 25%).

Cold infusion: 1–2 teaspoons in a cup of cold water, allowed to steep overnight. 1 cup three times a day.

Decoction: 1–2 teaspoons in a cup three times a day.

Syrup: 1–2 teaspoons three times a day.

Infusions, tinctures, compresses, and ointments for external use.

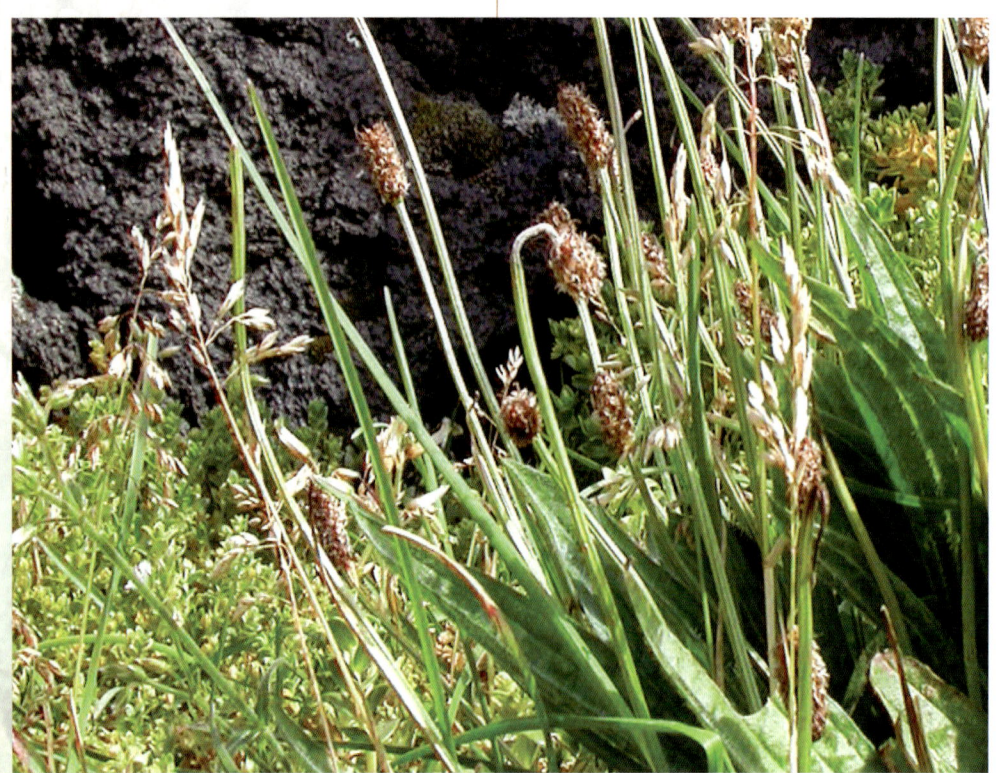

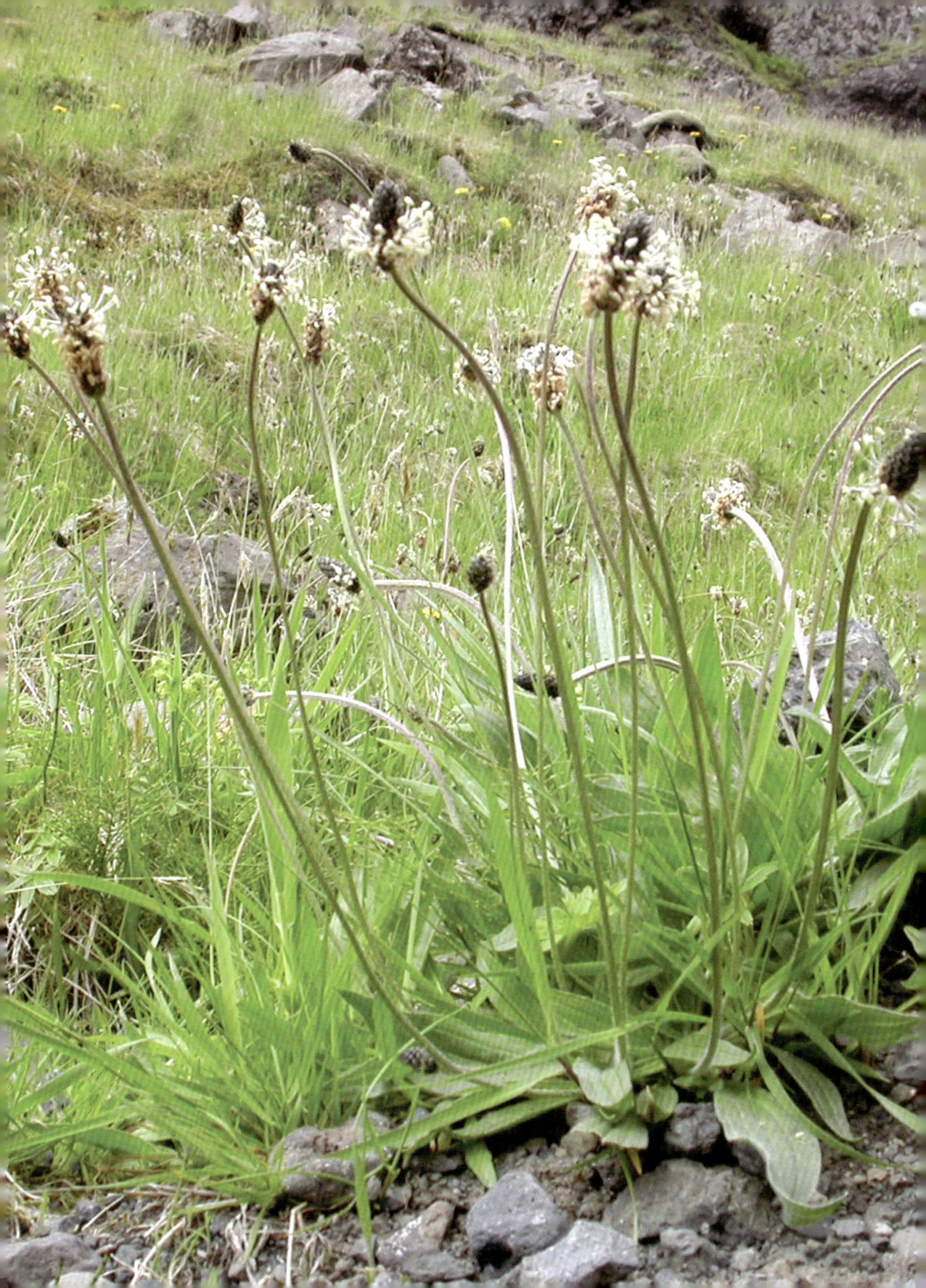

Rose Bay Willow Herb

Chamerion angustifolium
Onagraceae—Sigurskúfur

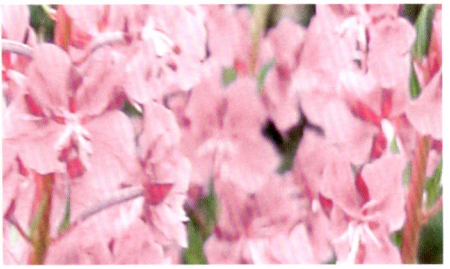

Habitat

Rose Bay Willow Herb grows all over Iceland but is not very common. It is mainly found on cliffs, sunny hillsides, and wasteland.

Parts Used

The entire plant is used, including the root.

Harvesting

The plant is collected at the start of bloom in July. The roots are harvested in spring.

Constituents

Tannins, flavonoids, mucilage, pectin, vitamins A and C.

History

The leaves of Rose Bay Willow Herb were readily used in the past instead of traditional black tea and they were fermented for this reason. In Siberia it has been used in a blend with Fly Agaric toadstools to brew an alcoholic drink. Native Americans traditionally used it for both healing and cooking. For instance, they have used the roots or leaves of the herb for diverse problems such as coughs, abscesses, wounds, bruises, pains, tuberculosis, cystitis, throat infections, gastritis, and colitis, as well as for drawing out splinters. The roots, leaves, and stalks have been used for food, either raw, fried, or boiled, both in Iceland and in many other countries.

Action

Astringent, demulcent, vulnerary, anti-inflammatory, antibacterial, and antifungal.

Uses

Rose Bay Willow Herb is first and foremost anti-inflammatory and is thought to work well for inflammation in the digestive system, such as ulcerative colitis and colitis. It is an astringent and is therefore good for diarrhea. It is also used for throat infections, mouth ulcers, hemorrhoids, and cystitis, and is reputedly a remedy for fungal infections, both in the vagina and in the digestive system. Used externally, Rose Bay Willow Herb heals skin problems and wounds. In Germany and Austria it has been popular for inflammation of the prostate gland.

Research

In vitro research on Rose Bay Willow Herb has shown it to be antibacterial,[1,2] antifungal,[1,3] and to have a strengthening effect on the immune system.[4] It also shows antioxidant properties[5,6] and a possible inhibiting effect on the growth of cancer cells in the prostate gland.[7-10] *In vitro* tests show that it is anti-inflammatory,[11,12] analgesic,[13] and has a beneficial effect on benign enlargement of the prostate gland.[14]

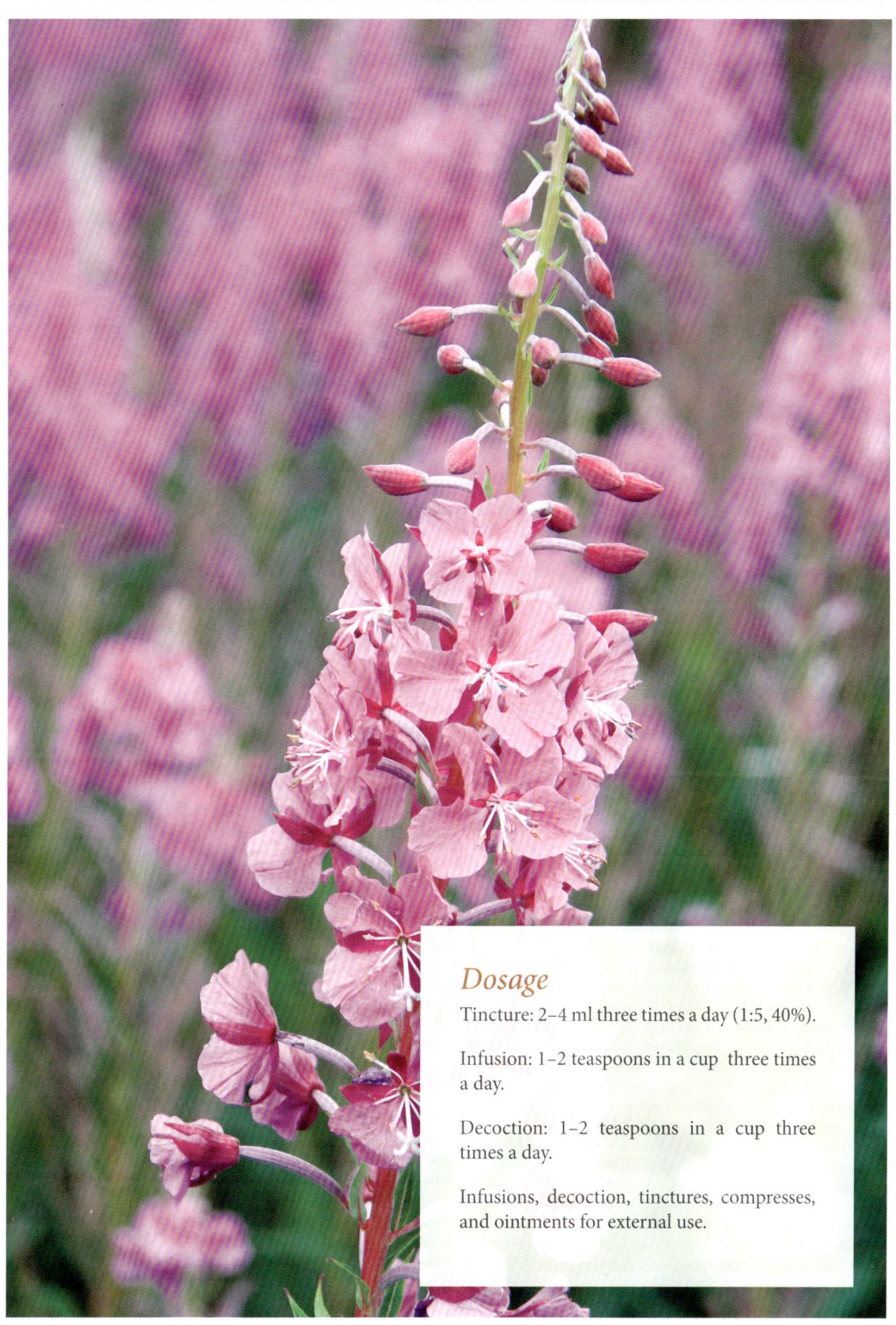

Dosage

Tincture: 2–4 ml three times a day (1:5, 40%).

Infusion: 1–2 teaspoons in a cup three times a day.

Decoction: 1–2 teaspoons in a cup three times a day.

Infusions, decoction, tinctures, compresses, and ointments for external use.

Roseroot

Rhodiola rosea
Crassulaceae—Burnirót

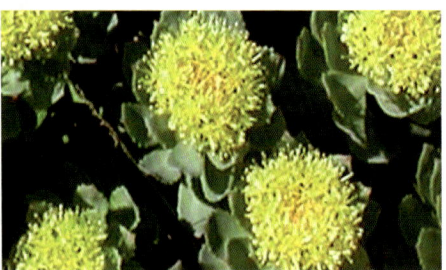

Habitat

Roseroot grows all over Iceland, but is sensitive to sheep grazing and has thus disappeared from large areas. It is also common in Icelandic gardens. Roseroot is dioecious; the male flower is yellow and the female is red.

Parts Used

Root.

Harvesting

The root is harvested in the autumn. It takes many years for Roseroot to mature, so harvesting in the wild is not recommended.

Constituents

Flavonoids, triterpenes, phenolic acids, salidrosides, rosin, rosavin, and rosarin.

History

In the old days, it was believed that Roseroot had protective powers and it was good to have it next to the body or to lay it at the bedside to ward off all evil. It was also considered good for a woman who was having trouble giving birth to put Roseroot in her bed so that it touched her. It was thought to be good for hair loss: other Icelandic names for Roseroot included "greiðurót" (comb root) and "höfuðrót" (head root). Another Old Icelandic name was "svæfla" (lull to sleep), which indicates that it was good for insomnia. It was also called "munnsviðarót" (mouth ulcer root). Many herbs that have similar astringent properties are used for sore mouth and mouth ulcers. The Native Americans used the flowers, roots, and leaves for stomach pains, colds, throat infections, tuberculosis, eye inflammation, and as an ointment for sores. The entire plant, including the root, was also used for cooking; for instance, the leaves were used fresh in salads or boiled as a vegetable.

Action

Astringent, sedative, vulnerary, increases physical and mental stamina, works against depression, anxiety, and insomnia.

Uses

The use of Roseroot in Western Europe and North America is fairly new. However, it has been used for generations as a medicinal herb in

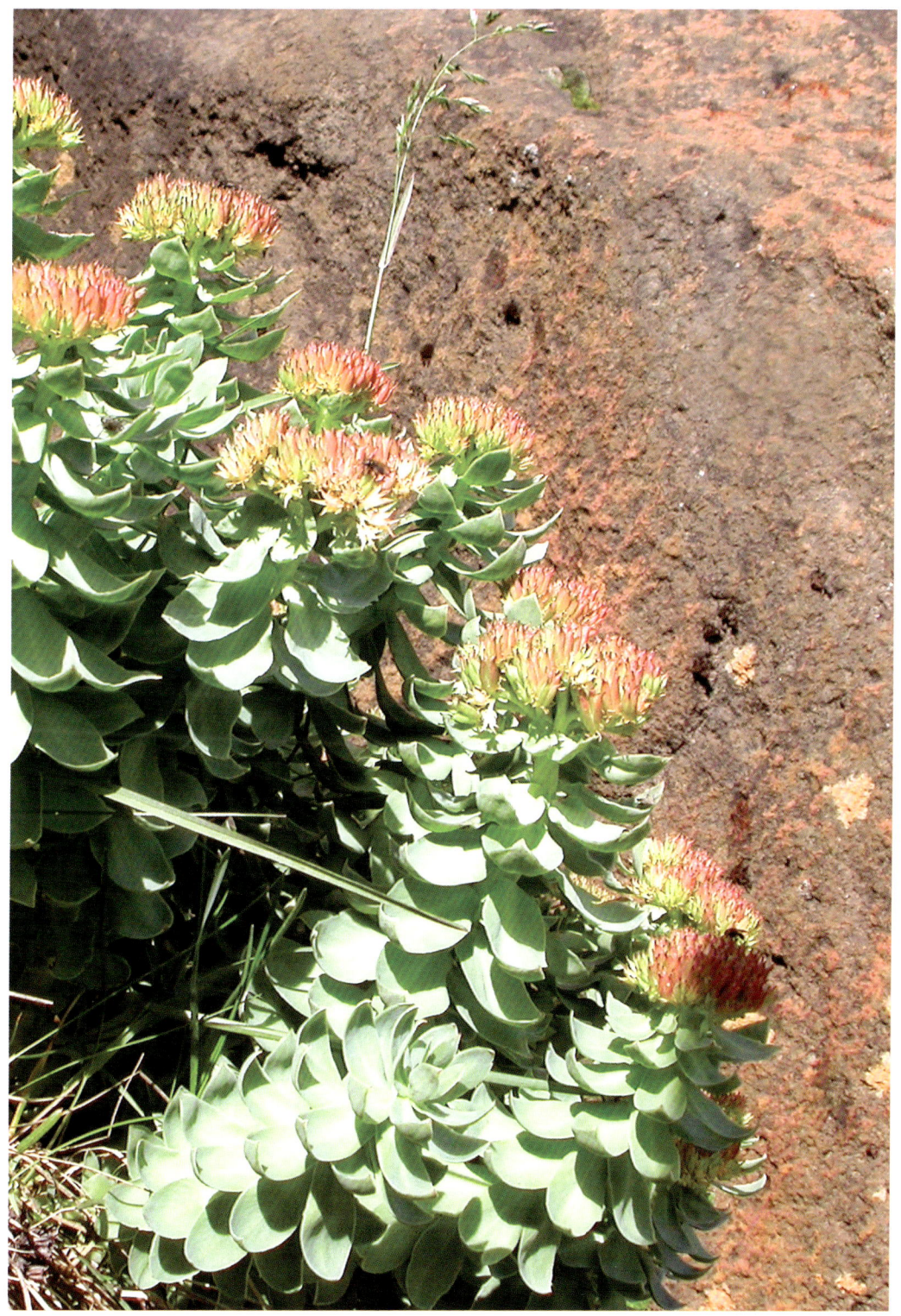

Eastern Europe and Asia. It is traditionally used to increase physical stamina and in Tibet it is used for lack of oxygen (e.g., to prevent altitude sickness). Roseroot is also traditionally used for psychological stress, restlessness, anxiety, fatigue, depression, and insomnia. Roseroot is an astringent and so works well for diarrhea and as an ointment for inflammation and rashes. In Tibet, it is used to reduce fevers, ease coughs, and clean the lungs of bad odor. Moreover, Roseroot is used for pneumonia, colds and influenza, halitosis, and bad underarm perspiration.

Research

In the research, sometimes a conventional tincture or decoction is used and sometimes a standardized extract, but often only the active ingredient salidroside is researched.

Some research has been done on Roseroot with respect to human endurance and stamina. Most research indicates that Roseroot increases oxygen flow, physical performance and stamina, as well as decreasing fatigue after exertion.[1-7] *In vitro* and *in vivo* testing have shown similar results.[8-15] However, this research has been criticized for the methods used and the quality thereof has been questioned. Also, some research has shown negative results.[16-19]

Roseroot has also been tested on patients under mental stress, such as an anxiety disorder or depression, with promising results.[20,21] Clinical research has been done on the efficacy of Roseroot on fatigue, exhaustion, lack of concentration, work phobia, and short-term memory, all with positive results,[22-26] while it has also been seen to have a positive effect on impotence and sleep.[23-27] In all of the above research studies, adverse reactions from Roseroot were found to be negligible. In addition, *in vivo* and *in vitro* tests have supported the theory that Roseroot has positive effects on psychological stress, depression, and anxiety.[12,28-36]

The effect of Roseroot on the heart has been researched through both *in vitro* and *in vivo* testing. It is thought to provide considerable protection against heart disease and has a positive effect on arrhythmia, hypertension, and atherosclerosis.[37-51] There are also indications that Roseroot has a positive effect on viral myocarditis.[52,53] In one case it has been argued that Roseroot might have caused rapid heartbeat in a patient who was taking medication for depression at the same time.[54]

Roseroot was shown to have anti-inflammatory properties through clinical and *in vivo* testing[5,55] and two research studies on patients who had undergone chest surgery indicate that Roseroot decreases the danger of surgery and speeds up recovery.[56,57]

There has been one small study in connection with bladder cancer in humans and here Roseroot showed a promising effect.[58] Quite a few *in vitro* and *in vivo* tests have shown that Roseroot has an inhibiting effect on the growth and spread of cancer cells.[59-68]

Research has shown that Roseroot could be useful for various addictions as well as the stress of withdrawal (e.g., from smoking and drug use).[69,70,71] Similarly, it has shown promising results in the treatment of eating disorders, both anorexia and bulimia.[33,72]

In vitro tests have revealed the antioxidant properties of Roseroot.[11,30,35,73-77] The effects of Roseroot on neurological diseases have been researched both *in vitro* and *in vivo* and have shown that Roseroot could be useful in the treatment of Alzheimer's and Parkinson's diseases.[78-83] *In vitro* testing has also shown that Roseroot can lower blood sugar and can therefore be useful for diabetes and could possibly protect against the complications of diabetes.[44,84-86] Clinical research shows evidence that Roseroot slows down loss of moisture and can therefore protect the skin against dryness.[87] Research has revealed the possibility of using Roseroot on patients with hypothyroidism who have had to temporarily stop taking their medication while undergoing treatment for cancer.[88] It has also been shown that Roseroot has an inhibiting effect on the influenza virus and *Staphylococcus aureus*.[62,89] Roseroot has shown protective properties against lead poisoning[90] and on the liver.[91,92]

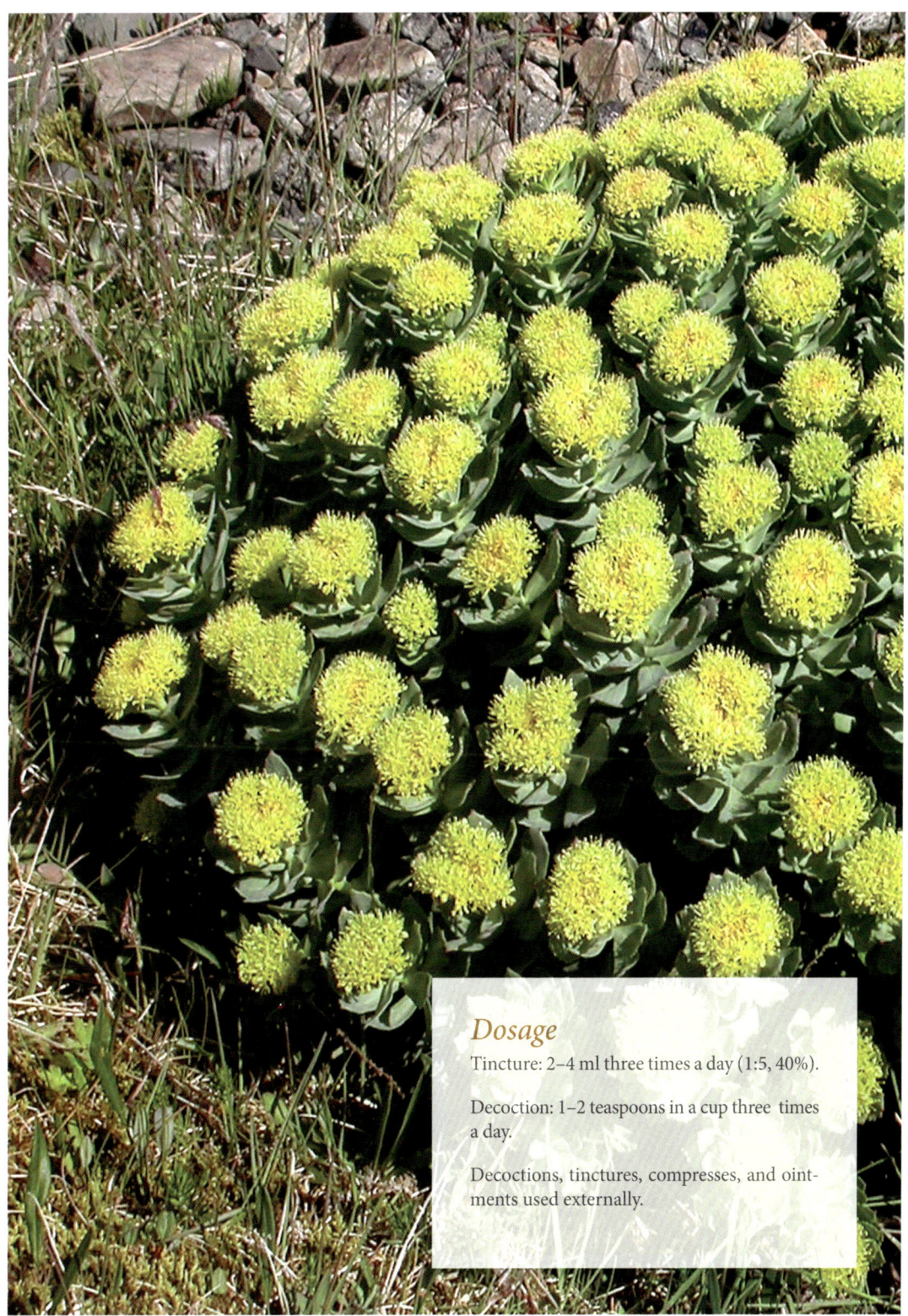

Dosage

Tincture: 2–4 ml three times a day (1:5, 40%).

Decoction: 1–2 teaspoons in a cup three times a day.

Decoctions, tinctures, compresses, and ointments used externally.

Rowan

Sorbus aucuparia
Rosaceae—Reynir

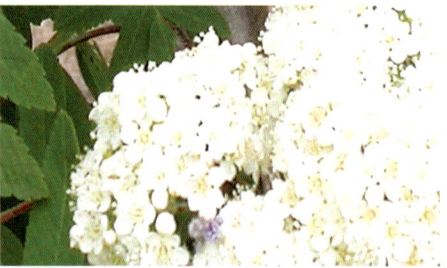

Habitat

Rowan grows sparsely in Birch forests all over Iceland and is also common in gardens in towns and the countryside.

Parts Used

The berries are used.

Harvesting

The berries are collected in autumn.

Constituents

Tannins, sorbitol, malic acid, sorbic acid, fructose, and vitamin C. The seeds of the berries contain a glycoside that forms cyanide if it comes into contact with water.

History

In the Scottish highlands there was a belief that the Rowan tree protected against witchcraft. This is why the trees were planted close to dwellings and why cow herders used Rowan tree sticks, as these were supposed to protect the animals against evil. In Icelandic folklore, the Rowan tree was believed to have nine good qualities and nine bad ones. It was considered unlucky to use Rowan wood for carpentry and it would also cause fights and arguments if it was used as firewood. However, if a married couple frequently quarreled, it was recommended for them to sleep on Rowan wood as it promoted better harmony. Native Americans believed that an infusion of Rowan leaves would help colds, diphtheria, coughs, and pneumonia. The leaves are reputed to induce vomiting and thus to heal

The Rowan berry dries, draws together and balances blood-letting and diarrhea. [...] The juice of the berry cleanses well and heals edema. [...] Despite all these good qualities, it has not been able to keep good grace with the ignorant people of this country. The devil among us, who wants to make us suspicious of God's gifts, has called the Rowan an unlucky tree. For example, Rowan wood may never be used for oarlocks, except on both sides; otherwise the boat will capsize. And another: Rowan may not be used for the nails in the stern except if there is one in the bow as well. A third example: neither woman nor any mammal will be able to give birth in a house where Rowan is planted. Then there is the fourth example: that friendship between two persons will end if they sit on opposites sides of a fire in which Rowan has been used for firewood.

Björn Halldórsson, Uses of Herbs, *1783*

This herb is astringent, diuretic and strengthening, so it is good against blood-letting, diarrhea and bladder stones. The jelly of new berries is to be taken 2 teaspoons at a time. The decoction of the berries is drunk in cups, three times a day. Dried berries, eaten 10 in the morning and 10 in the evening, are a good medicine for bladder stones.

Oddur Jónsson Hjaltalín,
Icelandic Botany, *1830*

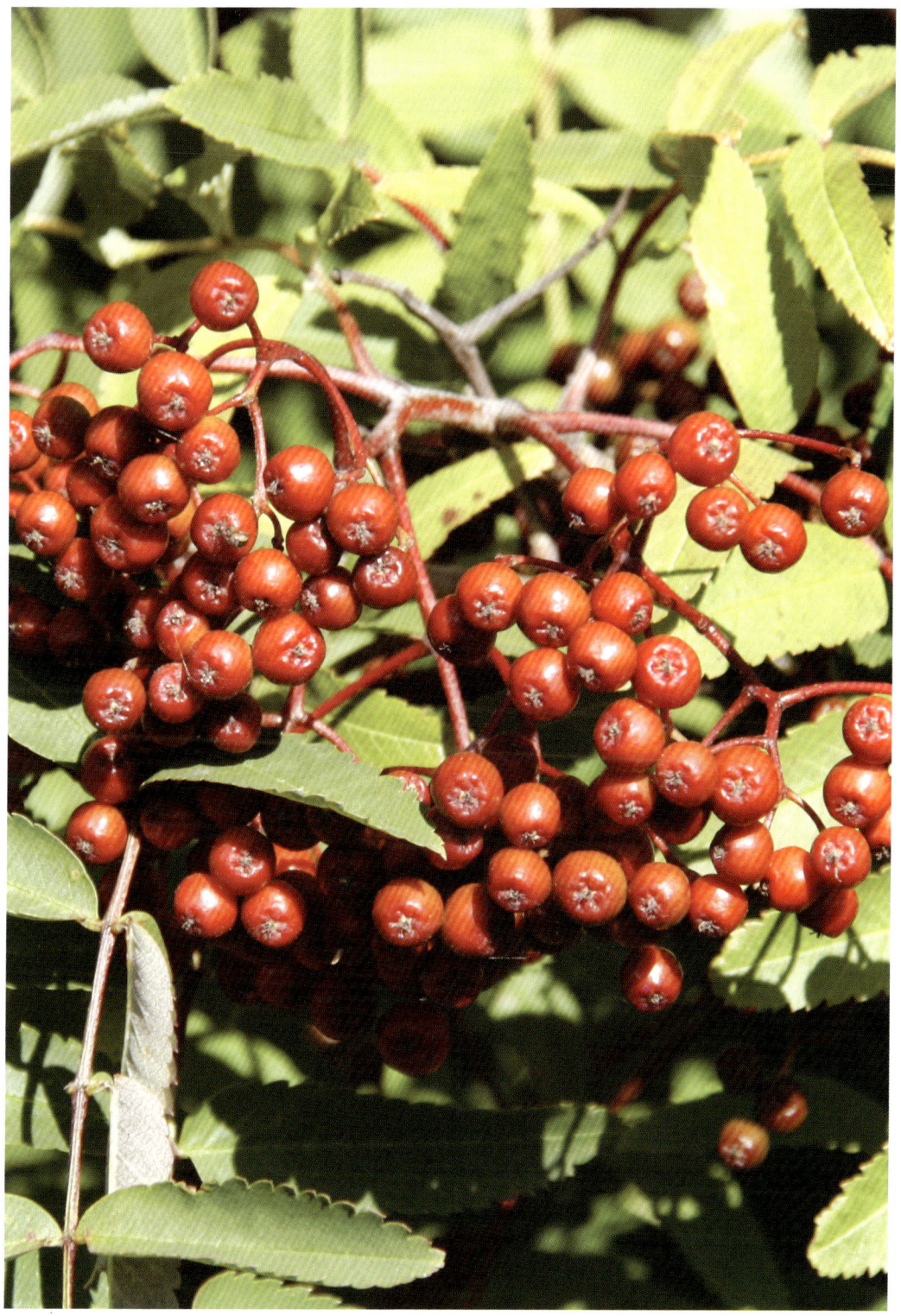

the aforementioned diseases. Rowan was used for woodwork and to tan leather, brew ale, and dye yarn. It has also been dried and ground into flour for baking.

Action

Astringent and antibacterial.

Uses

The fresh juice of the berries is mildly laxative, but if the berries are dried or boiled in a jelly, they are astringent and good for diarrhea and hemorrhoids. They are also beneficial as a mouthwash for sore throats, and externally for hemorrhoids and white vaginal discharge. The berries are thought to be good for arthritis, menstrual pain, and urinary tract infections. Rowan bark contains a high proportion of tannin and a decoction of the bark is considered good externally for cleansing wounds and for vaginal discharges.

Research

In vitro tests on the flowers, berries, and leaves of Rowan have shown its antioxidant properties.[1,2]

Dosage

Juice: 1 teaspoon of fresh juice as needed.

Jelly: 1 tablespoon of jelly three to five times a day.

Cold decoction: 1 teaspoon of dried berries in a cup of cold water; allow to stand overnight. 1 cup a day.

Warning

The seeds of the berries contain a glycoside that forms cyanide if in contact with water, so the seeds should always be removed from the berries if the latter are to be used for cooking or medicinal purposes. The leaves of the Rowan tree also contain this glycoside, so they are not recommended for medicinal use.

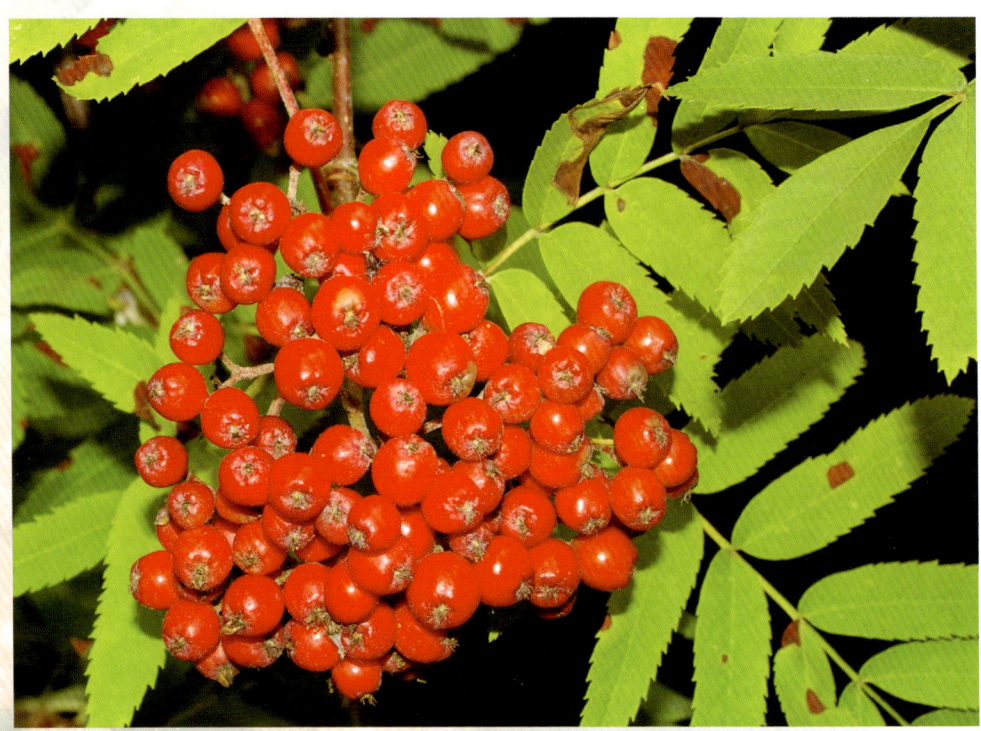

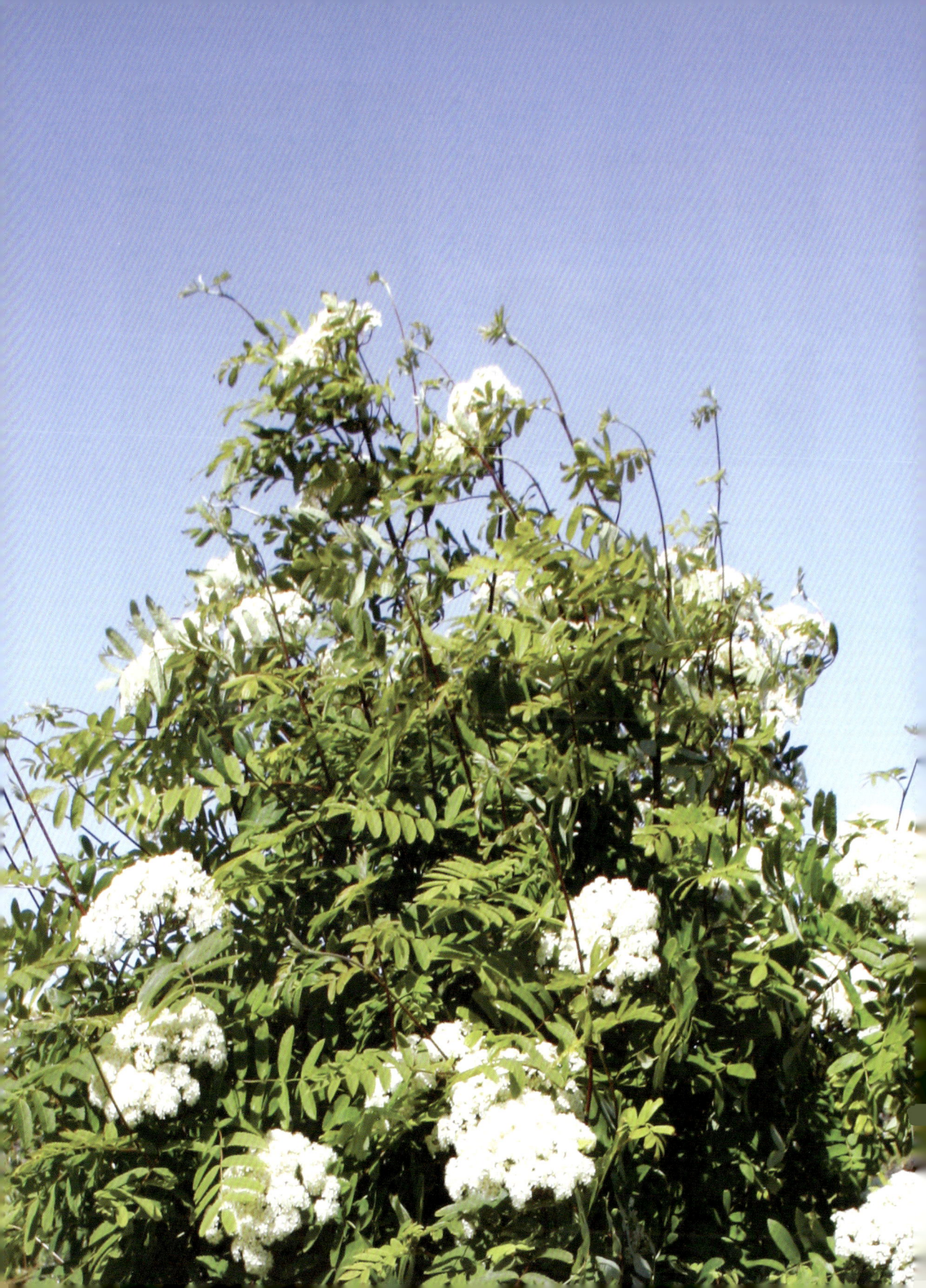

Scurvy Grass

Cochlearia officinalis
Brassicaceae—Skarfakál

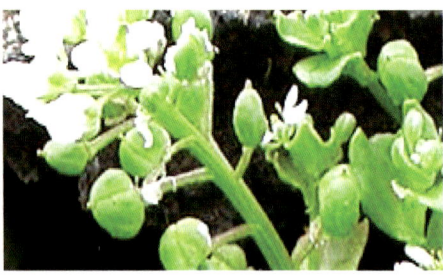

Habitat

Scurvy Grass grows mainly on rocks and sea cliffs. It is quite common along the Icelandic coastline.

Parts Used

The entire plant is used, except for the root.

Harvesting

Scurvy Grass is collected just before bloom in May–June.

Constituents

Glucosinolates, alkaloids, flavonoids, tannins, essential oils, vitamin C, and minerals.

History

Scurvy Grass is rich in vitamin C and, in the past, was thought to be a good preventive for scurvy, which is caused by a lack of vitamin C. It was very popular for use among sailors. The name Scurvy Grass is a direct indication of its use against scurvy. Another Icelandic name for it, "skyrbjúgsjurt," also means scurvy grass. In the past, it was not unusual for Scurvy Grass to be used in salads or cooking.

This herb is considered one of the best against scurvy. It is good for easing menstrual bleeding in women. Porridge is made from Scurvy Grass as with other greens. It may also be salted for cooking and storage. It is also possible to make a good, healthy salad with it. To blend spirits, French or Danish, or otherwise French wine, with the blossoms of Scurvy Grass, makes a healthy drink given on an empty stomach, especially for those at risk of getting scurvy. It is also good to rinse the mouth for halitosis. A good French spirit in which the flowers of Scurvy Grass have been soaked, rather than the leaves, for about three months, is good to rub on arthritic inflammations and all such cold which is found in specific places on the body as it stiffens the blood. It is even better to wet a soft cloth in the same liquid and lay it over the cold areas.

Björn Halldórsson, Uses of Herbs, 1783

Action

Nourishing, antibacterial, diuretic, and a mild laxative.

Uses

Scurvy Grass is rarely used in Western herbal medicine nowadays. It is best used fresh, and is thought to be good for edema and mild constipation while also being useful when undernourishment is present. The juice from the plant is considered to be a good mouthwash for mouth ulcers, and used externally it is beneficial for acne.

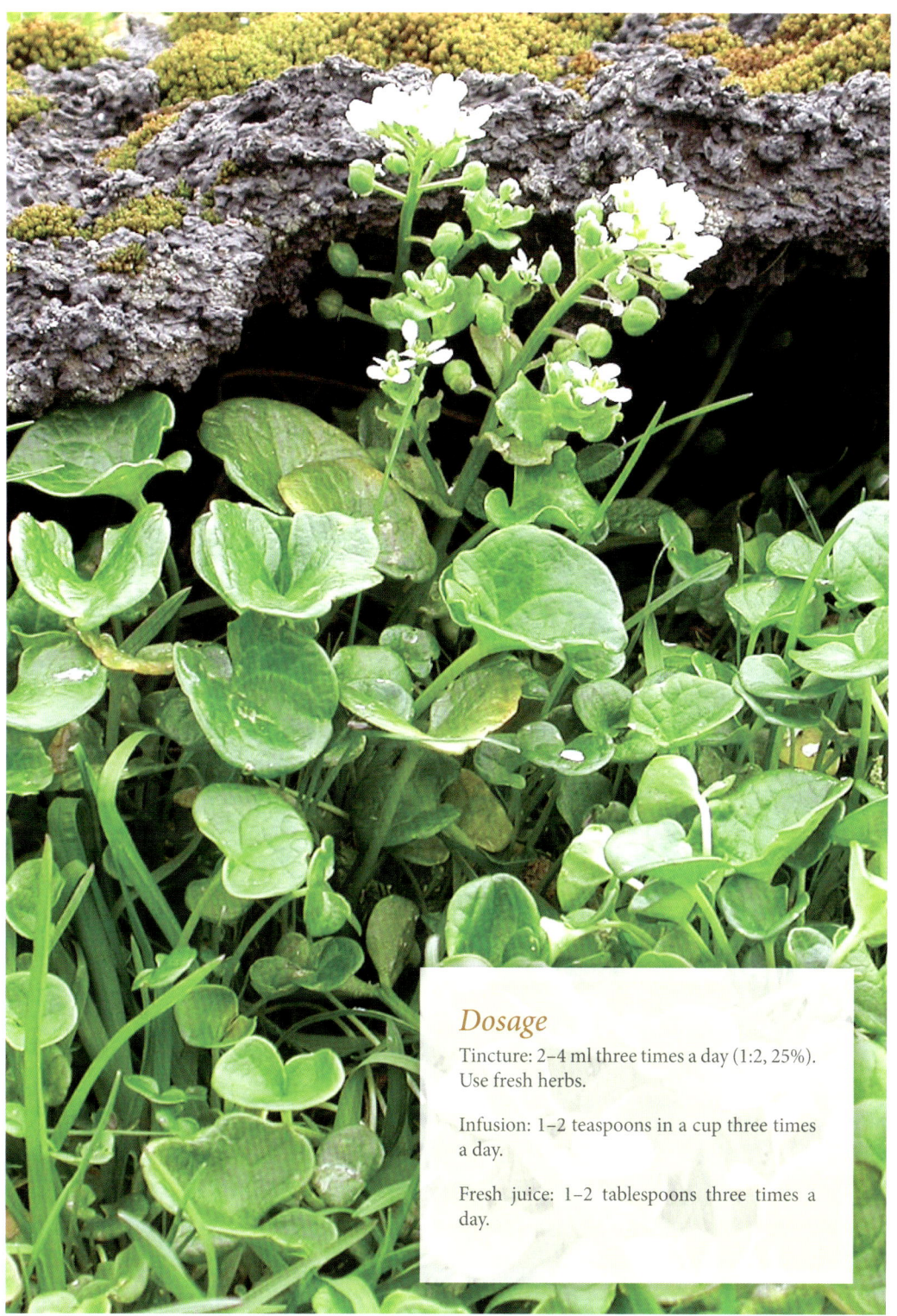

Dosage

Tincture: 2–4 ml three times a day (1:2, 25%). Use fresh herbs.

Infusion: 1–2 teaspoons in a cup three times a day.

Fresh juice: 1–2 tablespoons three times a day.

Sea Mayweed

Tripleurospermum maritimum
Asteraceae—Baldursbrá

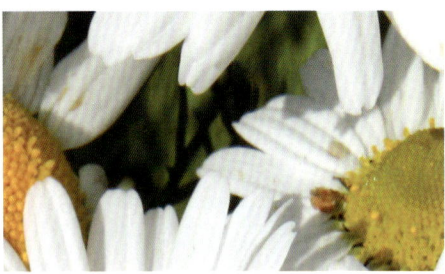

Habitat

Sea Mayweed grows all over Iceland, especially close to houses, as well as on roadsides and beaches.

Parts Used

Flowers.

Harvesting

Collected in July when in bloom.

Constituents

Essential oils and flavonoids.

History

Sea Mayweed is closely related to Chamomile (*Chamomilla recutita*), which is a renowned ancient healing herb and for which a great amount of research and documentation exists to prove its healing powers. As Chamomile does not grow wild in Iceland, Sea Mayweed has been used instead, the healing powers of which are reportedly similar to Chamomile. The old genus name for Sea Mayweed and Chamomile was *Matricaria*, meaning mother's love; aptly, Chamomile is well known as a treatment for various gynecological problems. Icelandic sources report the use of Sea Mayweed for women. From ancient times, this herb has been connected to Icelandic folklore (e.g., the belief that if one sleeps with Sea Mayweed under the pillow, the thief's identity will be revealed in the dream).

Action

Anti-inflammatory, sedative, analgesic, carminative, antispasmodic, and antiviral.

Uses

Nowadays, Sea Mayweed is not used much as a healing herb in the Western world. It has been considered beneficial for digestive problems (i.e., flatulence and stomach cramps, as well as gastritis). Sea Mayweed is also used for period pains and to ease symptoms of menopause. It is said to calm digestion, ease anxiety, and improve sleep, and is used externally to heal wounds.

Research

In vitro tests show the inhibiting effect of Sea Mayweed on poliovirus type 2 and herpes simplex virus 1.[1]

Dosage

Tincture: 2–6 ml three times a day (1:5, 40%).

Infusion: 1–2 teaspoons in a cup three times a day.

Infusions, tinctures, compresses, and ointments used externally.

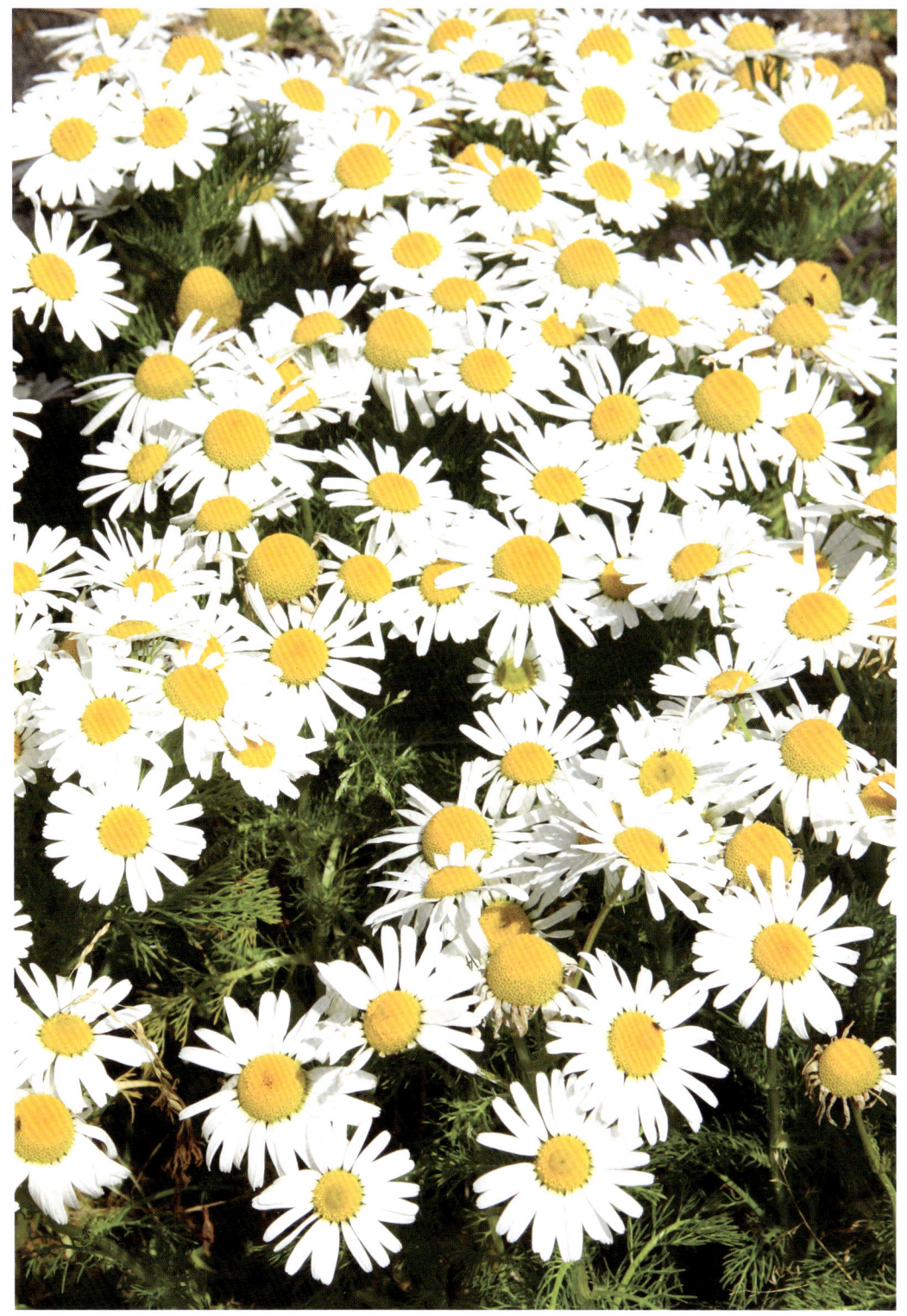

Self-heal

Prunella vulgaris
Labiatae—Blákolla

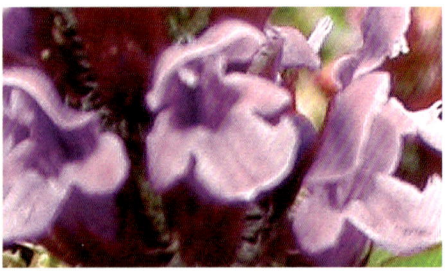

Habitat

Self-heal grows mainly in South and West Iceland, but also in Fljótsdalur district in the Northeast and Eyjafjörður in the North. It grows best in geothermal areas and where the air is warm.

Parts Used

The entire plant is used, except for the root.

Harvesting

Self-heal is collected in bloom in June–July.

Constituents

Triterpenes (betulin, ursolic, and oleanolic acids), flavonoids (rutin), phenolic acid (rosmarinic acid), coumarin, and essential oils.

History

Self-heal is an ancient medicinal herb and has been used for centuries. The name itself reflects the belief in its healing properties over time. Gerard, a renowned 16th-century English herbalist, said that no herb equals Self-heal for healing wounds. In Ireland, it was a very popular medicinal herb and was mainly used for lung and heart diseases and to stop bleeding.

Self-heal was highly praised by Native Americans, who believed it worked well for strengthening the heart, eyes, and womb, as well as being effective against throat infections, diarrhea, fever, colic, hemorrhoids, tuberculosis, venereal diseases, and any sores or skin rashes. It was also recommended for improving attention and concentration before hunting and for those sick with grief. Self-heal was considered a good culinary herb too, its leaves being used raw in salads or boiled as a vegetable.

Action

Vulnerary, astringent, hemostatic, hypotensive, diuretic, anti-inflammatory, antibacterial, and antiviral.

Uses

In the past, Self-heal was a popular medicinal herb, but it is not used much nowadays. Traditionally it has been used as a gargle for sore and infected throats. It is also used to stop internal bleeding and for diarrhea. Externally, it is considered good for hemorrhoids and vaginal discharges, and for healing wounds. In China, Self-heal is still a very popular herb and has been used since time immemorial. It is thought to be good for dizzy headaches, conjunctivitis, tuberculosis in the lymph nodes, hypertrophy of the thyroid gland, mastitis, hypertension, fever, edema, anxiety, gout and arthritis, tinnitus, infected and swollen cervical lymph nodes, and cancer. In Korea, Self-heal is traditionally used for edema, nephritis, glandular fever, and hypertrophy of the thyroid.

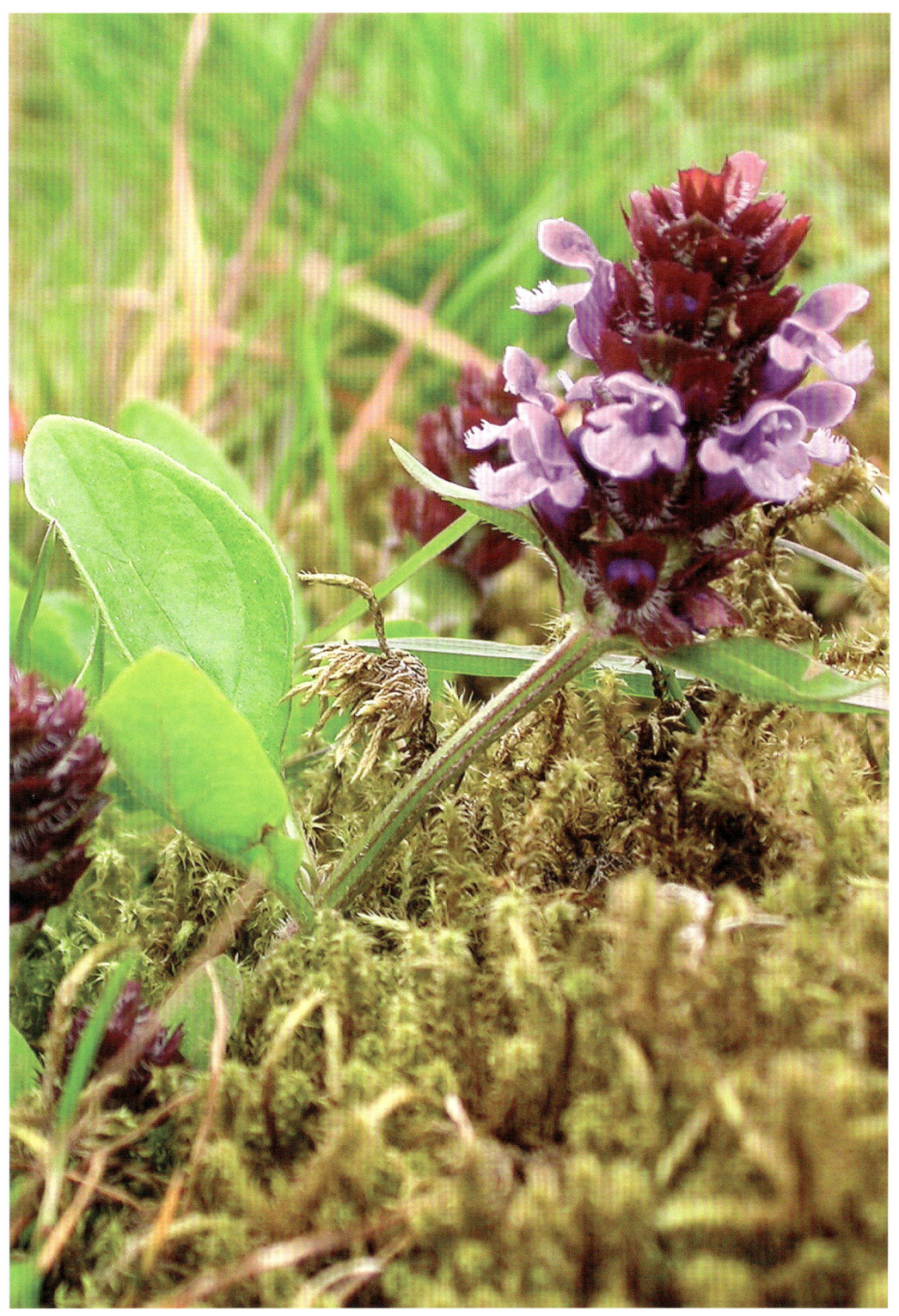

Research

Self-heal has been the subject of extensive research, mainly in Asia, where it has been traditionally used for centuries as a medicinal herb. Clinical research on a standard preparation, which contained Self-heal and two other Korean herbs, revealed that this blend had as much analgesic power as the painkiller Celecoxib for arthritis.[1] In another clinical trial in Korea with the same preparation, the effects of Self-heal on osteoarthritis were noted.[2] Clinical research in the Czech Republic on the effects of a preparation containing Self-heal and other medicinal herbs on gingivitis showed the activity of this preparation.[3] *In vitro* testing also showed the effects of Self-heal on gingivitis.[4] A few *in vitro* and *in vivo* tests show the antibacterial and antiviral effects of Self-heal,[5–8] and specific tests have been carried out against the herpes simplex virus 1 and 2 and HIV.[15–21] In addition, Self-heal is also thought to be active against the EIAV virus (Equine Infectious Anemia Virus).[22]

Many *in vitro* tests demonstrate the anti-inflammatory effect of Self-heal.[4–6, 23–26] Self-heal is also considered to stimulate the immune system,[5,6,25,27] work against autoimmune diseases,[24] and have antioxidant properties.[7,28,29] Furthermore, it is thought to protect the heart[30] and lower blood pressure;[31] have a positive effect on diabetes type 2;[32–34] work against allergies,[26,35,36] tuberculosis, and acute hepatitis;[31] and be good for women with endometriosis.[37,38] Self-heal is believed to protect the skin from the damaging effects of the sun,[39,40] act like a diuretic,[41] improve osteoarthritis,[42] and possibly work against amnesia.[43] Last but not least, it is thought that Self-heal inhibits the growth of various cancer cells.[26,27,37,41,44–52]

Dosage

Tincture: 1–5 ml three times a day (1:5, 25%).

Infusion: 1–2 teaspoons in a cup three times a day.

Syrup: 1–2 teaspoons three times a day.

Infusions, tinctures, compresses, and ointments used externally.

Warning

It is known that Self-heal can cause allergies, but this is rare. Allergic reactions can take the form of itching, swelling in the mouth, nausea, diarrhea, and vomiting.

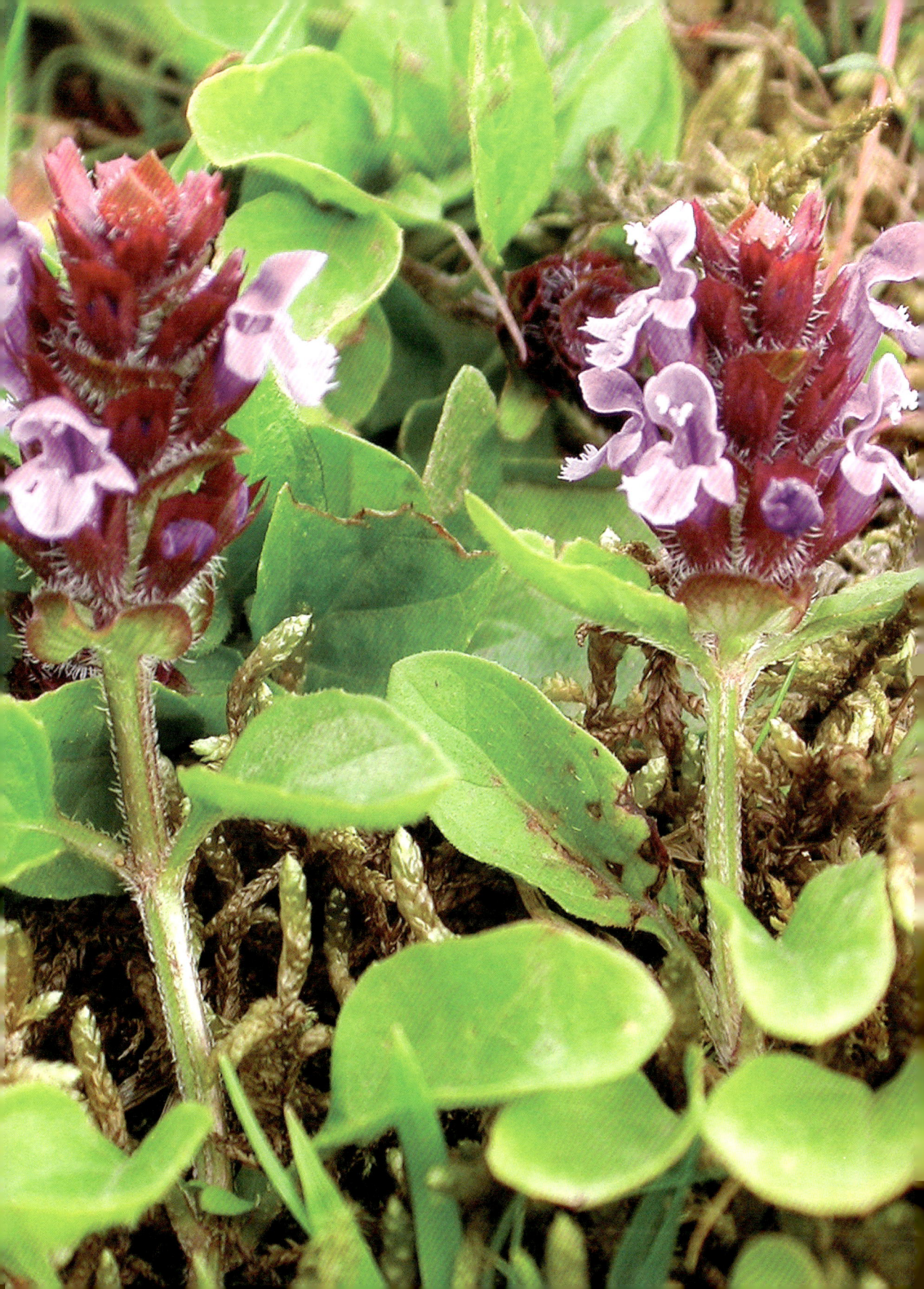

Sheep's Sorrel

Rumex acetosella
Polygonaceae—Hundasúra

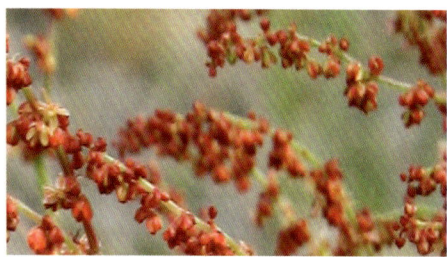

Habitat

Sheep's Sorrel is common all over Iceland except in the North. It grows well in gravel and sandy soil.

Parts Used

The entire plant is used, including the root.

Harvesting

The leaves are collected in May–June, before blooming, and the roots are harvested in autumn.

Constituents

Anthraquinones, flavonoids, oxalic acid, tannins, minerals, and vitamins.

History

The Native Americans placed the fresh and boiled leaves of Sheep's Sorrel onto wounds, warts, and corns. Sheep's Sorrel has mainly been used as a food, both in Iceland and elsewhere. The root has been used to dye yarn. Wood Sorrel (*Oxalis acetosella*) has been used in a similar way to Sheep's Sorrel and Sorrel, but it is a protected plant in Iceland. Similar references exist concerning the uses of Mountain Sorrel (*Oxyria digyna*).

Action

Diuretic, anti-inflammatory, mild laxative, cooling, diaphoretic, and febrifuge.

Uses

Sheep's Sorrel is first and foremost used fresh. The juice is deemed to be good against constipation and edema. Used externally, the fresh leaves are said to be cooling and good for rashes. The plant is also used for fever, inflammations, and scurvy. The root of Sheep's Sorrel has been used for diarrhea and to reduce menstrual bleeding. Sheep's Sorrel is one of the herbs in the well-known formula Essiac, which originates from the Native Americans and is thought to be effective against cancer.

Research

In vitro testing on the Essiac formula, which contains Sheep's Sorrel along with *Rheum palmatum, Ulmus fulva,* and *Arctium lappa,* reveals its antioxidant properties.[1] Other research indicates that Sheep's Sorrel could suppress the growth of cancer cells.[2]

Dosage

Fresh juice: 1 tablespoon three times a day.

Infusion: 1 teaspoon in a cup three times a day.

Decoction: 1 teaspoon in a cup three times a day.

Infusions and compresses for external use.

Warning

Sheep's Sorrel can have toxic effects if taken in large doses. Those with kidney stones, osteoarthritis, gout, or excessive gastric acid should not use Sheep's Sorrel.

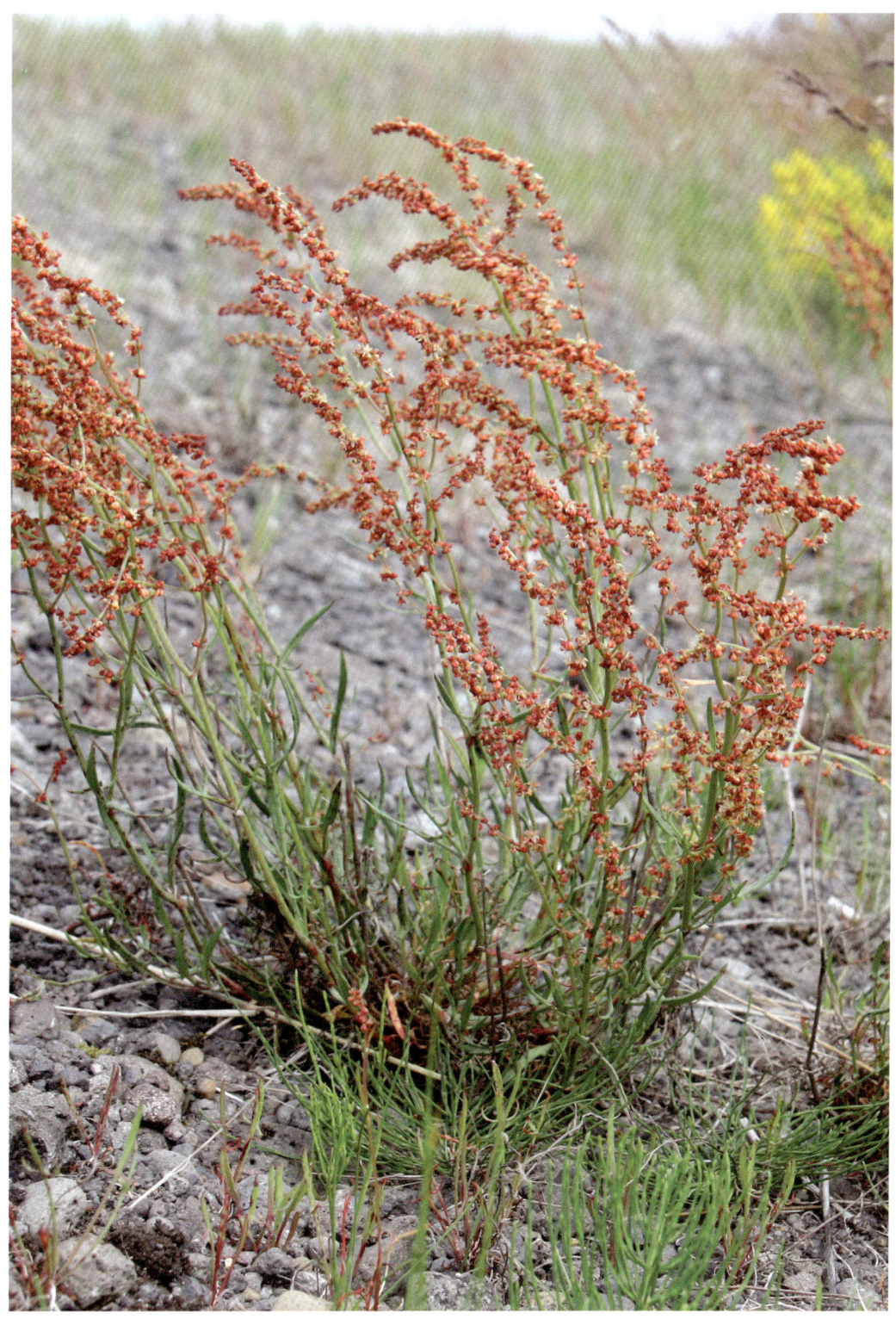

Shepherd's Purse

Capsella bursa-pastoris
Brassicaceae—*Hjartarfi*

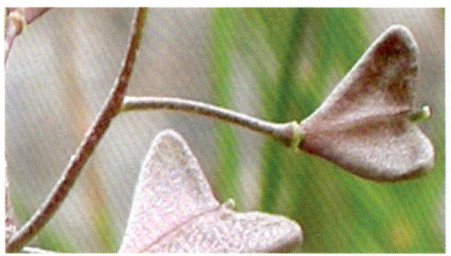

Habitat

Shepherd's Purse is common all over Iceland and grows mainly close to farmhouses and cultivated fields.

Parts Used

The entire plant is used, except for the root.

Harvesting

Shepherd's Purse is collected at the end of flowering when the seeds start to form in May–June. The dried herb does not keep well and it can be expected to lose potency after 6 months. Do not collect Shepherd's Purse if there are signs of white fungus on it.

Constituents

Flavonoids (quercitrin), glucosinolates, alkaloids, essential oils, and polypeptides.

History

The pods of Shepherd's Purse are heart-shaped and resemble that of an old-fashioned leather purse. The Latin name *bursa-pastoris* means Shepherd's Purse and refers to the shape of the seed pods. The same can be said for the Old Icelandic names "smalapungur" (herder's pouch), "töskugras" (pouch herb), "pungarfi" (pouch weed), and "prestapungur" (priest's pouch). Shepherd's Purse was used with good results in World War I to stop the bleeding of soldiers' wounds. Prior to then, it was used instead of quinine as a febrifuge for malaria. The leaves were a popular vegetable and evidence of this can be found in references to the Native Americans as well as to the people of Tibet, Nepal, and China. In China, Shepherd's Purse is sold in markets like other vegetables. The Native Americans have used Shepherd's Purse a lot as a medicinal herb, particularly for dysentery, diarrhea, stomach cramps, and intestinal worms. They have also used the herb as a vegetable, both fresh and cooked, and crushed the seeds for baking. In Iceland in the old days, people believed that nosebleeds could be stopped by holding Shepherd's Purse in the hand until it got warm.

Action

Astringent, hemostatic, diuretic, anti-inflammatory, antibacterial, antifungal, stimulates uterine contractions, and increases blood flow to the limbs.

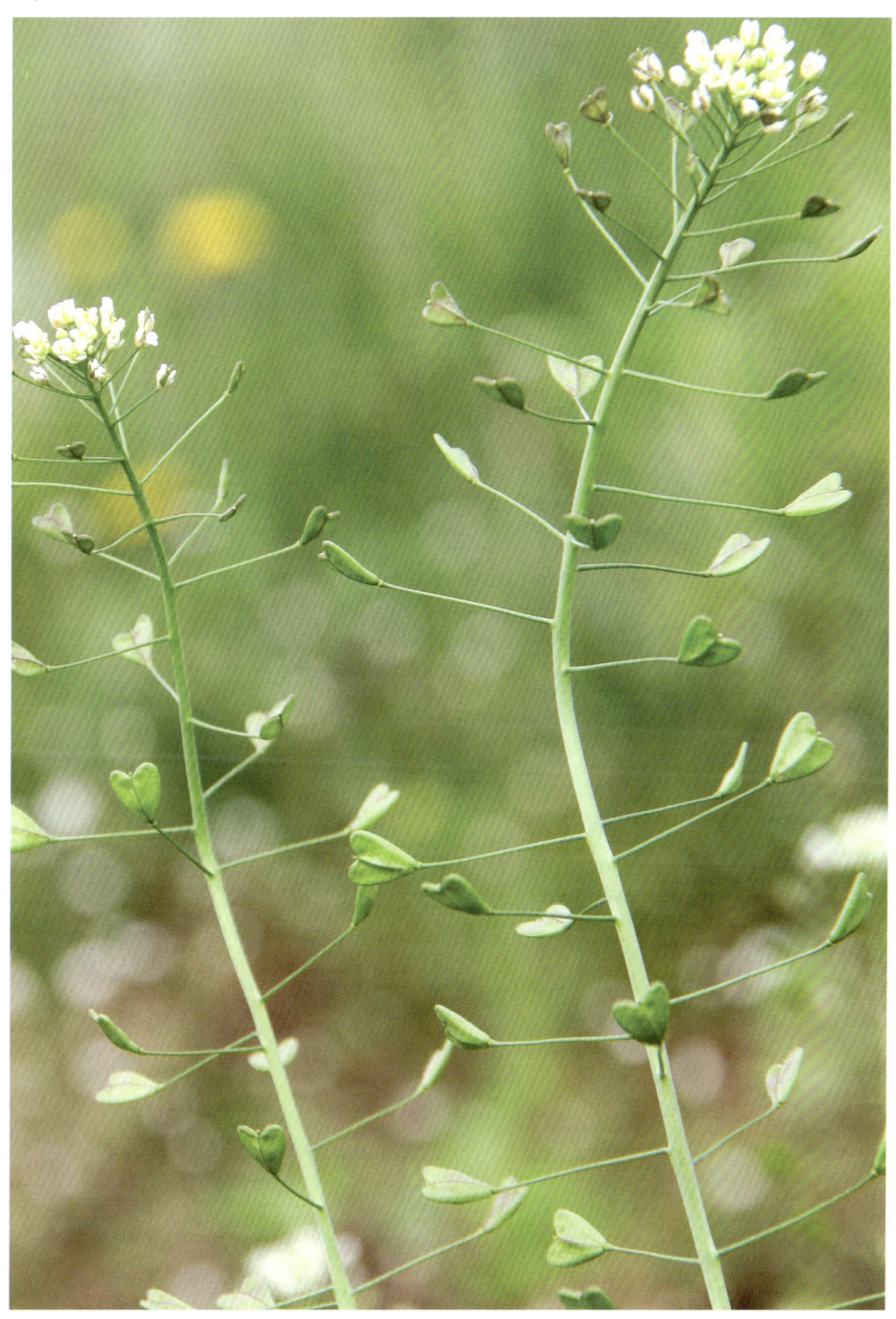

Uses

Shepherd's Purse is considered to be one of the best herbs for stopping bleeding, especially heavy menstrual bleeding, spotting, and bleeding due to benign tumors in the uterus or endometriosis, but also for all kinds of other bleeding, from nosebleeds to bleeding in the urethra. Shepherd's Purse is also used for cystitis and hemorrhoids, and to stop diarrhea. Externally, Shepherd's Purse is good for stopping bleeding and for healing wounds. The Chinese have long used it as a medicinal herb in a similar way to the Europeans. Shepherd's Purse ranks seventh among the Chinese medicinal herbs that are considered to be good contraceptives. In North America, Shepherd's Purse has been used in childbirth to increase contractions after full dilation of the cervix. In Tibet, Shepherd's Purse is thought to be good for nausea and vomiting, kidney and lung diseases, neurological diseases, and edema.

Research

In vitro testing has revealed the antibacterial and antifungal effect of Shepherd's Purse,[1,2] as well as its diuretic and anti-inflammatory effects.[1] Shepherd's Purse also increases muscle contraction in the uterus and thus strengthens it.[1,3] Research has shown that Shepherd's Purse promotes blood coagulation, increases blood flow to the limbs, has a dilating effect on coronary arteries, hinders capillary leakage, and has a short-term effect on lowering blood pressure.[1] Shepherd's Purse also inhibits the growth of cancer cells,[1,4,5] has a soothing effect on wounds, and can lighten skin.[6]

Dosage

Tincture: 1–5 ml three times a day (1:5, 25%).

Infusion: 1–2 teaspoons in a cup three times a day. With heavy menstrual bleeding it is good to start to drink this just before menstruation starts and then at 1–2 hour intervals while bleeding is heaviest.

Infusions, tinctures, compresses, and ointments for external use.

Warning

When menstruation is abnormally heavy, it is imperative to rule out malignant changes before using Shepherd's Purse or other herbs for the problem. Do not use Shepherd's Purse during pregnancy. Those with kidney stones should not use Shepherd's Purse, and large doses for extended periods of time should also be avoided.

Tea for Heavy Menstrual Bleeding

2 parts Shepherd's Purse

1 part Knotgrass

1 part Lady's Mantle

3–4 tablespoons of the herb blend is placed in a 750 ml vacuum flask filled with boiling water. Strain the herbs when pouring into a cup, then put them back into the flask and let it stand the whole day. Drink from the flask throughout the day.

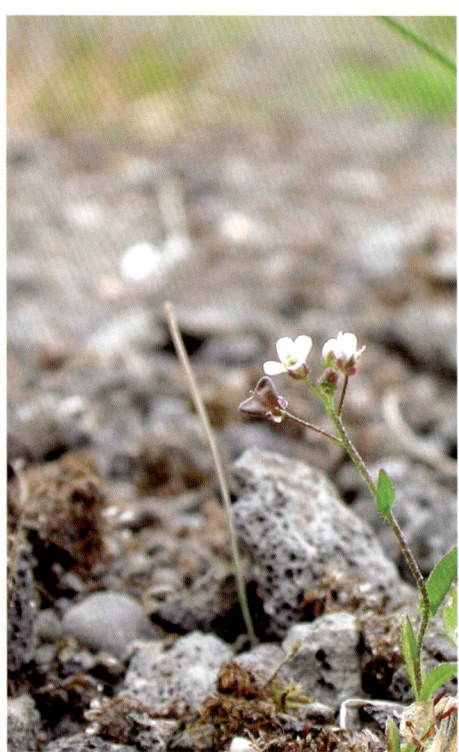

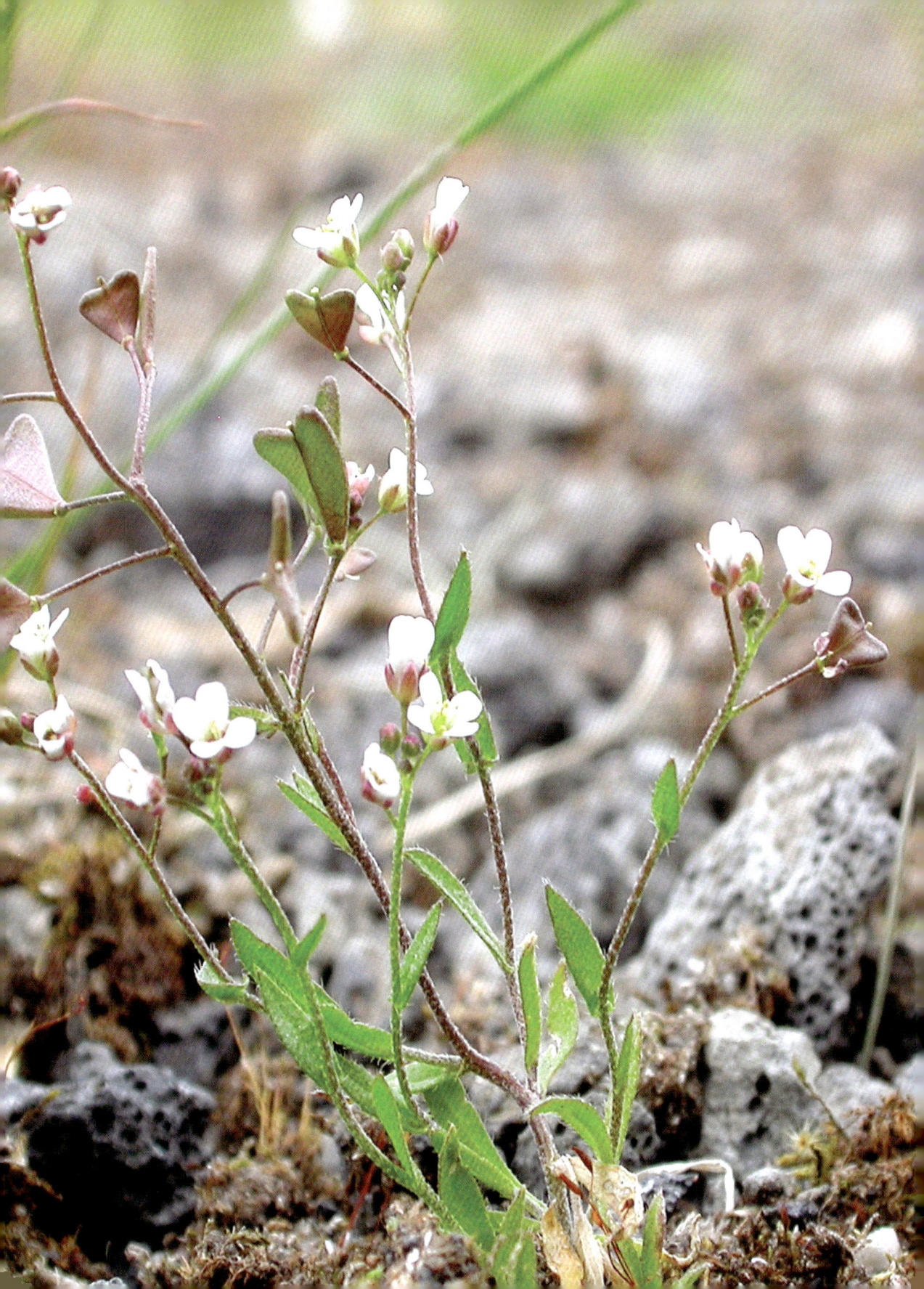

Silverweed

Argentina anserina
Rosaceae—Tágamura

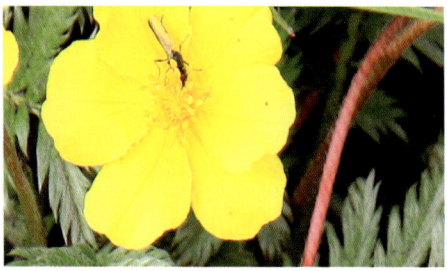

Habitat

Silverweed is common all over Iceland and grows in sandy soil and close to beaches.

Parts Used

The entire plant is used, including the root.

Harvesting

Silverweed is collected in bloom in June and the roots are harvested in autumn.

Constituents

Tannins, flavonoids (quercitrin) and coumarin.

History

The Latin name *Argentina* is drawn from the word "argentum," meaning silver. Silverweed is also called "silfurmura" in Icelandic, and the English name is associated with silver as the undersides of the leaves have a silverish color. The name *anserina* is drawn from the word "anser," meaning goose, as geese are fond of Silverweed. The older generic name *Potentilla* is drawn from "potent," which refers to the powerful medicinal properties of Silverweed and other plants of the Rosaceae family. The

This herb is astringent, cooling and healing. It regulates the bleeding of women, if it is carried in the hand or placed under the heel in a sock. This last suggestion has recently helped one woman completely. The herb is placed over wounds, bruised and heated in a pot, then made into a poultice. [...] Silverweed with vinegar is said to strengthen the teeth. The decoction, ingested, dissolves clotted blood and heals internal wounds and blood spitting, almost as well as Yarrow. It regulates the bleeding of women, heals white discharge and diarrhea and also back pain. The same decoction can be sniffed up the nose, for those with heavy nosebleeds, and a cloth moistened with the decoction can be laid on the forehead; this regulates blood circulation. [...] Silverweed, bruised with salt and vinegar and laid over the instep of the foot, heals dysentery and diarrhea.

Björn Halldórsson, Uses of Herbs, *1783*

Argentina species were eaten in the past, as one old Icelandic rhyme states: "had children and clothes, dug up roots and silverweed." Silverweed was also used to dye yarn and tan leather. In the past, water distilled from Silverweed was a very popular beautifier that was supposed to eliminate freckles and pimples as well as take the sting out of sunburn.

The Native Americans used Silverweed a great deal, both as food and medicine. The whole herb was thought to be good for diarrhea and the leaves were diuretic. Externally, Silverweed was put on wounds and inflammation. The Native Americans of Canada held Silverweed in high esteem as a medicinal herb and the roots were, for example, a valuable wedding gift. The Chief owned the area in which Silverweed grew and restrictions were placed on how much the public could pick. Silverweed was considered in the past to be antispasmodic and good for menstrual

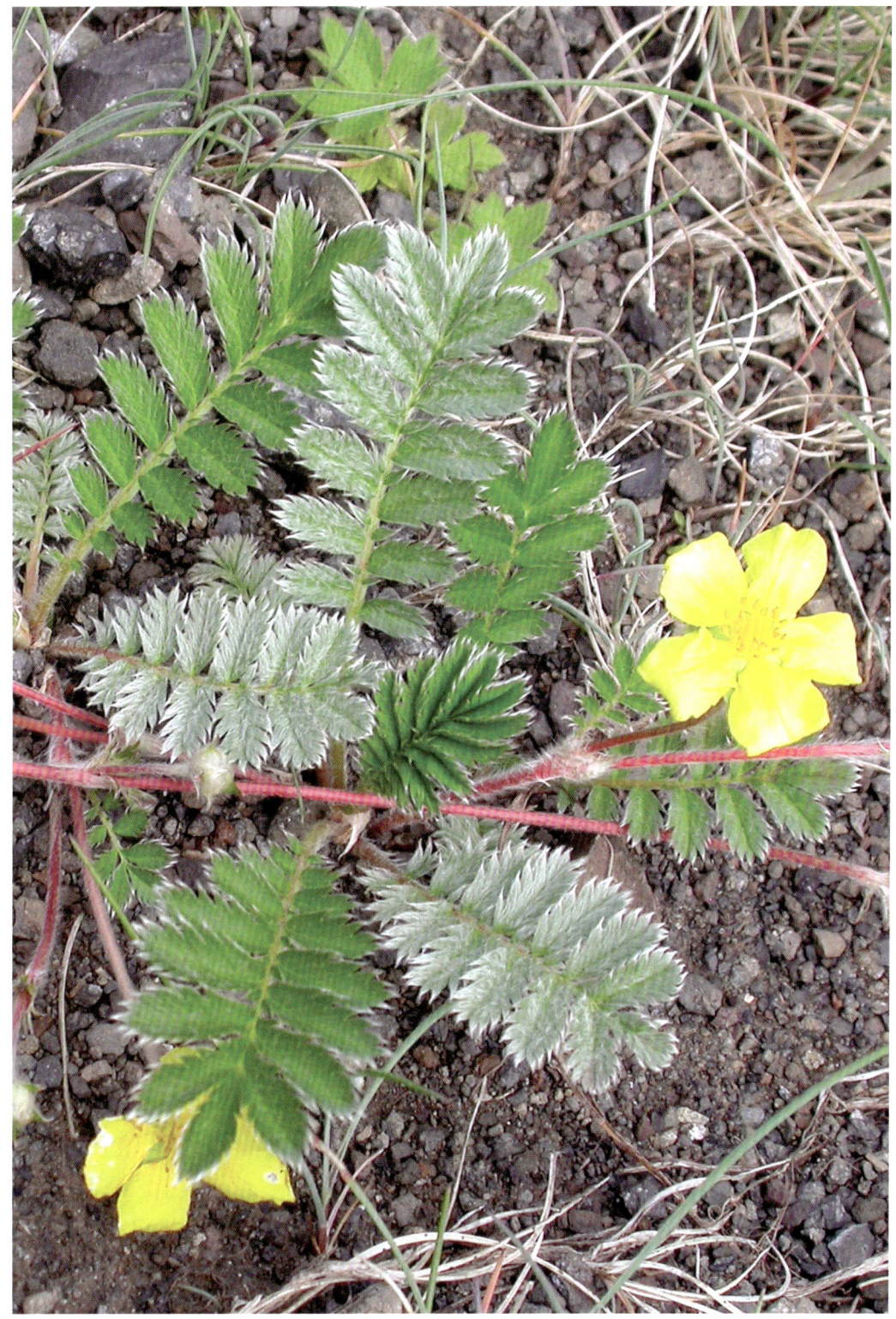

pain and gastritis, but now herbalists are doubting these actions. Tormentil (*Potentilla erecta*), which is protected in Iceland but is common in other countries, also has a long history as a medicinal herb. It contains high levels of tannins and is therefore even more astringent than Silverweed. Eged's Silverweed (*Argentina egedii*) has also been used as a medicinal herb similar to Silverweed, but it is also very rare in Iceland.

Action

Astringent, anti-inflammatory, antibacterial, antiviral, antifungal and haemostatic.

. . . .

Uses

Silverweed is thought to be an excellent mouthwash for gingivitis, mouth ulcers, and sore throats. It has also long been used for gastritis, stomach ulcers, diarrhea, and fevers. Externally, Silverweed works well for bleeding hemorrhoids and vaginal discharges, as well as for healing wounds. In China there is a long tradition of using Silverweed for hepatitis B.

Research

Silverweed has shown, through *in vitro* tests, to be antibacterial and antifungal, especially in cases of infection of the gums. It also showed effectiveness against *Helicobacterium pylori*, which causes gastritis and stomach ulcers.[1,2]

Both *in vitro* and *in vivo* tests on isolated compounds of Silverweed show antiviral action on hepatitis B[3] and possible stimulation of the immune system.[4] Clinical research on Tormentil (*Potentilla erecta*) showed a positive effect on ulcerative colitis.[5] Research on Tormentil also reveals that it is anti-inflammatory,[6] antibacterial,[7] and has an inhibitory effect on the growth of cancer cells.[8]

Dosage

Tincture: 2–4 ml three times a day (1:5, 40%).

Infusion: 1–2 teaspoons in a cup three times a day.

Decoction: 1–2 teaspoons in a cup three times a day.

Infusions, decoctions, tinctures, compresses, and ointments for external use.

Mouthwash for Ulcers

1 part Silverweed

1 part Water Avens

1 part Creeping Thyme

Put 1 tablespoon of the blend in a cup, pour boiling water over, and cover. Allow to steep for 30 minutes. Strain the herbs. Rinse the mouth and drink the remainder as an infusion. 3–4 cups a day.

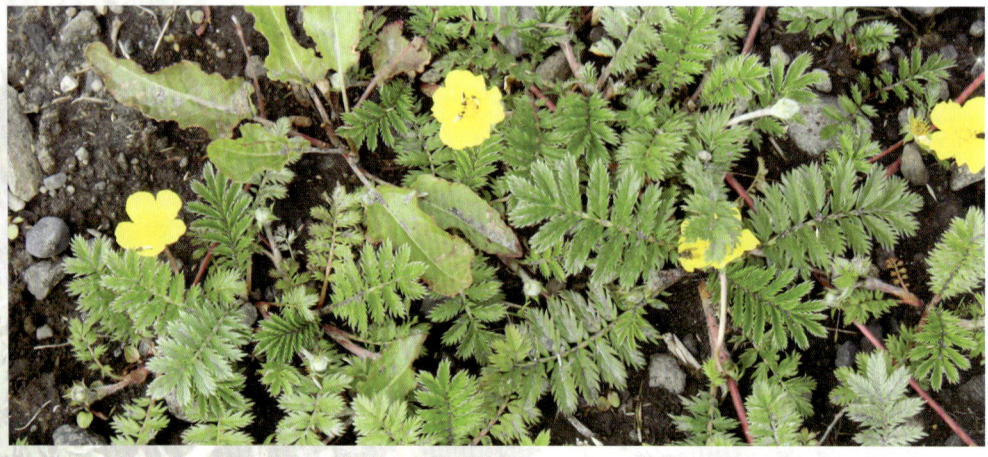

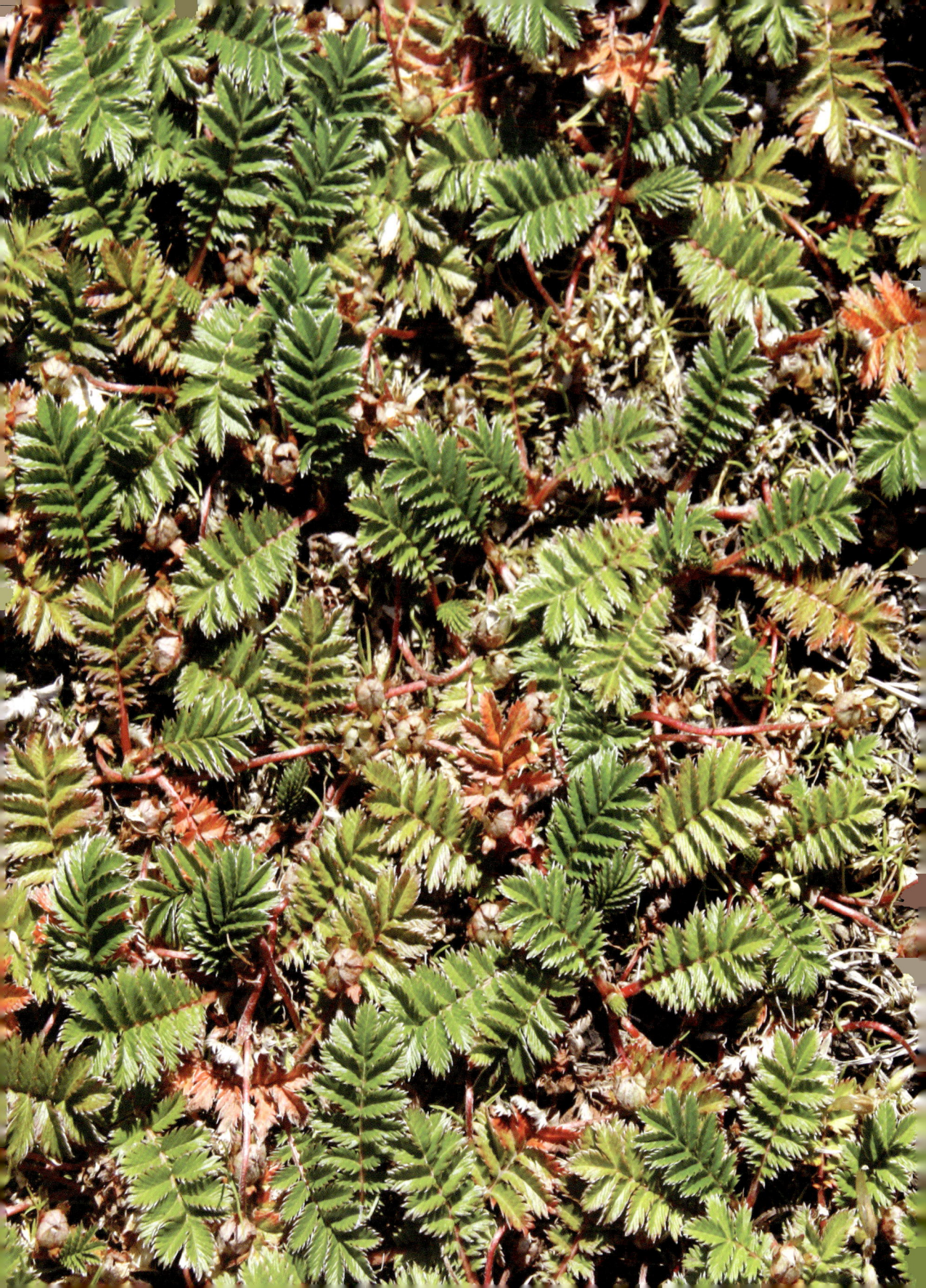

Sorrel

Rumex acetosa
Polygonaceae—Túnsúra

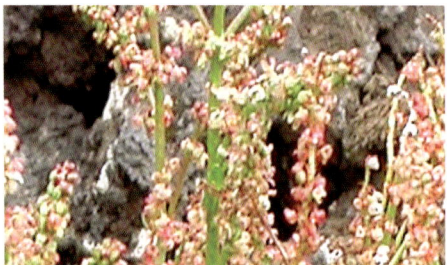

Habitat

Sorrel is common all over Iceland in fields and on heaths.

Parts Used

The entire plant is used, including the root.

Harvesting

The leaves are collected before bloom in May–June and the roots are harvested in autumn.

Constituents

Flavonoids, oxalic acid, vitamins, minerals, and anthraquinones.

History

In the past, the leaves and roots were used to reduce bleeding. Sorrel root is used to dye yarn and an infusion of the stems and leaves was used to polish silver and bast furniture. The juice from Sorrel was also used to remove stains from clothes. Sorrel and other closely related species have been much used in cooking, both in salads and in soups and sauces. The Old English name for Sorrel is Green Sauce, as an English tradition was to make a blend of Sorrel, vinegar, and sugar to have with cold meats.

Action

Mild laxative and diuretic, febrifuge, and cooling.

Uses

Sorrel is not used much in Western herbal medicine nowadays. The leaves of Sorrel are thought to be cooling and both infusions and the fresh juice of the herb are good to drink for fevers. It can also be used for constipation and edema. Sorrel contains vitamin C and was used for scurvy in the past. In China, Sorrel is thought to be powerful against worms, scurvy, fevers, stomach pain, diarrhea, and skin diseases. In Nepal, compresses of Sorrel root are use for dislocations (e.g., when a limb is out of joint, like a shoulder, for instance).

Research

In vitro tests on isolated constituents in Sorrel showed its inhibiting effect on the growth of cancer cells.[1,2]

Dosage

Fresh juice: 1 tablespoon three times a day.

Infusion: 1 teaspoon in a cup three times a day.

Decoction: 1 teaspoon in a cup three times a day.

Infusions and compresses for external use.

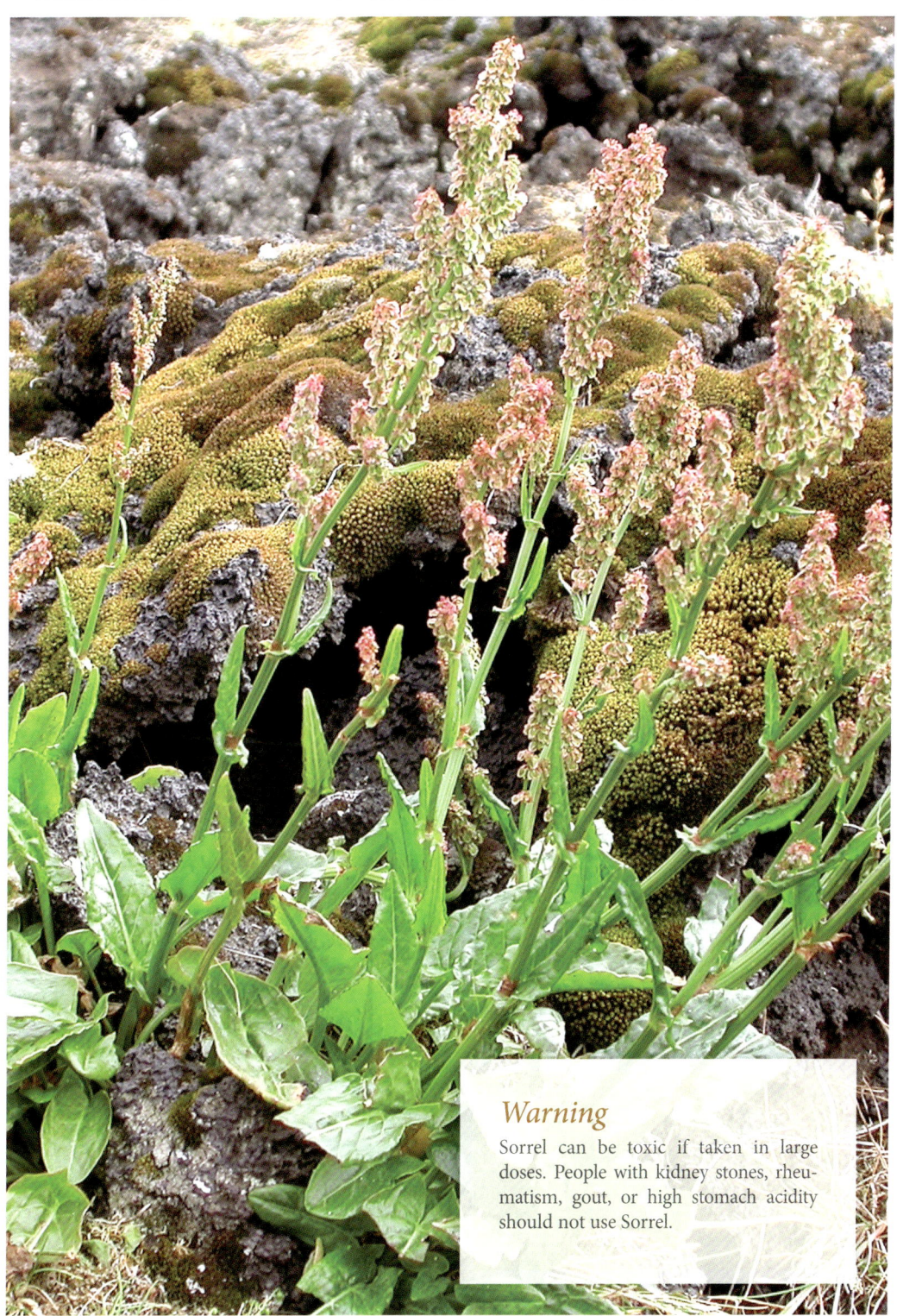

Warning

Sorrel can be toxic if taken in large doses. People with kidney stones, rheumatism, gout, or high stomach acidity should not use Sorrel.

Speedwell

Veronica officinalis
Scrophulariaceae—Hárdepla

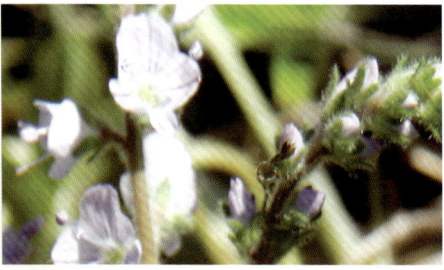

Habitat

Speedwell grows mainly in South and West Iceland in grassy hollows and ravines.

Parts Used

The entire plant is used, except for the root.

Harvesting

Speedwell is harvested just before bloom in July.

Constituents

Iridoids (aucubin), acetophenone glucosides, flavonoids, and saponins.

History

Speedwell was considered an important medicinal herb in Europe in the 16th and 17th centuries. It was thought to be both a diuretic and expectorant and was often used for coughs, tuberculosis, skin diseases, exhaustion, kidney diseases, and arthritis, as well as for healing wounds. In 1935, however, a well-known French herbalist by the name of Leclerc declared that the medicinal power of the tea made from Speedwell was similar to that of the hot water used for the tea. Its use subsequently declined.

The Native Americans also used Speedwell for various ailments, such as coughs and ear infections and for healing wounds. They used the root of Speedwell to ease birth and a decoction was drunk against witchcraft. In Iceland the herb was called a panacea, which indicates that it was a much-valued medicinal herb. *V. chamaedrys, V. serpyllifolia,* and *V. anagallis-aquatica* have also been used in a similar way to Speedwell. *V. anagallis-aquatica* is a rare plant in Iceland and should not be picked.

Action

Stomachic, mild expectorant, mild diuretic, and vulnerary.

Uses

Speedwell is not used much in herbal medicine today and does not rank highly among medicinal herbs. It is thought to stimulate digestion, loosen mucus from the respiratory tract, and heal sores and skin rashes. Speedwell was also considered to be good for the spleen, kidneys, and urinary system, for arthritis, for strengthening the nervous system, and for curbing foot perspiration.

Research

In vivo tests revealed that Speedwell lowered cholesterol in animals that were given cholesterol-rich fodder. When it was given to animals that were fed on fodder with little cholesterol, however, there was no effect.[1] The vulnerary effect of Speedwell on stomach ulcers in animals has also been demonstrated.[2]

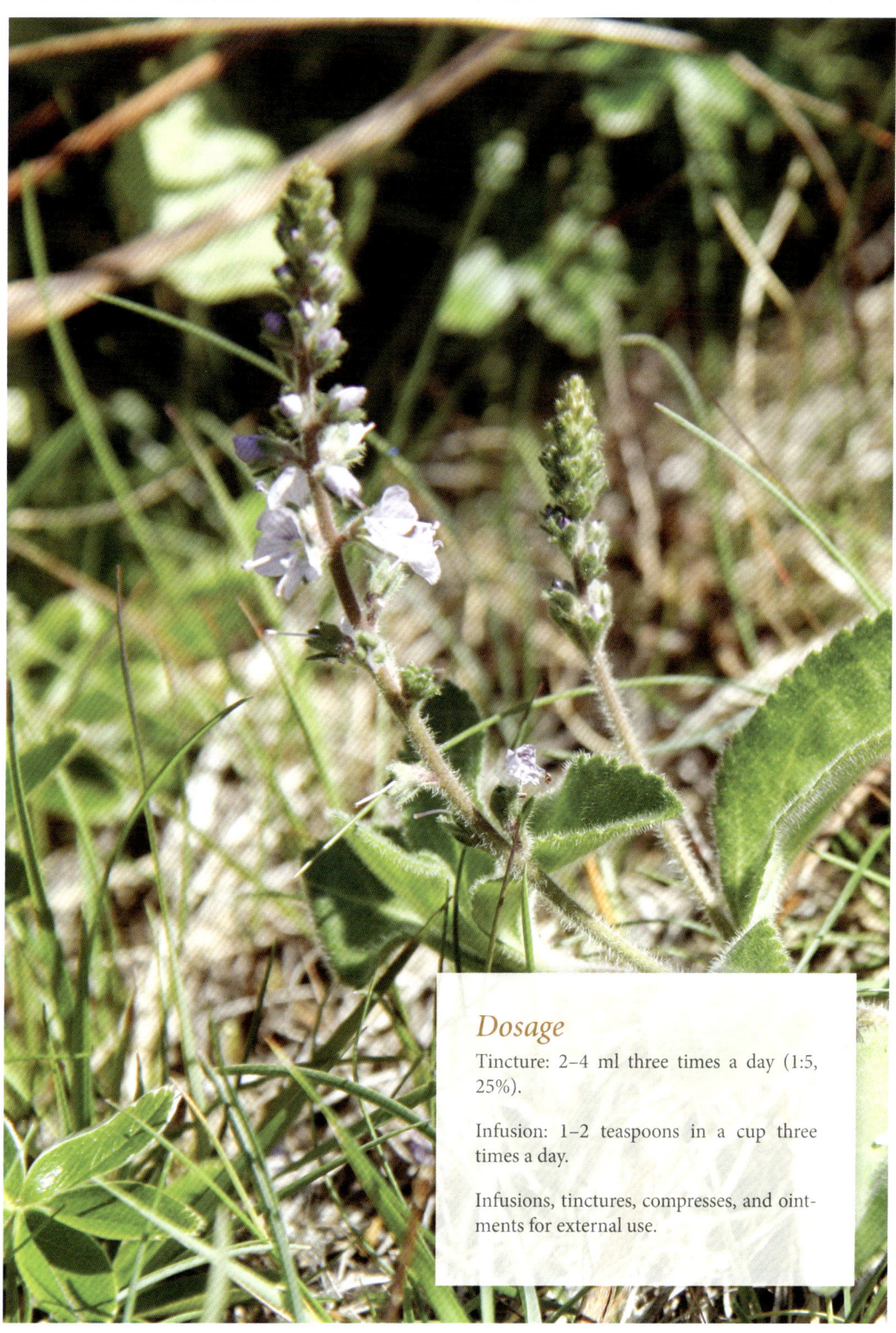

Dosage

Tincture: 2–4 ml three times a day (1:5, 25%).

Infusion: 1–2 teaspoons in a cup three times a day.

Infusions, tinctures, compresses, and ointments for external use.

Spotted Orchid

Dactylorhiza maculata
Orchidaceae—Brönugrös

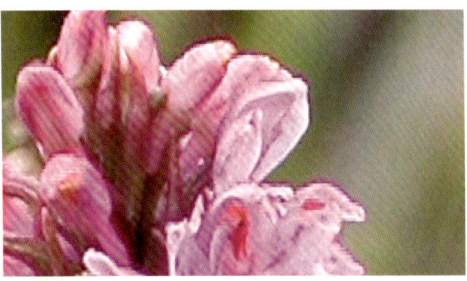

Habitat

Spotted Orchid is found all over Iceland, especially in the South.

Parts Used

Roots.

Harvesting

The root is dug up in autumn and dried.

Constituents

Mucilage, starch, and protein.

History

The former species name for the Spotted Orchid in Latin is *Orchis maculata*, "orchis" meaning testicles in Greek and manhood in Latin. This name refers to the tuberous roots, which are common in the Orchidaceae. The reason for the analogy is because Spotted Orchid, together with other Orchidaceae species, is said to cause sexual arousal and increased fertility. The Old Icelandic name for Spotted Orchid is "elskurót" (love root) or "graðrót" (horny root). Other Icelandic herbs of the Orchidaceae family associated with sexual arousal and fertility are "couple's grass" (*Pseudorchis staminea*) and "love grass" (*Platanthera hyperborea*).

A flour called Salep is made from the roots of Spotted Orchid and related species. This is boiled in milk and honey and is considered to be very nourishing. The word "salep" comes from the Arabic and means fox testicles. Salep was a common drink in England in the 17th and 18th centuries and is still drunk in Turkey and Greece. Salep is one of the ingredients in Turkish Delight.

Action

Nutritive, demulcent, and vulnerary.

Uses

Nowadays, Spotted Orchid is only used occasionally in Western herbal medicine, and then mainly for stopping diarrhea and upset stomachs. It is also thought to strengthen nerves and works well for fatigue.

This herb has great power to strengthen fertility in both men and women, especially the root which increases male arousal, preserves women's menses and ensures a timely birth. The herb is aromatic, especially at night. The new tubers under this herb, lain on evil sores, cleans them well and stops them from decaying further. These same tubers, when boiled in wine, reduce female menses and stimulate urination. The root has tubers of which one sinks and the other floats above. Those who wish to use this herb should steep the harder tuber in fine wine for a while before drinking. Others cook the tubers or eat them raw in milk, and some mix them with sugar like other spices. Ointment can be made from the herb to cure rashes. Internally it is good for gripe and dysentery.

Björn Halldórsson, **Uses of Herbs, 1783**

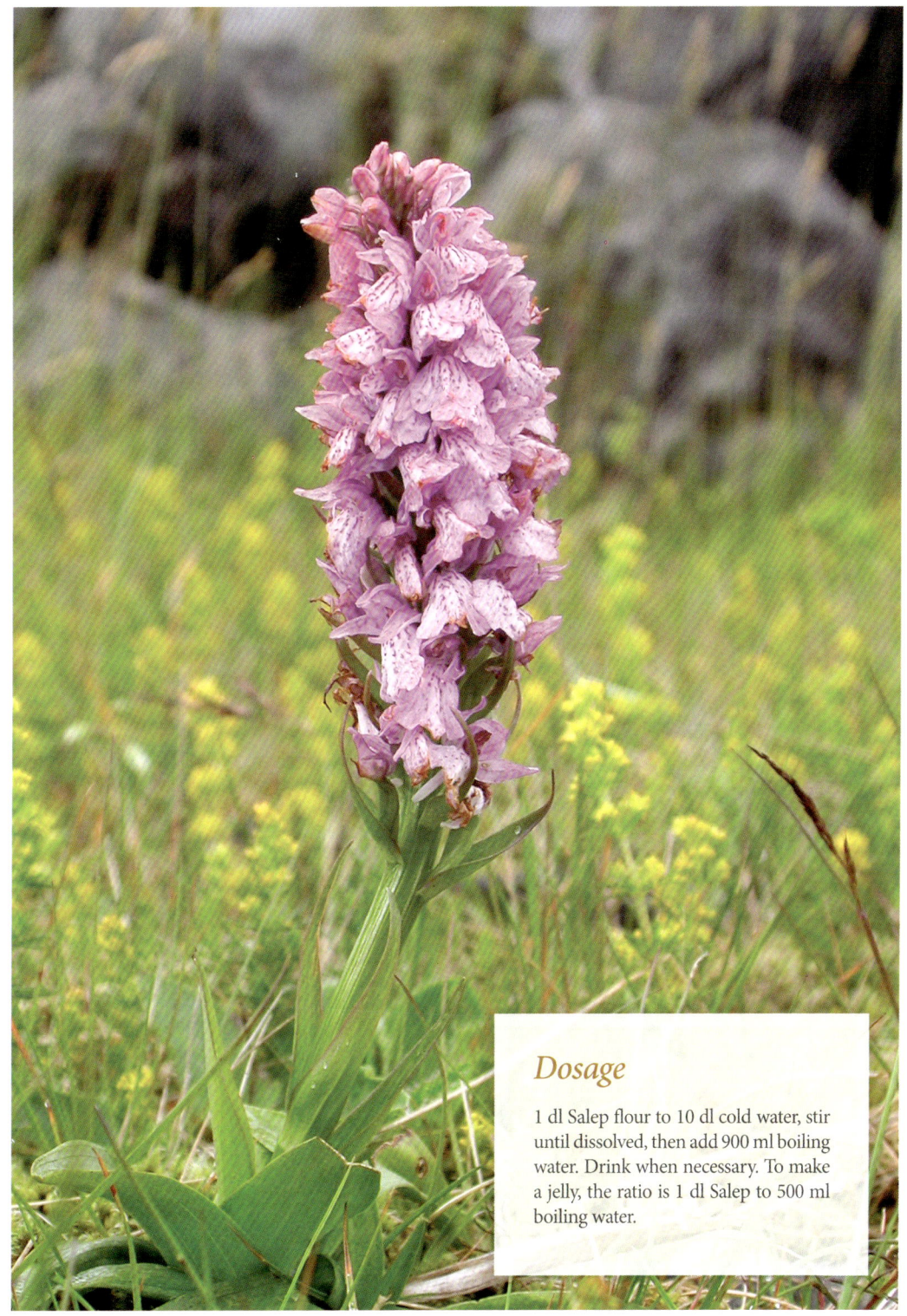

Dosage

1 dl Salep flour to 10 dl cold water, stir until dissolved, then add 900 ml boiling water. Drink when necessary. To make a jelly, the ratio is 1 dl Salep to 500 ml boiling water.

Stinging Nettle

Urtica dioica
Urticaceae—Brenninetla

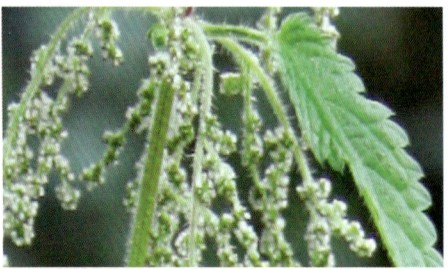

Habitat

Stinging Nettle is an imported species that grows only near farmhouses. It is rare in Iceland but is found in a few places.

Parts Used

The entire plant is used, including the root.

Harvesting

It is collected from early spring until it blooms in July. Gardening gloves are a necessity when harvesting.

Constituents

Leaves: Flavonoids, amines (histamine, choline, acetylcholine, serotonin), glucoquinone, calcium, potassium, silicic acid, and iron. Root: Phytosterols, phenols, and triterpenes.

History

The Latin genus name *Urtica* comes from the verb "urere," meaning to burn or sting, and refers to the burning caused by fresh Nettles. The use of Stinging Nettle as a medicinal herb is centuries old and documentation of its medicinal properties goes back to AD 1. Nettle is rare in Iceland

The root of this big nettle, boiled in wine and doctored with honey, is good for coughs and wheezing and all chest pains because it cleans the lungs well, destroys phlegm and spreads all mucus which has settled and stagnated in the chest. Two or three spoons should be taken evenings and mornings.

Björn Halldórsson, Uses of Herbs, *1783*

This herb promotes urination and has dissolving properties. It provokes women's courses and wet coughs. Of the decoction of the root, which is mixed with an eighth of honey, two spoons shall be taken at a time, 4 times daily. The leaves of the herb have stinging points upon their upper surface; with these it is very good to sting lifeless and insensible limbs of the body.

Oddur Jónsson Hjaltalín,
Icelandic Botany, *1830*

and grows in very few places. Creeping Thistle (*Cirsium arvense*) is often mistaken for Nettle because it stings as well. In fact, elderly Icelanders say that Creeping Thistle was called Nettle when they were young. However, Creeping Thistle does not resemble Nettle and should not be confused with it.

In the past, the fibers of Nettle, which are similar to those of flax and hemp, were used to weave cloth and make paper. They were also used in fish nets, both by the Native Americans and the British. When there was a shortage of cotton during World War I, Nettle fibers were used to make cloth in Europe. Nettle has a very long history as a culinary herb: countless recipes contain Nettle, and when boiled it is similar to spinach. Understandably, fresh Nettle is never used. It is also good for brewing beer, as a dye, and as food coloring.

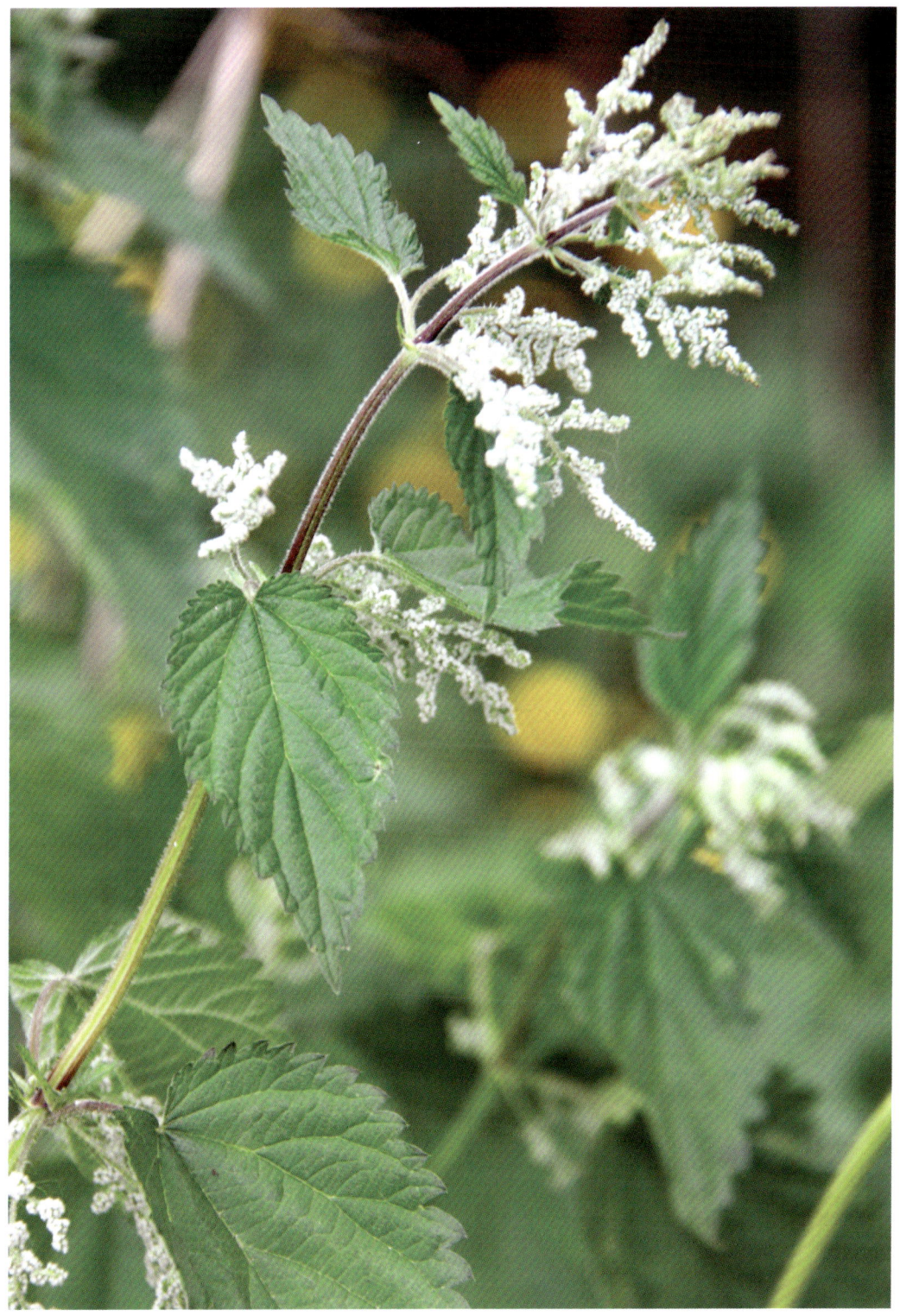

Nettle is considered to be a weed in most countries. It is easy to grow and so is used in gardening, both to repel insects and to make compost. In England, a good home remedy is to rub the leaves of Yellow Dock on Nettle burns in order to counteract the sting quickly. An old remedy for arthritis is to rub fresh Nettle leaves on the painful, swollen area. By doing this, blood flow is stimulated, the area becomes hot as it burns, and after a while the pain in the joints diminishes.

Nettle is used as a medicinal herb all over the world. In Africa, it is traditional to use it for nosebleeds and to stop both menstrual bleeding and internal bleeding. The Native Americans have long used Nettle for arthritic diseases, gynecological diseases, colic, urinary retention, and colds, as well as for stopping bleeding and stimulating hair growth. Old Icelandic folklore says that a safe remedy against magic consists of whipping the wizard with a Nettle wand.

Action

Diuretic, astringent, nourishing, anti-allergic, galactagogue, anti-inflammatory, hemostatic, hypoglycemic, hypotensive, reduces frequent urination, and lowers cholesterol.

. . . .

Uses

Nettle has been a popular medicinal herb since time immemorial and has extremely diverse properties. It is considered to be cleansing and is often used internally for skin problems, while it is thought to be especially good for infantile eczema. Nettle is also reported to be effective for arthritic diseases, especially when edema occurs due to malfunctioning kidneys, as it is a diuretic. It is also excellent for allergies such as hay fever, asthma, skin rashes, itching, and insect bites.

Nettle reduces excessive menstrual bleeding and bleeding after childbirth and is strengthening during menopause. It is also used for urethral inflammation and to prevent small kidney stones. It is thought to be excellent for sores and inflammation in the gastrointestinal tract, as well as for bloating and diarrhea. Nettle is full of minerals and is said to work against anemia and

to stimulate lactation, as well as being a tonic for those who are recuperating after a long illness. Nettle is also thought to lower blood sugar, blood pressure, and cholesterol.

Nettle root is reputed to be excellent for enlarged prostate gland, the symptoms of which include urination that is frequent, nocturnal, or painful or inability to urinate. Externally, Nettle is used for nosebleeds, vaginitis, sciatica, bleeding hemorrhoids, sores, and burns. Another traditional use is to wash hair with the tea or fresh juice, as this is said to stimulate hair growth, prevent hair loss, prevent dandruff, and give the hair a beautiful shine.

Research
Stinging Nettle Root

The effect of Nettle root on the symptoms of benign prostatic hyperplasia (BPH), (e.g., frequent urination and nocturnal urination), has been extensively researched. Two large clinical trials on a total of 904 men with BPH showed positive results with Nettle root and no side effects.[1,2] Many other small clinical trials have also shown positive results.[3] In a few large open clinical trials without placebo, in which over 15,000 men participated, Nettle root showed positive results for frequent urination and nocturnal urination.[4] The effects of Nettle root blended with other herbs on BPH have also been well researched. Large clinical trials on Nettle root and Saw Palmetto (*Serenoa repens*) have shown positive effects on BPH,[5–9] and so has clinical research on Nettle root, avocado oil, and soy oil[10] and Nettle root, Saw Palmetto, and Maritime Pine (*Pinus pinaster*).[11] Similarly, many *in vitro* and *in vivo* tests have shown positive results with Nettle root on BPH.[12,13] Nettle root is also thought to be powerful against chronic bacterial infections in the prostate gland[14] and both the leaves and the root have possible inhibiting effects on cancer cells in the prostate gland.[15–18]

Stinging Nettle Leaves

Five open clinical trials without placebo were done in which the effects of Nettle on arthritic diseases were tested. In these, 10,368 patients participated for 3 weeks to 12 months. In each trial some patients continued to use conventional painkillers while others took only Nettle leaves. 80–95% of the patients evaluated the effects of Nettle as good or very good and 93–95% said they tolerated it well.[4] Other *in vitro* and *in vivo* trials on the anti-inflammatory properties of Nettle showed positive action for arthritic diseases.[19-22] Two clinical trials using Nettle, cod liver oil, vitamin E, and zinc have shown positive results on osteoarthritis.[23,24] A small clinical trial on the diuretic effect of Nettle showed positive results[4] and *in vivo* tests showed the same effects.[25] Positive results were also shown by clinical trials in which the fresh leaf was used externally to produce stinging in chronic joint pain in order to reduce the pain.[26-28]

Many *in vitro* tests have shown the antioxidant action of Nettle leaves[29-44] and have proved that the leaves kill bacteria[42,45] and viruses[46-52] as well as being effective against plant fungus.[53] Some research on Nettle shows its effects on lowering blood sugar,[4,54-61] blood pressure,[4,25,62-64] and cholesterol.[65,66] One study, however, showed that Nettle does not lower cholesterol.[67] Research also shows that Nettle has an anti-inflammatory effect[4,68,69] and a positive effect on colitis.[70]

Other research on Nettle showed it to have a stimulating effect on the immune system,[68,71] a positive effect on hay fever,[72,73] and an analgesic effect.[4] Nettle also has preventive action against heart and coronary disease[74] and protects liver cells in diabetes.[75]

Dosage

Tincture: 4–6 ml three times a day (1:5, 40%).

Infusion: 1–2 teaspoons in a cup three times a day.

Decoction: 1–2 teaspoons in a cup three times a day.

Infusions, decoctions, tinctures, compresses, and ointments used externally.

Warning

The leaves of Nettle have little hairs that sting and burn when touched. These hairs are destroyed by boiling or drying so it is safe to eat boiled nettle leaves or drink tea made with the dried leaves. Only young leaves picked just before bloom should be used for eating or medicinal purposes as the older leaves have particles that could irritate the kidneys. Fresh Nettle is not recommended during pregnancy.

Milk-stimulating Tea

2 parts Stinging Nettle

1 part Caraway seeds

Put 3–4 tablespoons of the blend into a 750 ml vacuum flask and pour boiling water into it. Strain the tea into cups and then put the herbs back into the flask and allow to stand the whole day. Drink from the flask throughout the day.

Stone Bramble

Rubus saxatilis
Rosaceae—Hrútaber

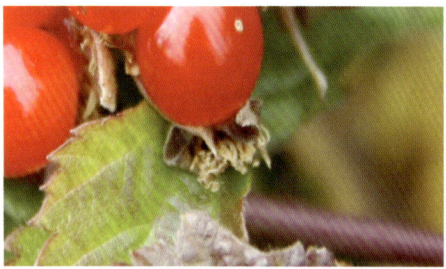

Habitat

Stone Bramble is quite common all over Iceland and grows well on forest floors.

Parts Used

The entire plant is used, including the root and berries.

Harvesting

The leaves are collected just before bloom in early summer, the berries are picked in August, and the root is harvested in autumn.

Constituents

Flavonoids and tannins.

History

Stone Bramble is used as food, mainly for making jam, and it has also been used to dye yarn. Many closely related species to Stone Bramble are used in herbal medicine; Raspberry (*R. idaeus*) is the best known of these. Raspberry leaves are used extensively for infertility and during pregnancy. References state that most of the other *Rubus* species used as medicinal herbs have a similar effect.

Action

Astringent and hemostatic.

Uses

Stone Bramble is not much used in Western herbalism nowadays. Both the dried berries and leaves are said to help with inflammation of the digestive system and diarrhea, but may also be used as a rinse for soreness in the mouth, throat, and vagina. In India, the herb is thought to be good for dysentery and bleeding; there, the root is also used for diarrhea and whooping cough.

Dosage

Tincture: 2–4 ml three times a day (1:5, 40%).

Infusion: 1–2 teaspoons in a cup three times a day.

Decoction: 1–2 teaspoons in a cup three times a day.

Infusions and tinctures used as a rinse.

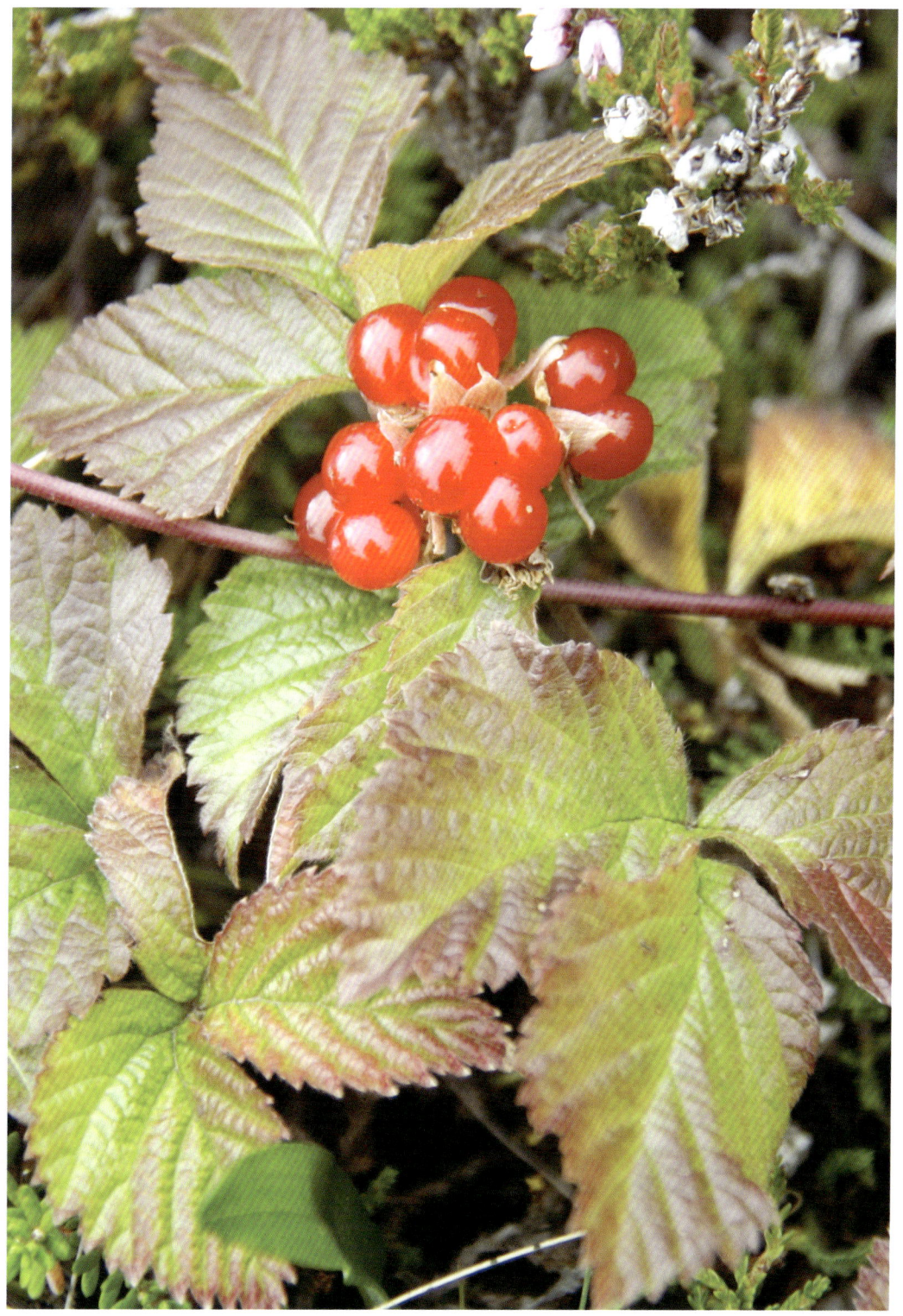

Sundew

Drosera rotundifolia
Droseraceae—Sóldögg

Habitat

Sundew is rather rare, but is found in wetlands in West and North Iceland.

Parts Used

Flowers.

Harvesting

Sundew is both small and rather rare so it is not recommended for picking.

Constituents

Naphthoquinones (plumbagin), flavonoids, enzymes, and essential oils.

History

The Latin name *Drosera* comes from the Greek, meaning dew. The reason for this name is because the drops on the leaves resemble dew but are actually sticky mucus that the leaves produce and use to catch insects. Sundew, like Butterwort, is an insectivorous plant. The Old English name is Lustwort, which refers to its use as an aphrodisiac, in particular for women. The Old Icelandic name is "hringormagras" (ringworm herb), which indicates that this herb was used to eliminate ringworm on the skin. The juice from Sundew has also been used to curdle milk. In the past, a cough syrup of Sundew and Thyme (*Thymus vulgaris*) was readily given to children, while English references from the 15th century reveal that Sundew was thought to be beneficial for sadness and depression.

Action

Antitussive, antibacterial, antifungal, antiviral, antispasmodic, expectorant, and anti-inflammatory.

Uses

There is a long tradition of using Sundew for coughs and lung diseases and it is thought to be especially good for whooping cough, dry cough, and asthma. When used fresh externally, it is also considered useful for warts and corns. Sundew has also been used for both gastritis and stomach ulcers. In China and Nepal a close relative, *Drosera peltata*, is used externally for lymphitis, dysentery, headaches, and arthritis.

Research

In vitro tests on Sundew have shown its antibacterial, antiviral, and antifungal properties.[1] Sundew has also shown anti-inflammatory[2-4] and antispasmodic effects in *in vitro* tests.[4]

Dosage

Tincture: 1–2 ml three times a day (1:5, 60%).

Infusion: ½ teaspoon in a cup three times a day.

Syrup: 1 teaspoon three times a day.

The fresh juice is used externally on warts and corns 1–2 times a day.

Warning

Sundew should only be used internally in small doses, and caution should be exercised when using Sundew externally on warts and corns.

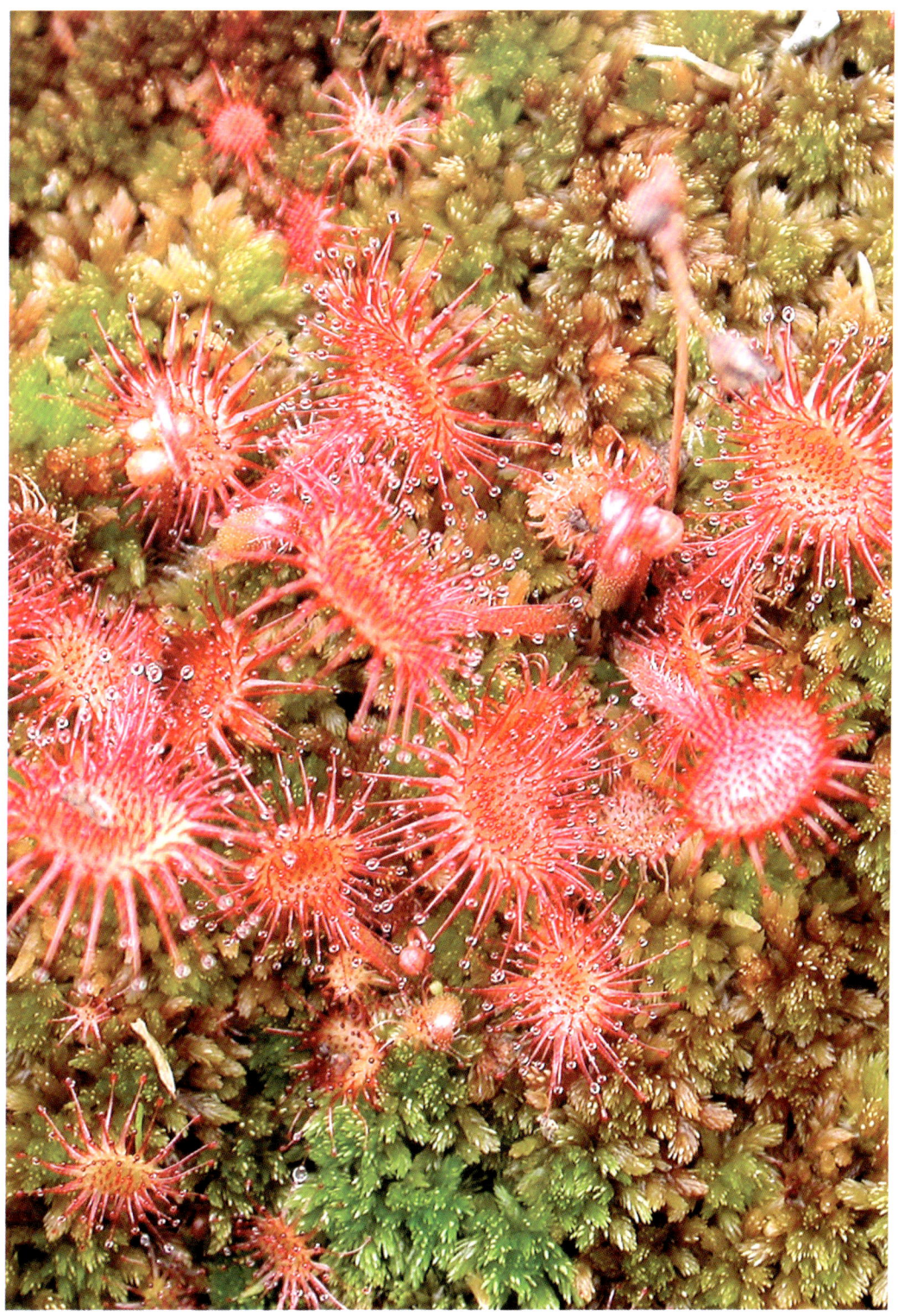

Sweet Cicely

Myrrhis odorata
Apiaceae—Spánarkerfill

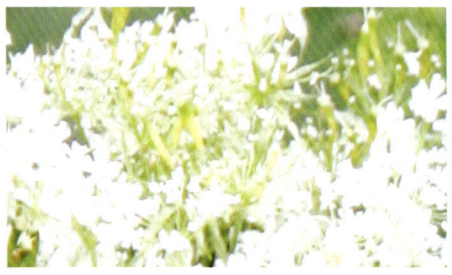

Habitat

Sweet Cicely grows near houses and alongside streams all over Iceland. It is easy to distinguish it from Cow Parsley because it has a strong anise smell and taste.

Parts Used

The entire plant is used, including the root.

Harvesting

The leaves are collected before bloom in June and the seed and roots in autumn.

Constituents

Essential oils and flavonoids.

History

The Latin name *Myrrhis odorata* indicates that Sweet Cicely has a strong smell reminiscent of myrrh. The taste of Sweet Cicely is that of anise and the smell is not unlike that of Lovage (*Levisticum officinale*). The leaves, roots, and seeds have all been used for cooking and the seeds and roots have also been used to flavor liqueur. Sweet Cicely was used as a preventive against the Black Death.

Action

Carminative, stomachic, expectorant, and mild diuretic.

Uses

Sweet Cicely is rarely used in Western herbal medicine nowadays. The decoction of the root is thought to be good for coughs and for releasing mucus, as well as for improving digestion and easing bloating and flatulence. Sweet Cicely is thought to be mildly diuretic and good for anemia and gout. In the past it was also thought to lower blood pressure, while externally Sweet Cicely was considered good for healing old and suppurating wounds. The root was used for snake and dog bites.

Dosage

Tincture: 2–4 ml three times a day (1:5, 40%).

Infusion: 1–2 teaspoons in a cup three times a day.

Decoction: 1–2 teaspoons in a cup three times a day.

Infusions, decoctions, tinctures, compresses, and ointments for external use.

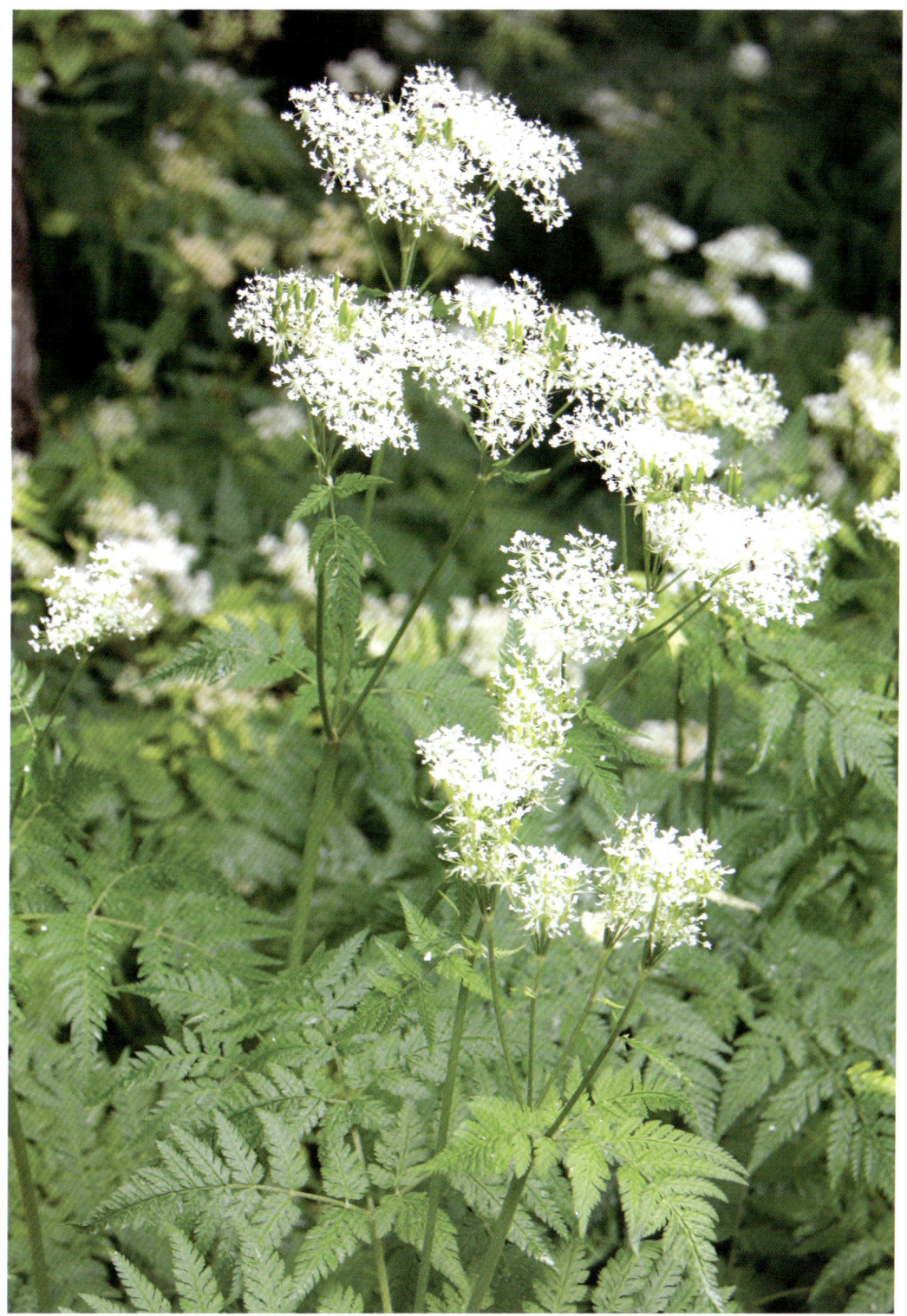

Sweet Grass

Hierochloe odorata
Poaceae—Reyrgresi

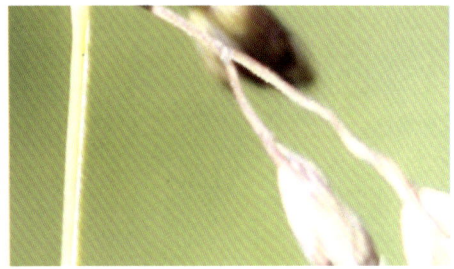

Habitat

Sweet Grass is common all over Iceland and grows in grasslands and on mountainsides.

Parts Used

The entire plant is used, including the root.

Harvesting

All summer.

Constituents

Essential oils.

History

Sweet Grass was used in the past by the Native Americans as incense for holy ceremonies. They also drank an infusion of Sweet Grass for coughs, throat infections, and genital diseases, as well as for stopping vaginal bleeding and for hastening placental birth. Another custom is to place Sweet Grass among clothes to give them a good smell and protect them against moths. The plant was also used as straw and as filling for pillows and mattresses. Sweet Grass leaves were woven into baskets and were also used as perfume and shampoo. The Latin name *odorata* refers to its aromatic quality.

Various common names for this plant (e.g., Sweet Grass and Vanilla Grass), refer to its aromatic nature, while the name Holy Grass refers to its use in holy ceremonies.

Uses

It is not known if Sweet Grass is used in Western herbal medicine nowadays. In the past, it was thought to be diuretic and also strengthened the heart and cleansed the blood, as well as being good for healing external wounds.

Research

In vitro tests have shown that Sweet Grass has antioxidant properties.[1–3]

Dosage

Not known.

Ointments for external use.

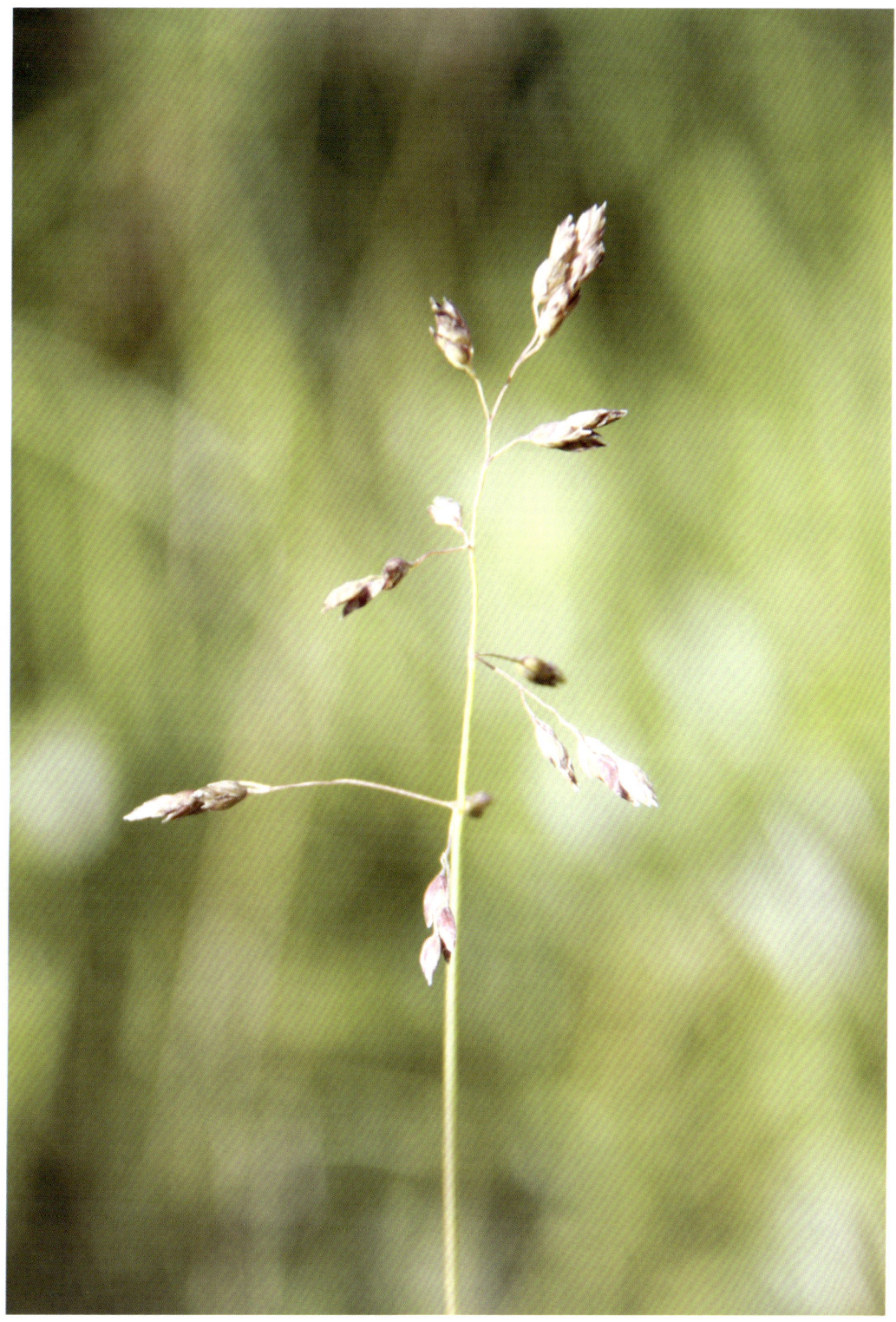

Sweet Vernal Grass

Anthoxanthum odoratum
Poaceae—Ilmreyr

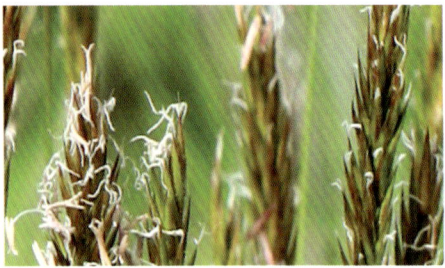

Habitat
It is common all over Iceland.

Parts Used
The entire plant is used, except for the root.

Harvesting
Sweet Vernal Grass is collected all summer after the pollen has fallen or the seeds have formed.

Constituents
Essential oils and coumarin.

History
The Native Americans have used Sweet Vernal Grass for basket-making and in rituals for a long time. During the plant's drying process, coumarin oils emit a characteristic smell as the Icelandic name "Ilmreyr" (scented hay) indicates. In the past, Sweet Vernal Grass was placed among clothes to make them smell good.

Action
Sedative, works against hay fever, and increases blood flow.

Uses
Sweet Vernal Grass is not used much in Western herbal medicine today, but in the past it was used for hay fever. A tincture was made that was sniffed when symptoms of hay fever were evident. Similarly, 3–4 drops of the tincture were taken with water every hour until the symptoms stopped. Sweet Vernal Grass has also been used for insomnia and exhaustion; it is either used externally in a bath or else a few drops of the tincture are taken internally. It is traditionally used as a compress or in a bath for muscle and joint pain and swelling of the hands or feet. Sweet Vernal Grass is part of a well-known blend of German hay, Graminis flos, that has traditionally been used in baths and compresses.

Dosage
Tincture: 3–4 drops every hour for hay fever symptoms (1:5, 25%). The tincture can also be sniffed for this purpose.

Compresses for external use.

Warning
Sweet Vernal Grass contains coumarin, which is a blood thinner and protects against blood clotting and thrombosis. Cases are known in which the coumarin in Sweet Vernal Grass has caused hemorrhaging in animals and even death.[1,2] It is not advisable to take more than 3–4 drops of the tincture at a time, and not more than four times a day.

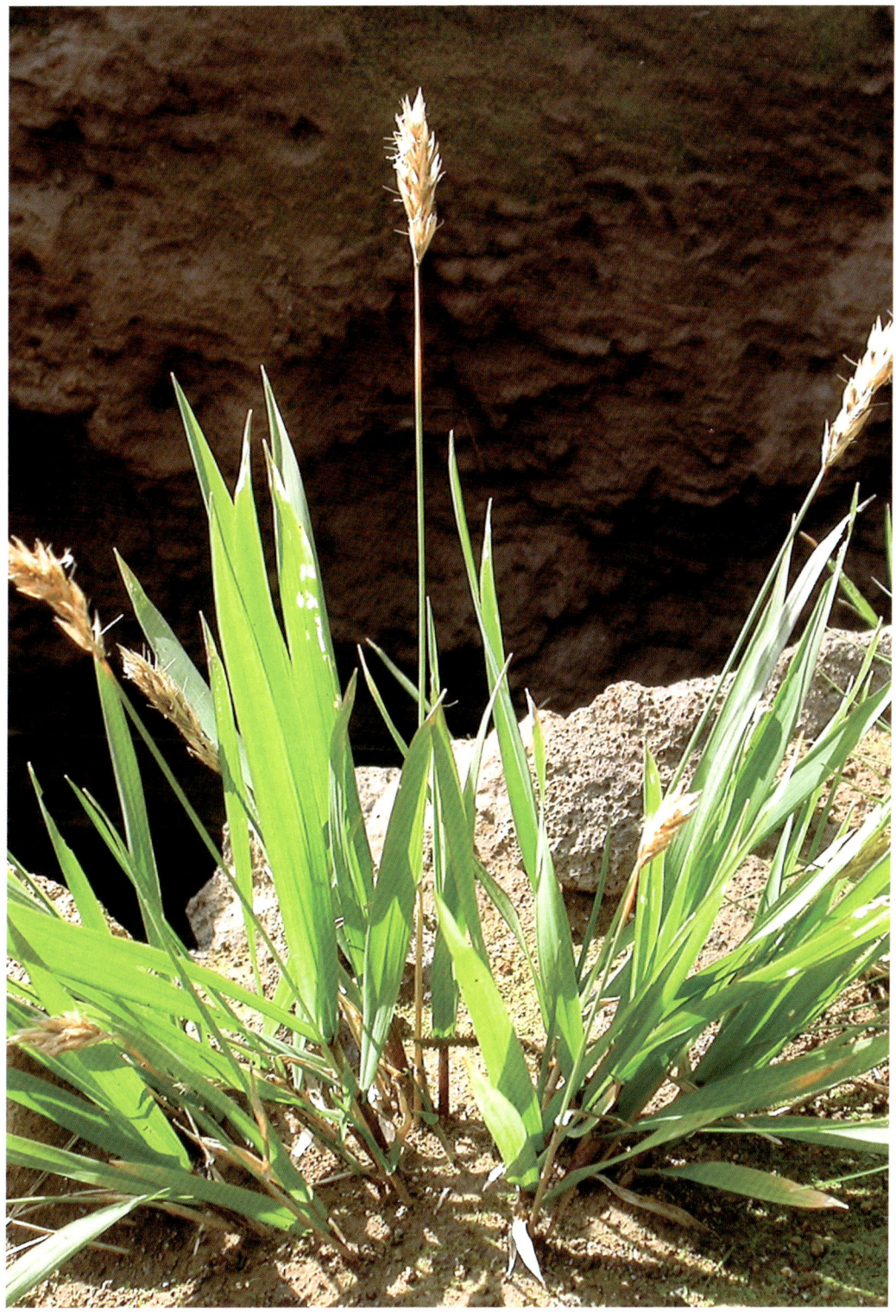

Valerian

Valeriana officinalis
Valerianaceae—Garðabrúða

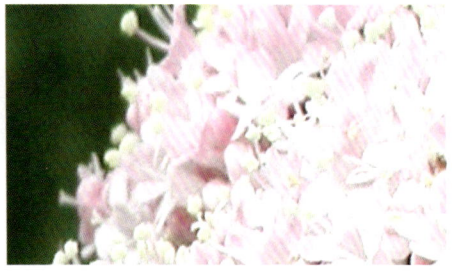

Habitat

Valerian is mainly grown in gardens and is rare as a wild herb.

Parts Used

Root.

Harvesting

The root is harvested in autumn.

Constituents

Essential oils, iridoids, and alkaloids.

History

Valerian has a long history as a medicinal herb, as sources dating back to the 4th century BC document its use for insomnia and its sedative effects. One common explanation of the Latin name *Valeriana* is that it comes from the word "valere," meaning "to be in good health."

A distinctive smell emanates from Valerian, particularly the root, and thus it was called Phu in the past. In the German children's tale about the pied piper from Hamelin, who cleaned the city of rats with his flute playing, it was said that he had Valerian in his pocket. Both rats and cats are very attracted to the smell and the Old Icelandic name for Valerian is "Kattarót" (Cat Root). When cats smell Valerian, they get extremely excited and their pupils dilate, thus it was considered good for eye problems, but it is also thought to increase sexual arousal in men and women. In Britain, Valerian was called All-heal in the Middle Ages as it was considered to be good for many diseases, including epilepsy. Species that are closely related to Valerian are also used all over the world as medicinal herbs.

Action

Sedative, nervine, hypnotic, antispasmodic, analgesic, carminative, and hypotensive.

Uses

Valerian has been used since time immemorial for anxiety and insomnia. It is especially effective for psychological stress, restlessness, hyperactivity, stress, and anxiety attacks. Valerian calms the nerves without disturbing concentration, does not cause sluggishness, and is not addictive. Valerian, taken just before sleep, is excellent for insomnia caused by worry and anxiety or for insomnia caused by muscle or joint pain. Valerian is also antispasmodic and is good for colitis, especially when this is caused by anxiety and stress. It is also good for muscle tension, menstrual cramps, and headaches caused by muscle tension and stress. Valerian

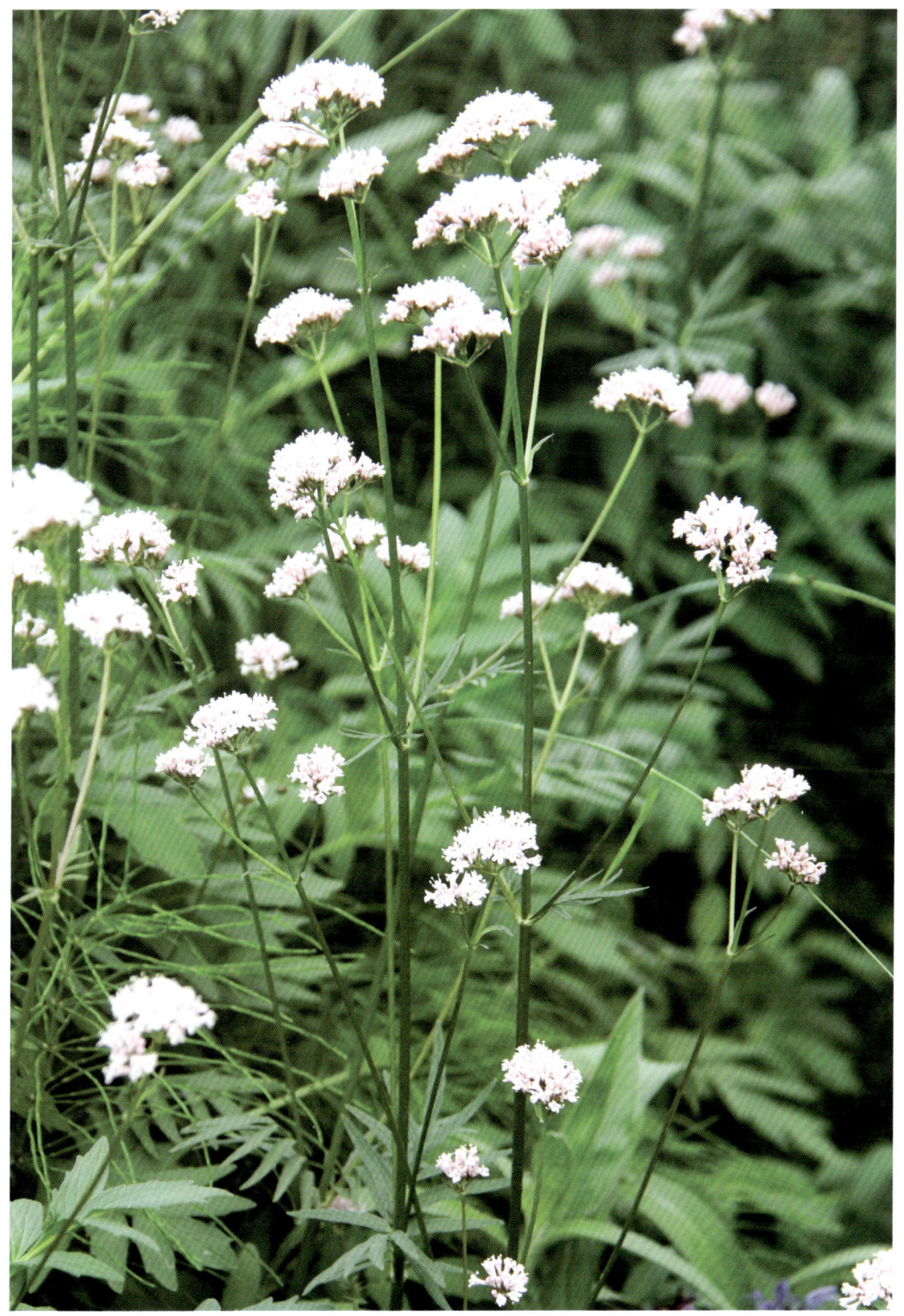

can be used in the bath or topically for muscle pain and it is considered to be a good disinfectant. It is known to lower blood pressure and calm rapid heartbeat.

Unlike many other medicinal herbs that have to be taken for a while before the effects are felt, Valerian works fast if taken in the correct doses and thus it is possible to use Valerian instead of conventional painkillers.

Research

Much of the research, including many clinical trials, reveals its efficacy against insomnia.[1–28] However, some research studies show no effectiveness whatsoever on insomnia.[29–35] Research on Valerian shows that it works well for anxiety and stress[10,11,13,17,18, 31, 36–47] though in one research trial the opposite is found.[48] Research has also demonstrated the usefulness of Valerian mixed with other herbs for insomnia and anxiety, namely Valerian and Hops (*Humulus lupulus*) or St. John's Wort (*Hypericum perforatum*).[13, 49–56] Clinical trials on 918 children under the age of 12 revealed the positive effects of Valerian and Lemon Balm (*Melissa officinalis*) for sleeplessness and restlessness.[57] Valerian it also good for depression,[31,58] epilepsy,[59] and Restless Leg Syndrome.[60]

In other research, Valerian is found to have antibacterial,[61,62] antifungal, and antioxidant properties.[61,63] It was also found to be an immune stimulant[64,65] and anti-carcinogenic.[66] Research has also shown that it has a relaxing effect on uterine muscles[67] as well as being a general muscle relaxant and vasodilator.[68–70] One research study, however, showed that it had no effect as a muscle relaxant.[31] Valerian is effective against angina,[71] can lower blood pressure[68] and can reduce withdrawal symptoms of morphine.[72] Clinical research shows that Valerian has no effect on male fertility[73] and does not damage animal fertility or animal fetuses.[13,74]

Dosage

Tincture: 2–6 ml three times a day (1:5, 40%).

Cold decoction: 1–2 teaspoons in a cup of cold water, allowed to steep overnight. 1 cup three times a day.

Decoctions, tinctures, compresses, and ointments for external use.

Warning

In some cases, Valerian can have the opposite effect (i.e., stimulate rather than sedate), and may cause insomnia.

Insomnia Remedy

1 tablespoon Valerian tincture or 1 cup of Valerian decoction. Take 1 hour before sleep.

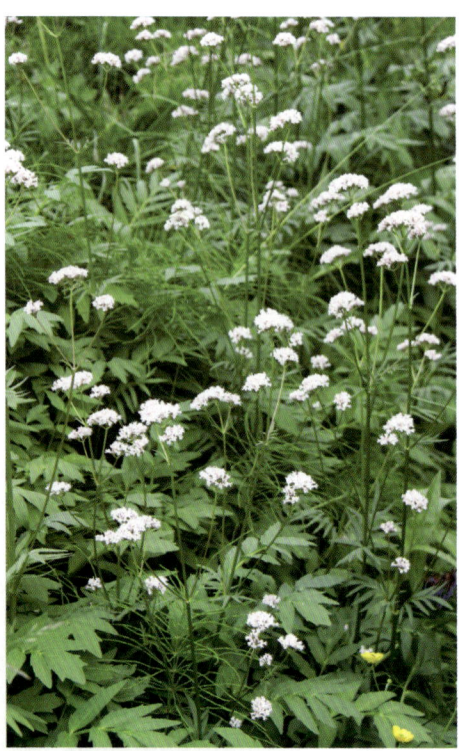

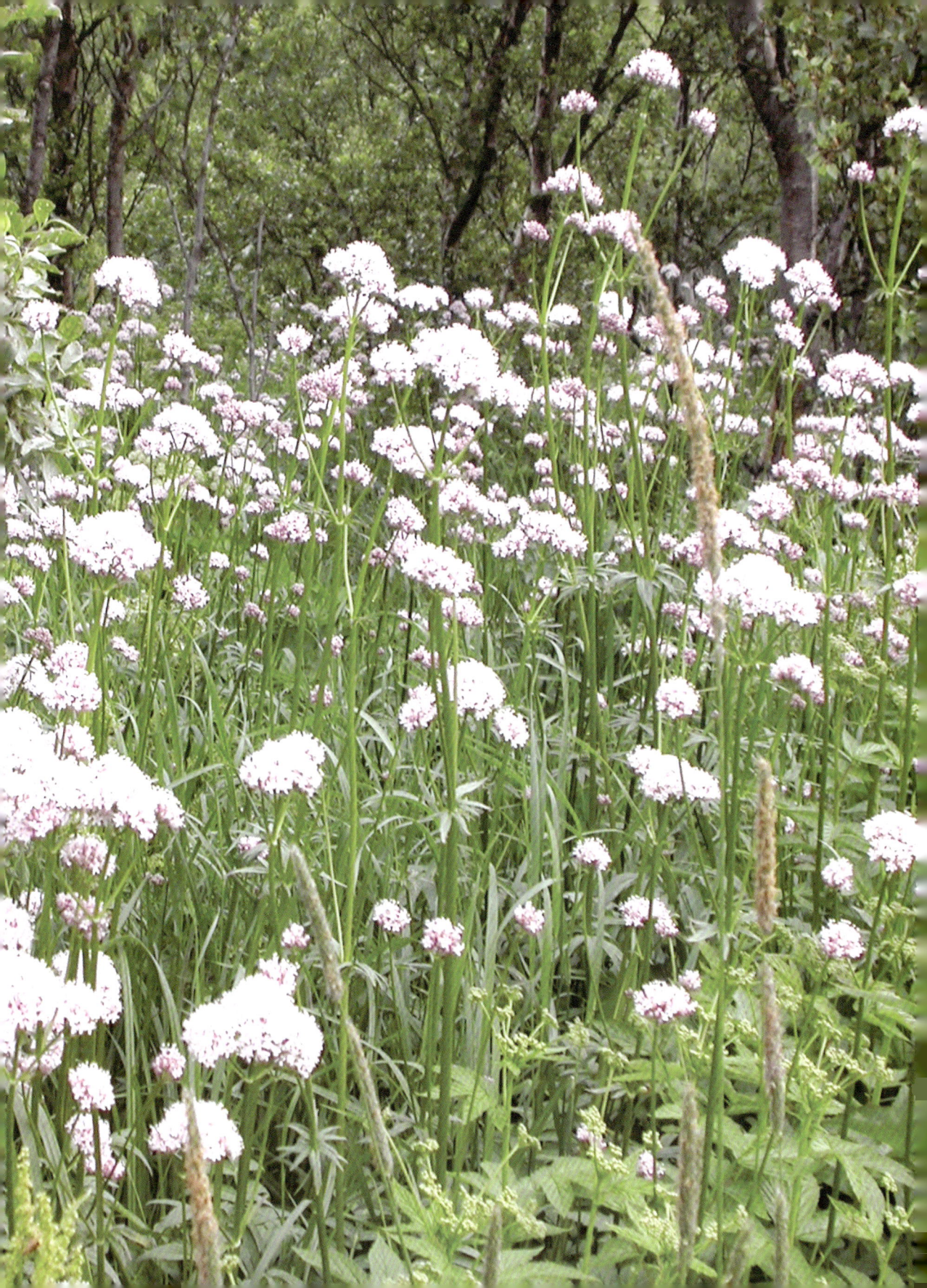

Water Avens

Geum rivale
Rosaceae—Fjalldalafífill

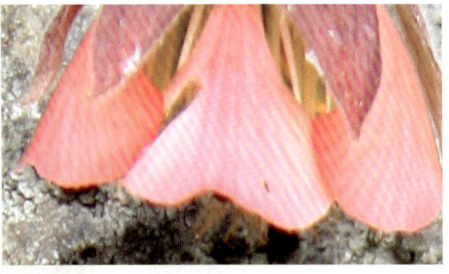

Habitat

Water Avens lives on damp heaths and in ravines and prefers moist earth. It is common all over Iceland except in the Southeast.

Parts Used

The entire plant is used, including the root.

Harvesting

Water Avens is picked while in bloom in June–July. The root is dug up in spring, as that is when the essential oils are most potent. It does not keep well and is best stored in vacuum-packed bags. It should only be ground when needed.

Constituents

Tannins, phenolglycoside, and essential oils.

History

The Latin genus name *Geum*, derived from the Greek word "geno," means aromatic. A pleasant smell reminiscent of clove emanates from the root when it is dug up in spring; this is due to the active substance eugenol, which is also found in clove buds. The Old Icelandic name for Water Avens is in fact "negulrót" (clove root). In North America, it has been called Indian Chocolate and Cure-All. The decoction from the root is thought to resemble the taste of chocolate, and was used quite a lot by the Native Americans, who often gave it to their children. It was considered good for diarrhea, dysentery, colds, coughs, and tuberculosis.

Action

Astringent, hemostatic, antibacterial, and anti-inflammatory.

Uses

Water Avens has been used to stop bleeding wounds and diarrhea for a long time. Usually the ground roots were used, although both the flowers and leaves were also used. Water Avens is good as a mouthwash for gingivitis and other inflammations of the mouth. The decoction is used in bath water for open wounds or hemorrhoids. Water Avens is also used for vaginal discharges, heavy menstrual bleeding, and spotting.

Research

In vitro testing has shown antibacterial and anti-inflammatory properties[2] of Water Avens.

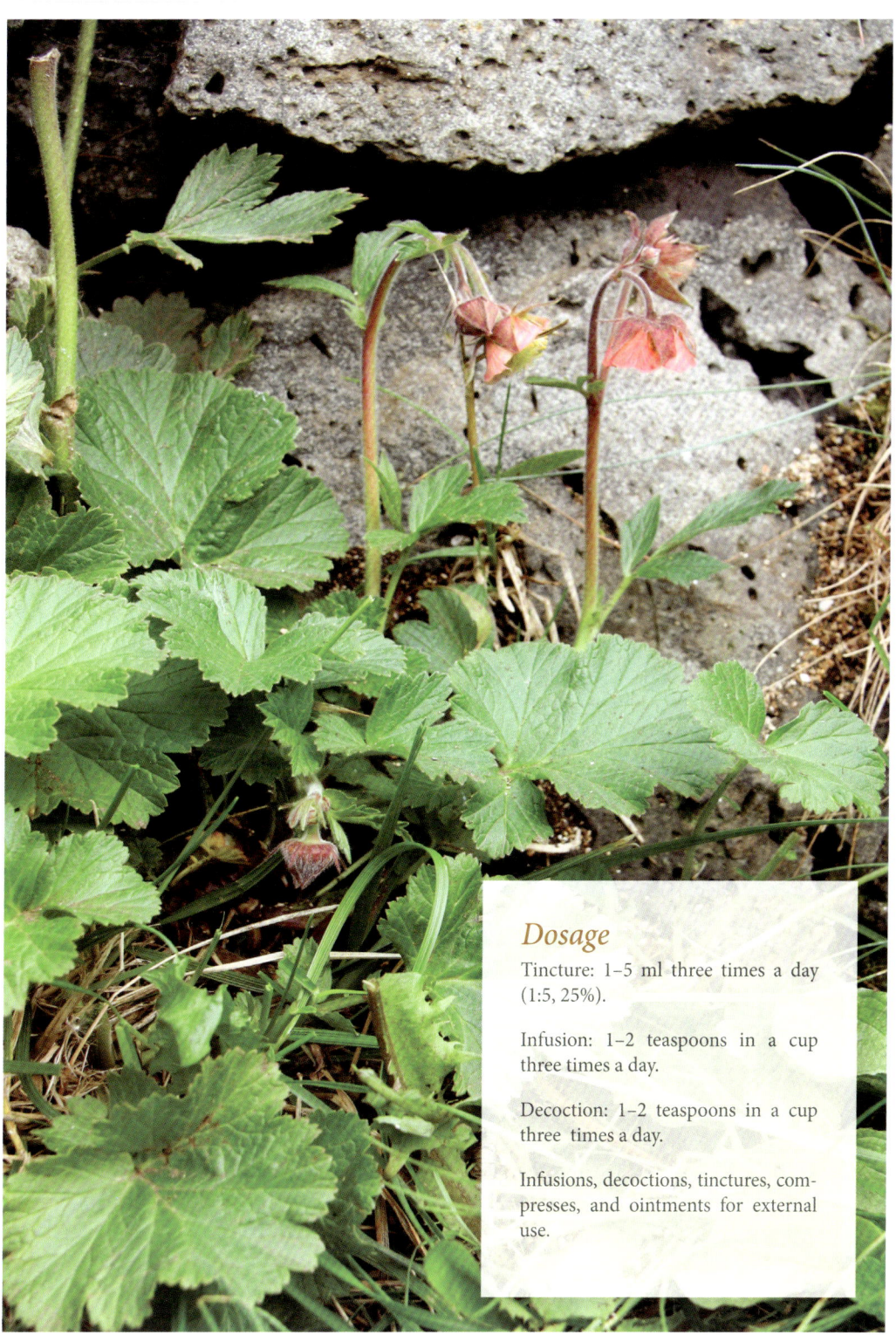

Dosage

Tincture: 1–5 ml three times a day (1:5, 25%).

Infusion: 1–2 teaspoons in a cup three times a day.

Decoction: 1–2 teaspoons in a cup three times a day.

Infusions, decoctions, tinctures, compresses, and ointments for external use.

Water Forget-me-not

Myosotis scorpioides
Boraginaceae—*Engjamunablóm*

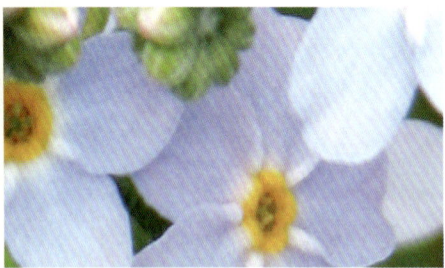

Habitat

Water Forget-me-not is originally an imported species and now grows alongside streams and rivers. It is rather rare and grows only in the northern part of Iceland.

Parts Used

The entire plant is used, except for the root.

Harvesting

It is collected in bloom in July.

Constituents

Not known.

Action

Expectorant.

Uses

Water Forget-me-not is seldom used as a medicinal herb in Western herbal medicine today. In the past, it was used in cases of lung diseases and whooping cough in syrup form. In France, it is considered to be beneficial as an external application for tired eyes, and internally for tiredness and sadness.

Dosage

Tincture: 2–4 ml three times a day (1:5, 25%).

Infusion: 1–2 teaspoons in a cup three times a day.

Syrup: 1–2 teaspoons three times a day.

Infusions and tinctures for external use.

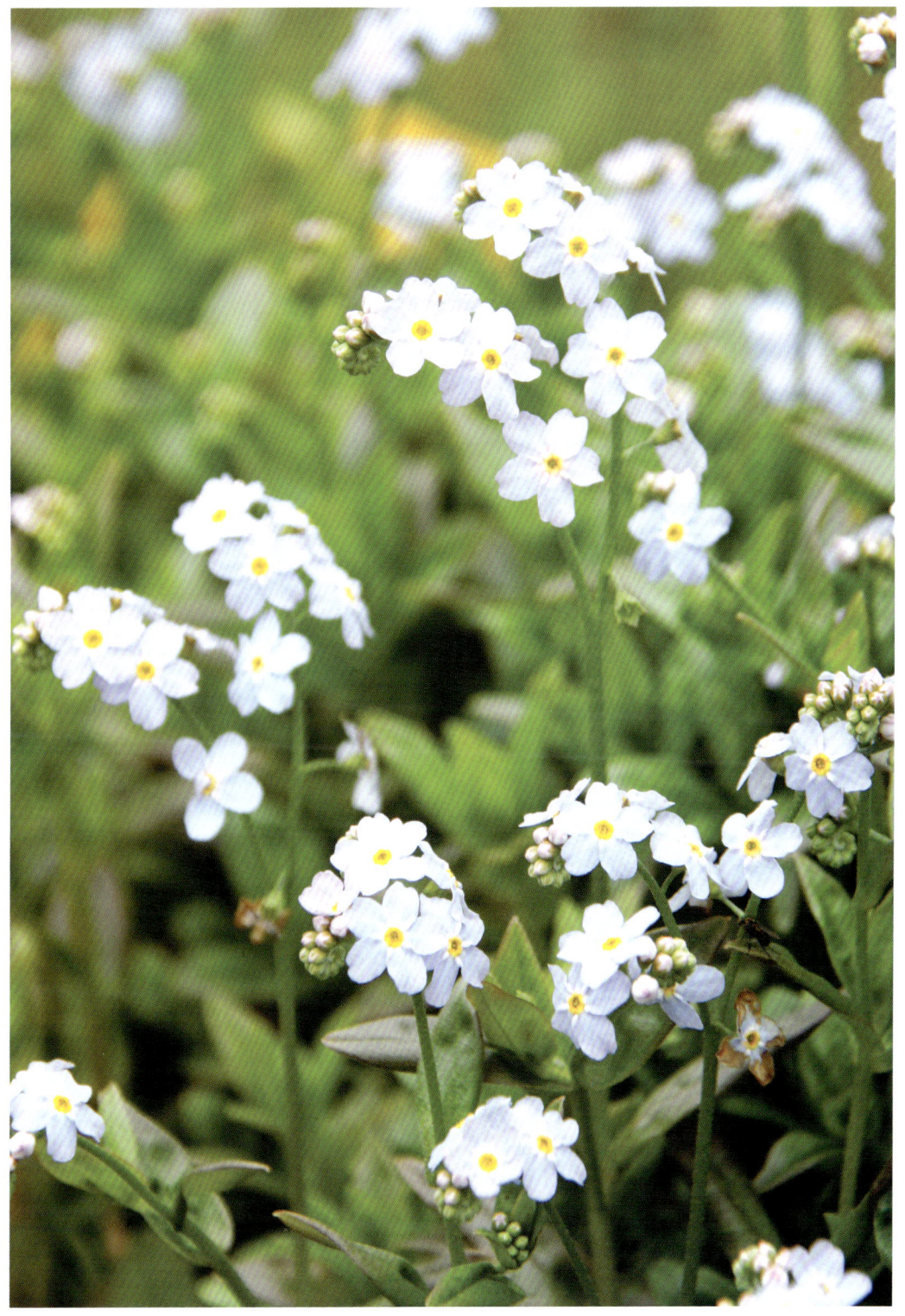

Water Speedwell

Veronica anagallis-aquatica
Scrophulariaceae—Laugadepla

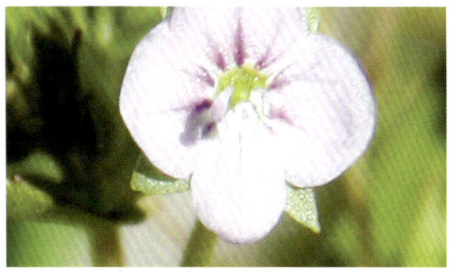

Habitat

Water Speedwell is rare and is only found in geothermal areas in Southwest Iceland.

Parts Used

The entire plant is used, except for the root.

Harvesting

Due to its rarity, collecting Water Speedwell is not recommended.

Constituents

Iridoid glycosides (aucubin) and phenylethanoid glycosides.

History

In old references, Water Speedwell was normally put in the same category as Speedwell as they were thought to have similar qualities.

Action

Astringent, anti-inflammatory, and vulnerary.

Uses

Water Speedwell is not used much in Western herbal medicine nowadays. In Turkey, it is thought to be good for arthritis, both as an anti-inflammatory and analgesic. In China, the root is used for fevers, hemorrhoids, and as a rinse for mouth and throat infections. In Korea, the root of Water Speedwell is considered good for beriberi, digestive disturbances, and white vaginal discharges. In India, the roots, leaves, and flowers are used against edema and to stimulate appetite, while the leaves are thought to be blood cleansing and effective against scurvy. In addition, the fresh, bruised leaves are considered to be vulnerary and are used externally on wounds, burns, and viral infections on the tips of fingers.

Research

In vitro testing of Water Speedwell in Turkey has indicated that it is both anti-inflammatory and analgesic. This is consistent with the Turkish traditional use of Water Speedwell for rheumatism.[1]

Dosage

Tincture: 2–4 ml three times a day (1:5, 25%).

Infusion: 1–2 teaspoons in a cup three times a day.

Infusions, tinctures, compresses, and ointments for external use.

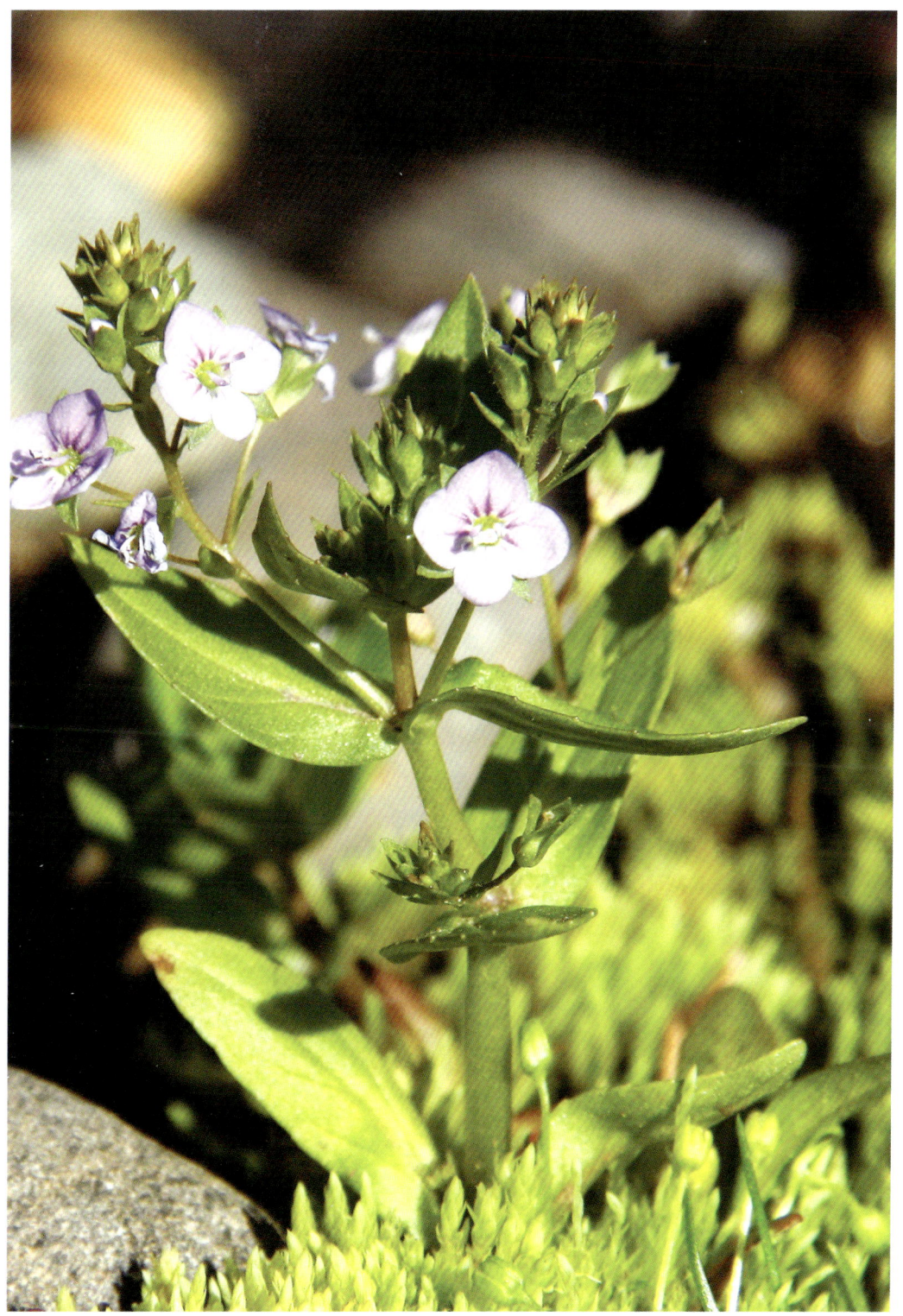

White Dead-nettle

Lamium album
Lamiaceae—Ljósatvítönn

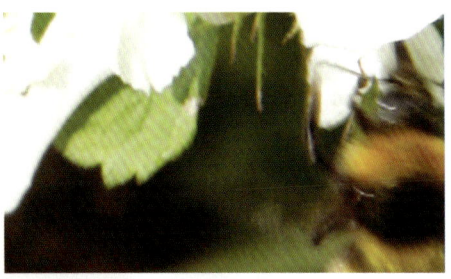

Habitat

White Dead-nettle is an imported species that is found near farms, mainly in Northwest Iceland.

Parts Used

The entire plant, except for the root.

Harvesting

White Dead-nettle is collected in bloom in June.

Constituents

Phenylpropanoids, iridoids, tannins, flavonoids, and saponins.

History

The name White Dead-nettle indicates that despite the leaves being similar to those of Stinging Nettle, they do not sting. It is closely related to Stinging Nettle and has long been used medicinally in a similar way. White Dead-nettle was considered especially good for gynecological diseases and there are references dating back to the Middle Ages to its use in such diseases. It is also used for cooking, in a similar way to spinach.

Action

Astringent, hemostatic, anti-inflammatory, diuretic, expectorant, mild sedative, demulcent, and vulnerary.

Uses

White Dead-nettle has been used for centuries, mainly to ease heavy menstrual bleeding, spotting, and post-partum bleeding. Similarly, it has been traditionally used, both externally and internally, for vaginal discharges caused by fungal and other infections as well as for menstrual pain and symptoms of menopause. White Dead-nettle is also said to be good for diarrhea and flatulence and, externally, for wounds, hemorrhoids, and varicose veins. It is thought to lessen mucus in the respiratory tract and is effective for bladder problems, insomnia, anemia, and inflammation of the prostate gland.

Research

In vitro tests on White Dead-nettle have revealed that it has antioxidant properties[1] and anti-inflammatory and diuretic action,[2] while also being a vulnerary for wounds.[3] Isolated constituents of the flowers of White Dead-nettle have shown antiviral effects against hepatitis C.[4]

Dosage

Tincture: 2–5 ml three times a day (1:5, 25%).

Infusion: 1–2 teaspoons in a cup three times a day.

Infusions, tinctures, compresses, and ointments for external use.

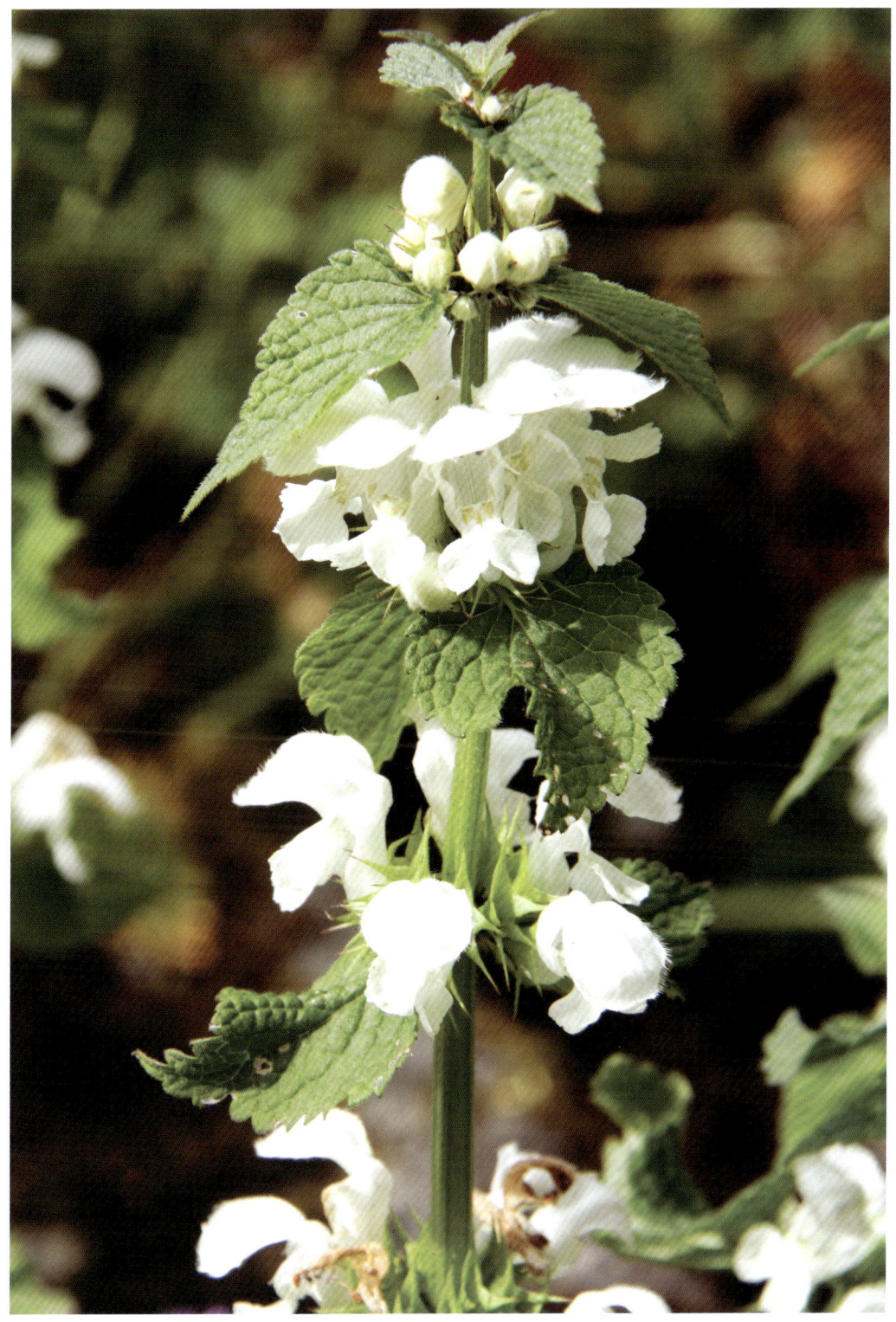

233

Wild Strawberry

Fragaria vesca
Rosaceae—*Jarðarber*

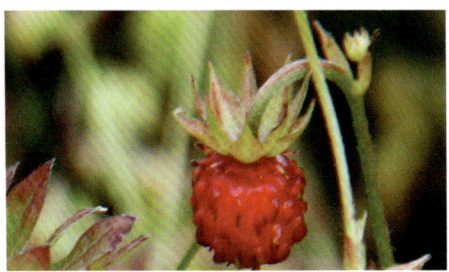

Habitat

Wild Strawberry is quite common all over Iceland and grows on sunny hillsides.

Parts Used

The entire plant is used, including stolons, roots, and berries.

Harvesting

The leaves and stalks are collected in May–June, the berries are picked in August, and the roots are harvested in autumn.

Constituents

Leaves: Flavonoids (quercitrin), tannins, essential oils. Berries: Fruit acids, essential oils.

History

Note that the strawberry plant discussed here is the plant that grows wild in Iceland and not the farmed varieties found in grocery stores. The farmed varieties are not considered to have the same qualities as Wild Strawberry. The Native Americans used the leaves and roots of Wild Strawberry for diarrhea but also ground them into a powder to put over wounds, both for disinfecting and for healing. They also placed a wad of leaves under the armpit as a deodorant. The berries were used in food. Wild Strawberry was considered a good tooth whitener and skin lightener and it was used to relieve sunburn.

Action

Mild astringent and diuretic.

Uses

Wild Strawberry is not used much in Western herbal medicine today. The roots and leaves of the plant are astringent and are used for diarrhea and dysentery, as a mouthwash for gingivitis and sore throats, and externally for minor wounds. The leaves and roots are thought to work well for vaginal discharges and have also been used for urinary tract infections. The berries are thought to have a diuretic and cooling effect as well as being a mild laxative. Both plant and berries are considered to be good for arthritis and gout. In Tibet, the plant is thought to be a febrifuge, is said to stop bleeding, and is typically used for respiratory diseases.

Research

Both *in vitro* and *in vivo* testing showed that Wild Strawberry leaves could lower blood pressure. Its action was thought to be similar to Hawthorn (*Crataegus oxyacantha*), which has been used for centuries to lower blood pressure.[1] The leaves of Wild Strawberry contain salicylic acid, which is anti-inflammatory,[2] while they are also considered to have considerable antioxidant properties.[3,4]

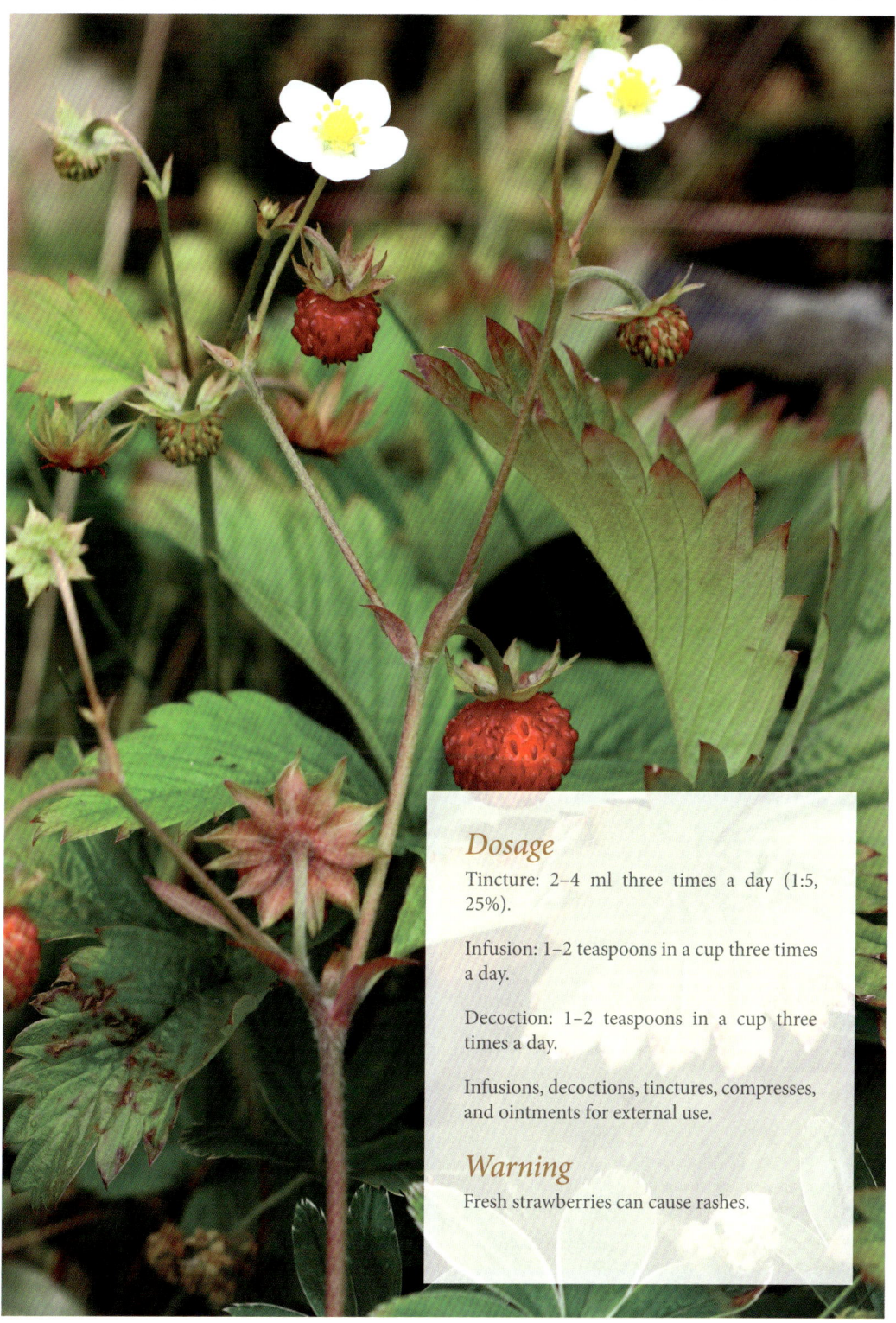

Dosage

Tincture: 2–4 ml three times a day (1:5, 25%).

Infusion: 1–2 teaspoons in a cup three times a day.

Decoction: 1–2 teaspoons in a cup three times a day.

Infusions, decoctions, tinctures, compresses, and ointments for external use.

Warning

Fresh strawberries can cause rashes.

Willow

Salix spp.
Salicaceae—Víðir

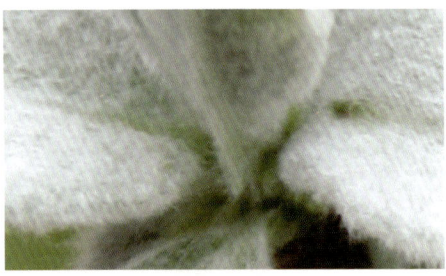

Habitat

Several Salicaceae species are very common in Iceland, namely Arctic Willow (*S. arctica*), Dwarf Willow (*S. herbacea*), Tea-leaved Willow (*S. phylicifolia*), and Woolly Willow (*S. lanata*). A few imported garden species have also spread, such as Alaska Willow (*S. alaxensis*) and Goat Willow (*S. caprea*). It is difficult to distinguish between the Willows as they are often very similar in appearance and cross-pollination is common between species.

Parts Used

Bark, leaves, and young branches.

Harvesting

Willows are collected in early summer before blossoming.

Constituents

Phenolic acids (salicylic acid), tannins, and flavonoids.

History

Of the many Willows that are used for medicinal purposes, the White Willow (*S. alba*) is the most well known and there are ancient references to its medicinal powers. In other references, mention is often made of *Salix* spp. or Willow in general, and no distinction is made between species regarding their medicinal powers. Willows contain salicylic acid, which is analgesic and anti-inflammatory and is the natural precursor of aspirin.

In the past, the seed fluff was used instead of cotton wool to cover wounds while the ash of the bark was used to remove warts, corns, and leg hair. Willow was also used to make ink, together with Bearberry. There are many references to the medicinal use of various Willow species among the Native Americans. They used Willow for diarrhea, fevers, and coughs, for increasing lactation, and for any sort of pain. Externally, Willow was thought to be good for bleeding wounds and hemorrhoids, as well as for leg cramps, sore eyes, broken bones, mouth ulcers, and blisters.

Action

Astringent, febrifuge, analgesic, antibacterial, anti-inflammatory, and reduces perspiration.

Uses

There is a long tradition of using Willow species for medicinal purposes. Willow is considered to be both analgesic and anti-inflammatory and it has been traditionally used, both externally and internally, for all kinds of arthritic disease as well as for muscle and back pain. It is also good for colds, influenza, fevers, headaches, migraines,

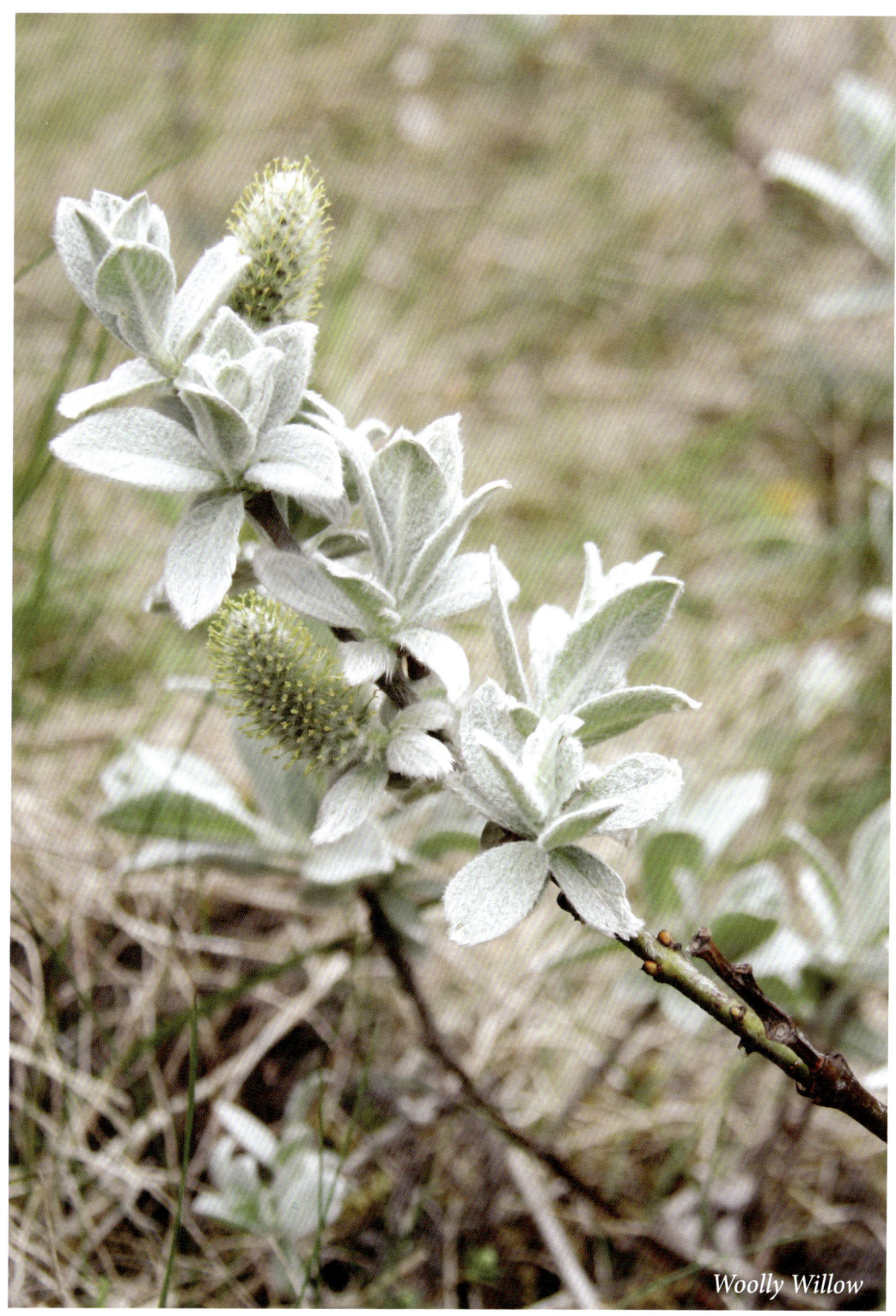

Woolly Willow

and other types of pain. Willow is thought to be a disinfectant and is used externally to clean and heal wounds. During menopause, Willow can reduce sweating, hot flashes, and night sweats. Willow is also astringent and was formerly used to reduce internal bleeding and diarrhea.

Research

Several clinical trials on *Salix alba* have revealed analgesic effects on chronic back pain, osteoarthritis, rheumatism, headache, and migraine. Further research on *S. alba* with both *in vitro* and *in vivo* tests shows anti-inflammatory, febrifugals, and blood-thinning action.[1] *In vitro* tests on *S. caprea* show that it is anti-inflammatory,[2] has antioxidant properties,[3,4] and can inhibit the growth of cancer cells.[4]

Dosage

Tincture: 3–6 ml three times a day (1:5, 25%).

Infusion: 1–2 teaspoons in a cup three times a day.

Decoction: 1–2 teaspoons in a cup three times a day.

Infusions, decoctions, tinctures, compresses, and ointments for external use.

Warning

It is known that Willows can cause allergies, especially in those who are allergic to aspirin. The use of Willow is not recommended for those on blood-thinning medication.

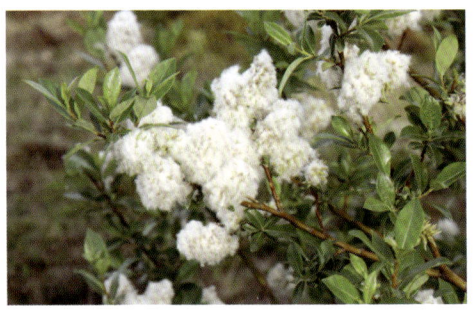

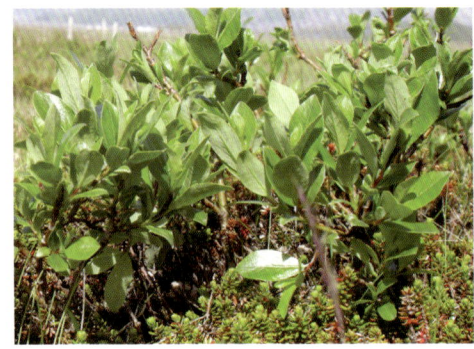

Tea-leaved Willow

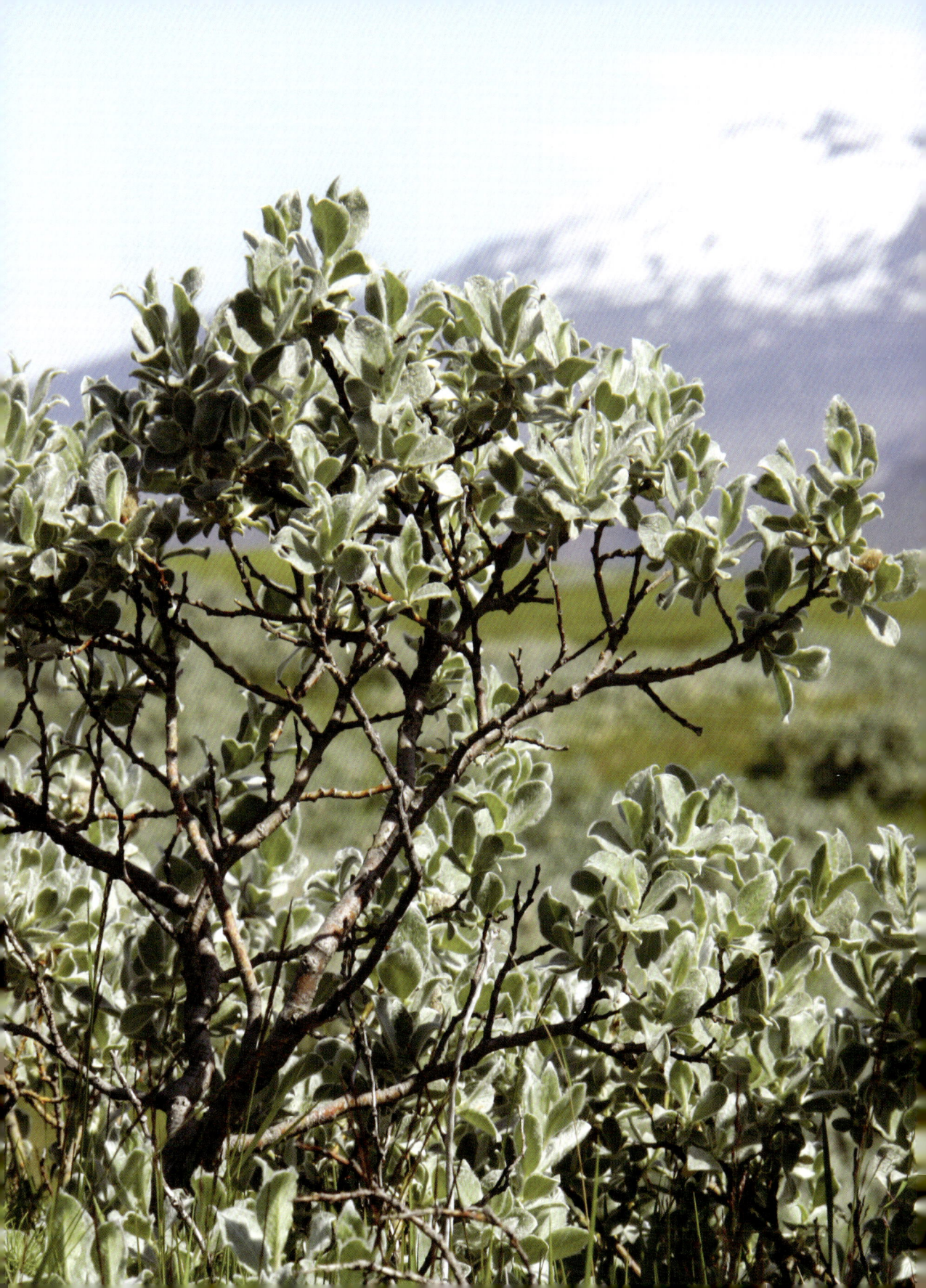

Wood Cranesbill

Geranium sylvaticum
Geraniaceae—Blágresi

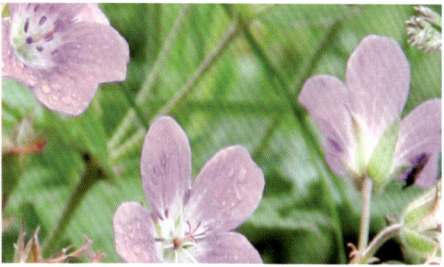

Habitat

Common all over Iceland, especially in Birch forests, hillsides, and grassy hollows.

Parts Used

The entire plant is used, including the root.

Harvesting

Collected while in bloom in June.

Constituents

Tannins, flavonoids, and essential oils.

History

The Latin genus name is *Geranium*, drawn from the Greek "geranion," meaning crane or birds from the Gruidae family. The fruit of the flowers of Wood Cranesbill is said to resemble a crane's beak, while Old Icelandic names are "storkanef" (stork's nose) and "storkablágresi" (stork geranium).

Action

Astringent, hemostatic, and vulnerary.

Uses

Wood Cranesbill is rarely used in Western herbal medicine nowadays. However, other Geranium species are extensively used all over the world. In Europe and North America, *G. maculatum* and *G. robertianum* have long been used for medicinal purposes, especially to stop diarrhea, internal and external bleeding, and vaginal discharges, and for healing wounds. In China, *G. wilfordii* and other species are considered good for gastritis, dysentery, and arthritis, as well as for strengthening bones and tendons. Externally it is used for wounds and skin rashes. In Tibet, it is thought that some Geranium species lower fever, relieve pain, and are anti-inflammatory, so they are used for pneumonia, influenza, pain, and inflammation of the limbs. Indian herbalists use it in a similar way.

Research

In Iceland, *in vitro* tests show that a blend of Angelica and Wood Cranesbill inhibits the breakdown of an important enzyme called acetylcholinesterase, which indicates that these herbs could help with amnesia.[1]

Dosage

Tincture: 2–4 ml three times a day (1:5, 25%).

Infusion: 1–2 teaspoons in a cup three times a day.

Decoction: 1–2 teaspoons three times a day.

Infusions, decoctions, tinctures, compresses, and ointments for external use.

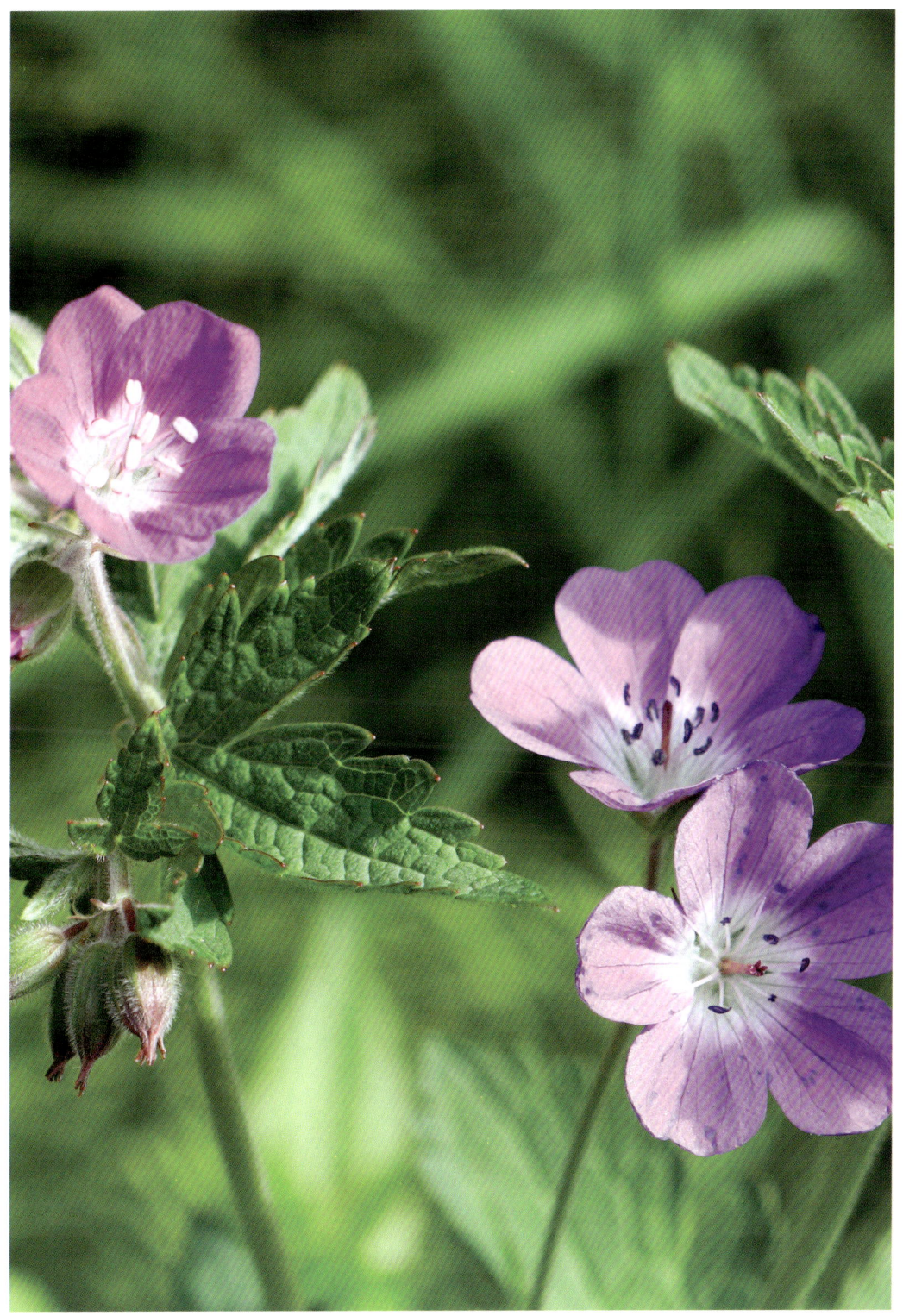

Yarrow

Achillea millefolium
Asteraceae—Vallhumall

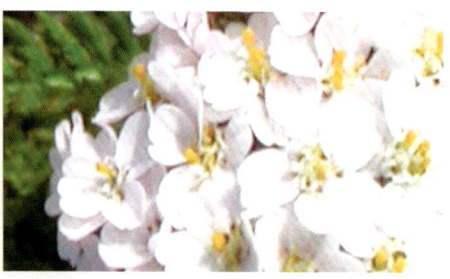

This herb is strengthening, demulcent, contracting, dissolving, blood cleansing, and improves cramps and stiffness of the body. It is good for all sorts of blood-letting, gripe, urinary retention, bloating, loss of appetite, coughs, jaundice and all sorts of internal inflammation.

Oddur Jónsson Hjaltalín,
Icelandic Botany, 1830

Habitat

Yarrow is common all over Iceland, especially near farmhouses but also in the mountains.

Parts Used

The entire plant, except for the root.

Harvesting

Yarrow is collected when the flowers have just emerged in June–July.

Constituents

Essential oils, sesquiterpenes, flavonoids (rutin, quercitrin), and alkaloids.

History

Yarrow is an extremely versatile medicinal herb that has a centuries-old history in herbal medicine. It is said that the genus name *Achillea* is drawn from the name Achilles, a Greek war hero who used Yarrow to heal the wounds of his soldiers; the Old Icelandic name is actually Achilles' herb. Other names connected to warfare were also used for Yarrow, as an ointment made from the herb was often used on soldiers' wounds. One indication that Yarrow was used to stop nosebleeds comes from an old name for the herb, Nosebleed, which was commonly used in previous times. Some references say, however, that Yarrow leaves were stuffed into the nose to bring about bleeding, since one ancient method of medical treatment involved taking blood from the patient. Yarrow also used to be known as Devil's Nettle, Devil's Plaything, and Bad Man's Plaything, all connected to Satan as the herb was also used for prophecy and magic. In China, the stems of Yarrow were used in the *I Ching,* which is a well-known book of divination. Yarrow was thought to be good for prophesying people's destinies (e.g., if Yarrow was put under the pillow, the following rhyme would evoke an image of the prospective spouse in the morning):

Thou pretty herb of Venus' tree, Thy true name it is yarrow; Now who my bosom friend must be, Pray tell thou me to-morrow.

(From Halliwell's *Popular Rhymes*)

It was also believed that a decoction of Yarrow eliminated wrinkles if used for cleaning the face, and if Yarrow was in a bride's bouquet, it guaranteed seven years of harmony. In the Middle Ages, honeymooners traditionally wore Yarrow to ensure a long and happy love life.

The leaves of Yarrow have been used in salads and the entire herb was used for making ale, as the Icelandic name indicates; "Vallhumall" means "hops of the valley." There are many documented references about the use of Yarrow by the Native Americans. They used Yarrow externally for inflammation, pulled muscles, and bruises and

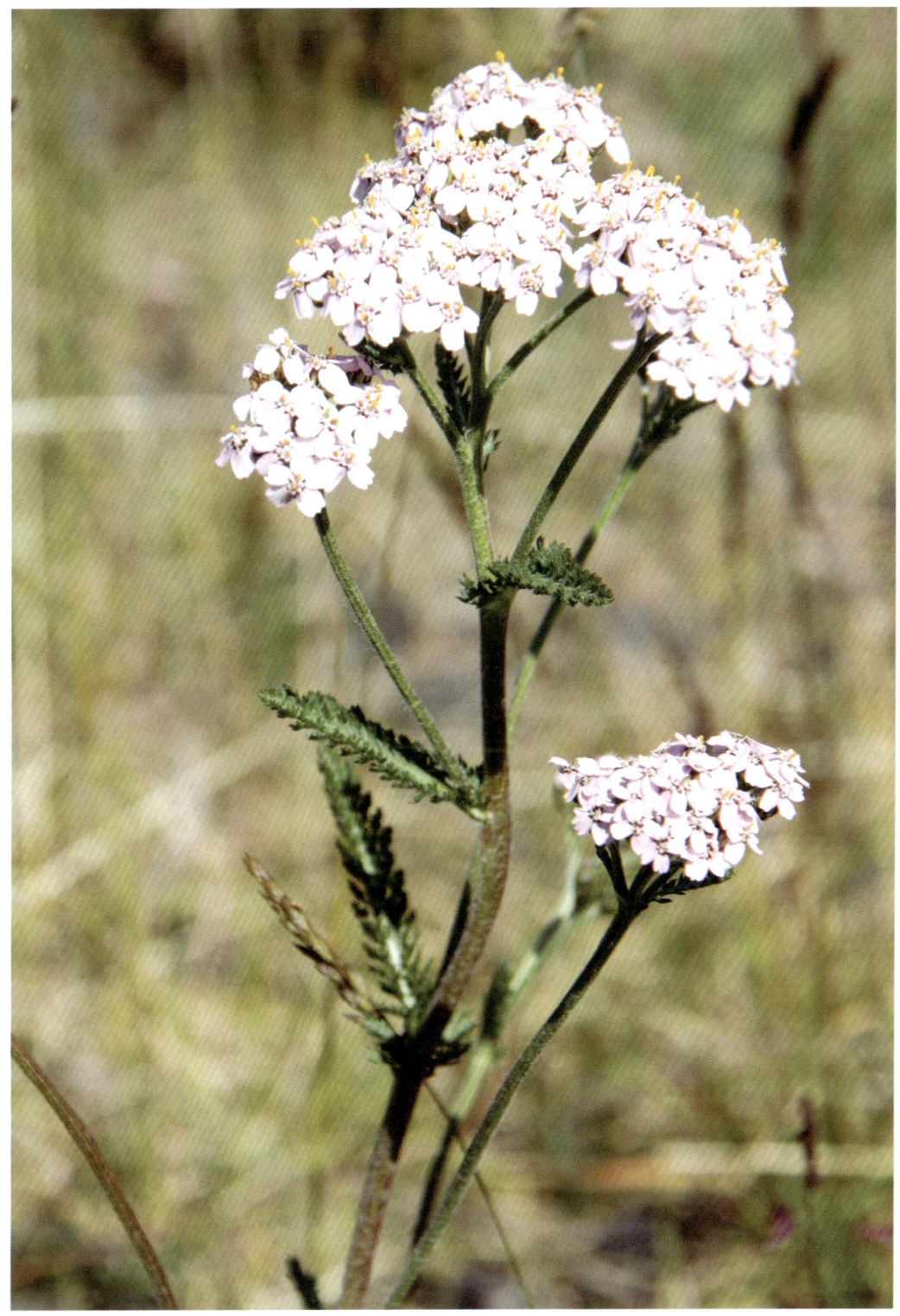

also for colds, influenza, and other respiratory diseases. It was used in powder form as a snuff for headaches and for any digestive disturbances.

Action

Astringent, diaphoretic, febrifuge, anti-inflammatory, hypotensive, antispasmodic, diuretic, cholagogue, hepatic, emmenagogue, antibacterial, hemostatic, anthelmintic, vulnerary, and strengthens the circulatory system.

. . . .

Uses

Yarrow is traditionally used to stop all kinds of bleeding, both internal and external, as well as for healing wounds and skin disorders; it is thought to be especially good for old sores that heal badly. It is also thought to increase appetite and to stop diarrhea, inflammation, and spasms in the digestive system. Yarrow is very useful for colds, sore throats, influenza, and fevers and is readily used for childhood diseases such as measles. It is used for regulating menstruation, for menstrual pain, and for too much or too little menstrual bleeding, as well as for vaginal discharges.

It is said to be able to lower blood pressure and to have a good effect on the venous system (e.g., on varicose veins and accompanying sores, phlebitis and hemorrhoids). Yarrow is also said to prevent blood clot formation, especially in the veins. It has always been a popular medicinal herb for arthritis, and in addition is thought to be diuretic and good for diseases of the urinary system. In China, Yarrow is used in a similar way to Europe and is thought to be good for menorrhagia, bleeding hemorrhoids, snake and dog bites, and any wounds. The Chinese also use Yarrow to improve digestion, for varicose veins, menstrual pain, hepatitis, and tuberculosis. In India, Yarrow is also thought to eliminate worms in domestic animals.

Research

Results from *in vitro* tests on Yarrow done at the University of Iceland indicate that Yarrow contains properties that could possibly relieve symptoms of autoimmune diseases.[1] *In vitro* tests have shown its antibacterial properties (e.g., against *Helicobacteria pylori*, which causes gastritis and stomach ulcers),[2–5] and its antiviral properties.[5] Research with *in vitro* tests has also revealed that Yarrow has antibacterial and antispasmodic effects.[5–8] Several research trials have shown the antioxidant effects of Yarrow.[5, 9–12] An infusion or juice of Yarrow has shown its febrifugal properties, but the tincture does not show such action.[5] Research has also revealed the positive effects of Yarrow on stomach ulcers[11] and an inhibiting effect on the growth of cancer cells.[13,14] Research has also shown its inhibiting effect on parasites,[15,16] insects,[17] and worms.[18] Yarrow appears to lower blood pressure, according to *in vivo* tests,[19] and reduces bleeding.[14] Research on Yarrow has revealed both temporary infertility in animals and no effect on fertility.[5,20]

Dosage

Tincture: 1–4 ml three times a day (1:5, 25%).

Infusion: 1–2 teaspoons in a cup three times a day.

Infusions, tinctures, compresses, and ointments for external use.

Warning

Do not use Yarrow when pregnant. It is known that herbs of the Asteraceae family, including Yarrow, can cause allergic reactions. Large doses of Yarrow are also known to cause nausea, headache, and dizziness, especially among the elderly. Simultaneous use of Yarrow with blood-thinning medication is not recommended.

Tea for Menstrual Pain

2 parts Yarrow

2 parts Lady's Mantle

Put 3–4 tablespoons of the blend into a 750 ml vacuum flask and pour boiling water into it. Strain the tea into cups and then put the herbs back into the flask and allow to stand the whole day. Drink from the flask throughout the day.

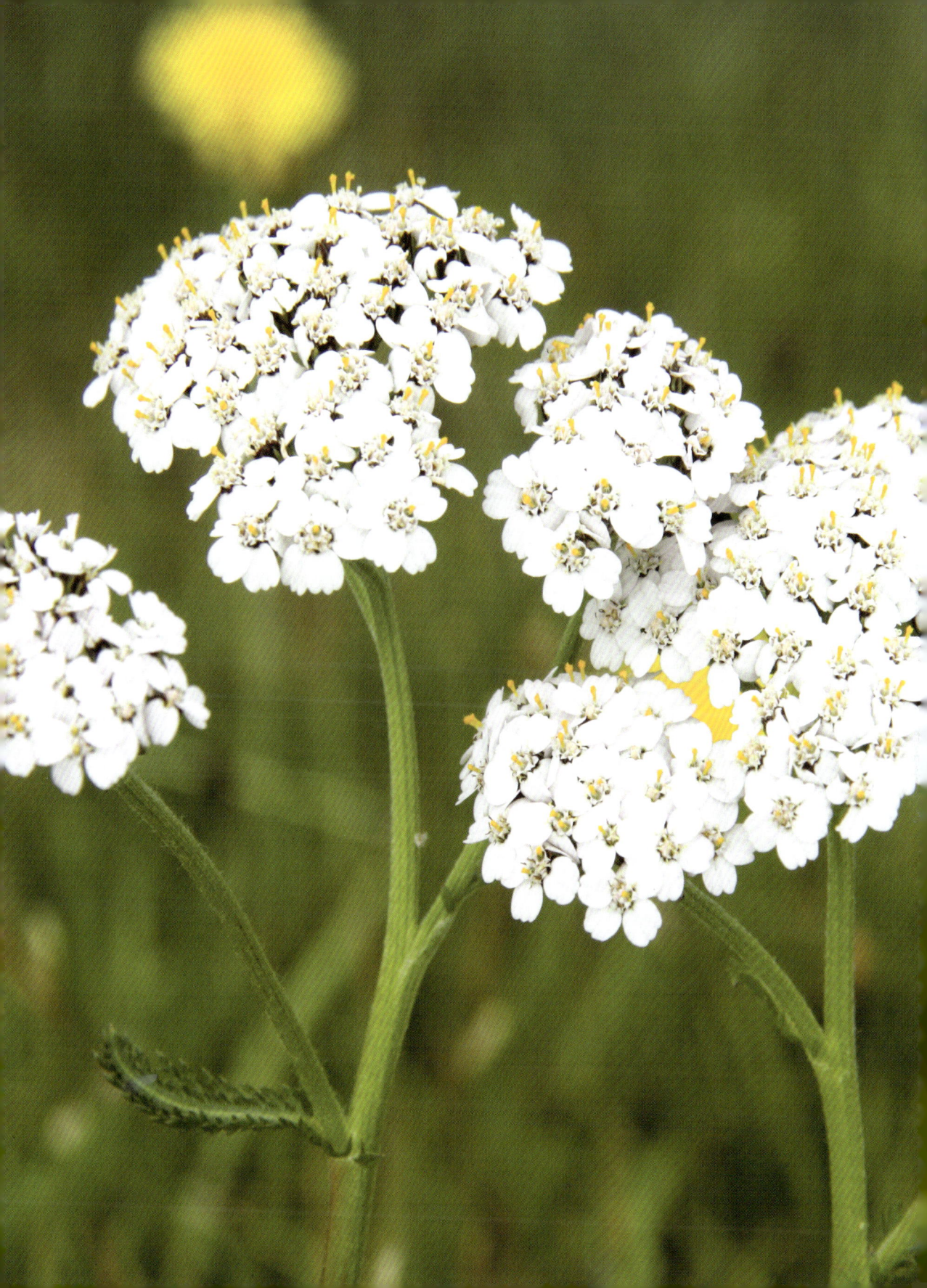

Yellow Rattle

Rhinanthus minor
Orobanchaceae—Lokasjóður

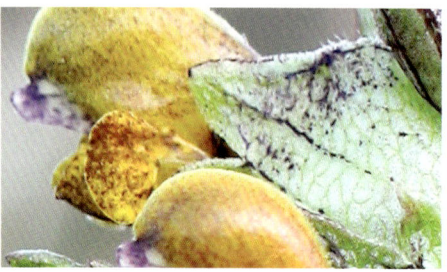

The decoction of this herb may be drunk for coughs. It is also said to be good to wash the weak eye. Germans eat this herb, young in spring, with cabbage or other vegetables. The seeds are used and cooked. The same are good for dysentery and jaundice.

Björn Halldórsson, Uses of Herbs, *1783*

Habitat

Yellow Rattle is common all over Iceland and grows in grasslands and meadows.

Parts Used

The entire plant is used, except for the root.

Harvesting

Yellow Rattle is harvested in early summer.

Constituents

Tannins and glycosides.

History

References from the 16th century indicate that Yellow Rattle has a good effect on eyes and functions similarly to Eyebright, which is a well-known medicinal herb for the eyes. At that time it was also considered to be good for colds and coughs. Yellow Rattle is also called Penny Grass, as children use the seeds as money in games. In addition, it has been used to dye yarn.

Action

Astringent.

Uses

It is not known if Yellow Rattle is used in Western herbal medicine nowadays. It was formerly thought to be strengthening for the eyes and was also considered to be effective for colds and coughs.

Dosage

Tincture: 1–4 ml three times a day (1:5, 25%).

Infusion: 1 teaspoon in a cup three times a day.

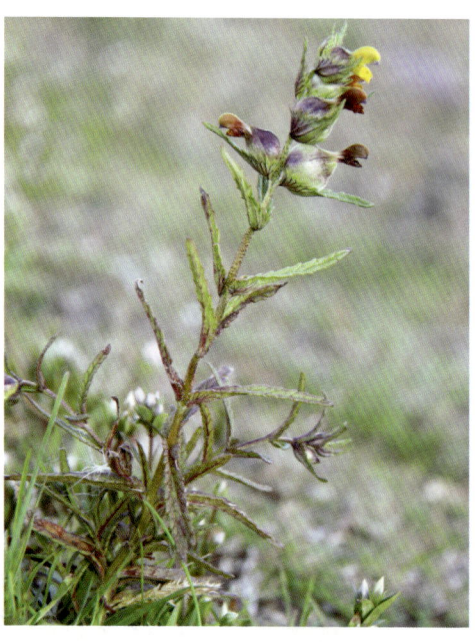

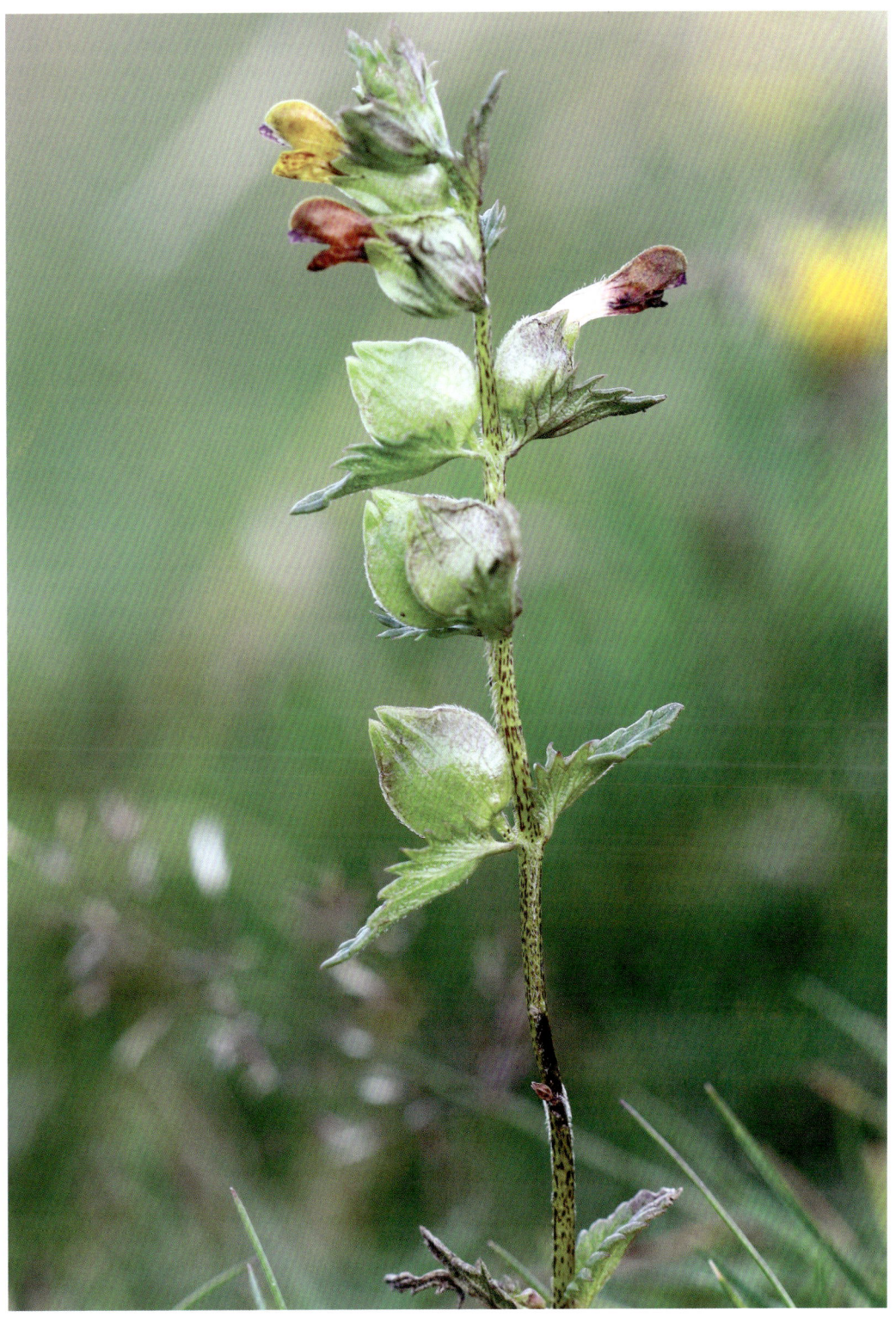

Glossary

The following explanations name the major actions of constituents of medicinal herbs, but are in no way exhaustive. Various unusual words and terms in this field are also explained.

Alkaloids are a diverse group of compounds, numbering about 10,000 in all. Many alkaloids—such as nicotine, caffeine, codeine, morphine, and heroin—are addictive and dangerous. Alkaloids can have various effects on the body; for instance, they can be analgesic, sedative, muscle relaxants, hypotensive, hypertensive, heart stimulants, and respiratory stimulants. Yarrow, for example, contains an alkaloid called betonicine, which is anti-inflammatory. Groundsel and Coltsfoot contain pyrrolizidine alkaloids, which cause toxic reactions, while Alaska Lupine contains lupine alkaloids, which can be toxic. Fir Clubmoss contains toxic lycopodium alkaloids.

Analgesic: pain reliever.

Anthelmintic: eliminates parasites from the gut.

Anthocyanin is the group of substances that give flowers, leaves, fruit and berries their pink, purple, blue, and red colors. They are considered to have antioxidant properties and strengthen the venous system. Blueberries and Crowberries are examples of plants containing anthocyanins.

Anthraquinones are found in many plants and usually have laxative properties. Icelandic medicinal herbs containing anthraquinones include Lady's Bedstraw, Sheep's Sorrel, Northern Dock, and Sorrel.

Anti-emetic: reduces nausea or vomiting.

Antioxidants are substances that inhibit or slow down the oxidation of other substances. Oxidation causes the formation of free radicals, which can damage living cells and spoil food. Antioxidants reduce the damaging effects of free radicals. Vitamins C, E, and beta-carotene, which are all found in vegetables, fruit, and herbs, are examples of antioxidants. Despite research being somewhat scientifically inconsistent, there are many indications that antioxidants can prevent disease and reduce the risk of cardiovascular diseases.

Antioxidants are also said to be able to reduce the risk of blood clots and atherosclerosis and stop wrinkle formation. Many flavonoids in medicinal herbs are antioxidant (e.g., the anthocyanins are found in large amounts in Bilberries and Crowberries).

Antitussive: reduces coughing.

Arbutin is a subgroup of phenols and is diuretic, antitussive, and antibacterial for the urinary system. Bearberry, Large-flowered Wintergreen, and Heather are examples of herbs that contain arbutin.

Astringent is an adjective used for the effect of medicinal herbs that contain tannins. See tannins.

Aucubin is one of the iridoid glycosides and has laxative and diuretic properties, among others. Herbs containing aucubin include Eyebright, Greater Plantain, and Speedwell.

Bitters or bitter substances are the terms used for the many ingredients in medicinal herbs that share the attribute of having a bitter taste. These compounds include iridoid glycosides, saponins, sesquiterpenes, lichen acids, and alkaloids. Bitters stimulate taste buds and increase salivation and digestive juices, so medicinal herbs containing bitter substances are used to stimulate appetite and strengthen digestion. Bitters stimulate pancreatic juices, duodenal juices and bile, as well as balancing the production of pancreatic hormones, which have an effect on blood sugar, insulin, and glucagon. Icelandic herbs containing bitters include Yarrow, Bogbean, Field Gentian, Dandelion, and Iceland Moss.

Caffeic acid belongs to the phenolpropanoids and is very common in medicinal herbs. Among other things, it is considered to be analgesic, anti-inflammatory, antibacterial, antifungal, and antiviral, as well as having antioxidant properties. Icelandic medicinal herbs that contain caffeic acid include Bilberry (leaves), Eyebright, Knotgrass, Speedwell, Butterwort, Dandelion, and Yarrow.

Carbohydrates, or saccharides, can be found in all plants in many different forms. The saccharides are divided into many subgroups; one subgroup is the polysaccharides, which includes inulin, pectin, glycosinolates, glycosides, and mucilage.

Carminative: eases flatulence and colic in the gut.

Cholagogue: stimulates the flow of bile from the liver.

Coumarins are a type of polyphenol and are found in over 700 herbs. Among other things, coumarins have antispasmodic and blood-thinning properties and increase light sensitivity of the skin. They are found in Heather, Self-heal, Sweet Vernal Grass, Silverweed, and Angelica.

Cyanogenic glycoside is a substance that is found, for instance, in the seeds of Rowan berries. It forms cyanide when in contact with water.

Demulcent: soothes irritated tissue, especially mucous membranes.

Diaphoretic: promotes perspiration.

Emmenagogue: promotes menstruation.

Essential oils are volatile oils that do not tolerate heat well, are often made up of many types of active substances, and have multiple functions. They give flowers their aroma and are distilled from many medicinal herbs. Essential oils often possess antibacterial, antiviral, and anti-inflammatory properties. Icelandic medicinal herbs that contain essential oils include Sea Mayweed, Self-heal, Creeping Thyme, Valerian, Caraway, Shepherd's Purse, Pineappleweed, Sweet Vernal Grass, Yarrow, and Angelica.

Expectorant: promotes expulsion of mucus from the respiratory tract.

Febrifuge: reduces fever.

Flavonoids are a very big subgroup of polyphenols and about 4,000 types are known. They are the pigments of flowers, fruit, and sometimes leaves. Flavonoids are divided into many subgroups such as flavonones, flavones, isoflavonoids, anthocyanins, flavanols, and flavonols. The active constituents within these groups are quercitrin, rutin, and genistein. Flavonoids have many diverse actions, including antioxidant properties, and are considered to be diuretic, anti-inflammatory, hypoglycemic, hypotensive, sedative, antibacterial, and antispasmodic. They also strengthen capil-

laries, have a mild estrogen effect, and stimulate the gallbladder and liver. Icelandic medicinal herbs containing flavonoids include Bilberry (leaves), Eyebright, Sea Mayweed, Heather, Downy Birch, Large-flowered Wintergreen, Wood Cranesbill, Self-heal, Knotgrass, Greater Burnet, Nettle, Roseroot, Juniper, Daisy, Greater Plantain, Lady's Bedstraw, Speedwell, Shepherd's Purse, Coltsfoot, Strawberry (leaves), Horsetail, Caraway, Lady's Mantle, Meadowsweet, Red Clover, Ribwort Plantain, Bearberry, and Silverweed.

Galactagogue: promotes milk flow.

Gallic acid is one of the phenolic acids and is thought to have diverse actions. It is known for being astringent, antibacterial, antiviral, antifungal, anti-inflammatory, and a muscle relaxant. Gallic acid can be found in Eyebright and Knotgrass.

Glucosinolates are mustard oil glycosides that exist only in mustard seeds, vegetables, and herbs of the Brassicaceae family. Glucosinolates can have antibacterial action, can stimulate blood circulation, and can protect against colon cancer. They are present in Scurvy Grass, Cuckooflower, and Shepherd's Purse.

Glycosides are polysaccharides that, when linked to other substances, form many diverse compounds that exist in medicinal herbs. They include cyanogenic glycosides, coumarin glycosides, anthraquinone glycosides, and saponins.

Hemostatic: reduces or stems bleeding.

Hepatic: enhances liver function.

Hypnotic: promotes sleep.

Hypoglycemic: lowers high blood-sugar levels.

Hypotensive: lowers high blood pressure.

Inulin is a polysaccharide that is found in vegetables and fruit but also in Dandelion root. Inulin is reputed to kill bacteria, lower blood sugar and cholesterol, inhibit the growth of cancer cells, and help absorb minerals in the body. Note that inulin is not the same as insulin, which is a hormone that is produced in the pancreas and lowers blood-sugar levels.

Iridoid glycosides are a group of substances that usually have a bitter taste and are found in many medicinal herbs. Bitter substances stimulate digestive juices and often play a major role in herbal medicine. Aucubin and asperuloside are examples of common iridoids. Of the Icelandic medicinal herbs that contain iridoid glycosides, Bogbean, which is very bitter, Eyebright, and Speedwell can be named.

Isoflavonoids number about 600 in total and contain active constituents that are said to have a mild estrogenic effect. Isoflavonoids can be found in Red Clover and Chickweed.

Minerals are found in most medicinal herbs and some have a high mineral content. Iceland Moss, Stinging Nettle, Dandelion, and Horsetail are examples of medicinal herbs that are rich in minerals.

Mucilage is a polysaccharide that, as the name indicates, forms mucus or a jelly-like substance when mixed with water. Mucilage protects the mucous membrane of the digestive tract from irritation and is especially good for indigestion, gastritis, and stomach ulcers. Mucilage can also have a laxative effect, while externally it works well in a compress. Iceland Moss, Irish Moss, Greater Plantain, Ribwort Plantain, Spotted Orchid, and Coltsfoot all contain mucilage.

Naphthoquinones contain a yellow pigment and also the substance plumbagin, which is antibacterial, antispasmodic, and antitussive. It exists, for instance, in Sundew and Common Sea-thrift.

Nervine: eases anxiety and tension.

Pectin is found in fruit and berries (e.g., Bilberry), and forms a jelly. Research has shown that pectin can possibly lower cholesterol and provide protection against colon cancer.

Phenolic acids are a subgroup of polyphenols and include gallic acid and salicylic acid. Herbs that contain phenolic acids include Eyebright, Downy Birch, Meadowsweet, and Willow species.

Phenols are a subgroup of polyphenols. They are common in medicinal herbs and are known for being antibacterial, anti-inflammatory, diuretic, and analgesic. Herbs that contain phenols include Bearberry, Meadowsweet, Large-flowered Wintergreen, Purple Marshlocks, and Willows.

Phenylpropanoids are a group of polyphenols that include substances such as caffeic acid, which is common in many medicinal herbs.

Polyphenols can be found in over 8,000 different herbs, and about half of them are flavonoids. Other subgroups of polyphenols include phenols, phenolic acids, phenylpropanoids, phenylquinones, cinnamic acid, coumarins, naphthoquinones, anthraquinones, and tannins.

Protoanemonin is a toxin found in Marsh Marigold. When dried or boiled, this toxin changes into anemonin and anemoninic acid and so loses its toxic effect.

Quercetin is a flavonol that affects many enzymes in the body and is considered to be anti-inflammatory, antiviral, and antioxidant, besides reducing allergic reactions and inhibiting growth of cancer cells. Bilberry (leaves), Heather, Downy Birch, Large-flowered Wintergreen, Lady's Bedstraw, Shepherd's Purse, Strawberry (leaves), Horsetail, Caraway, Lady's Mantle, Bearberry, and Silverweed all contain quercitin.

Quinones are divided into three subgroups: naphthoquinones, anthraquinones, and benzoquinones, but over 1,200 types of quinones have been identified. Quinones contain a high content of pigment, the most common of which are yellow, orange, and red.

Resin is an organic compound in various plants that hardens when dry and softens with heat. Resin is mainly found in trees, but is also found in small amounts in some medicinal herbs. Resin does not dissolve in water but is soluble in alcohol. Juniper, Purple Marshlocks, Grass of Parnassus, Fir Clubmoss, Male Fern, and Angelica all contain resin.

Rubefacient: irritant, produces redness of the skin.

Rutin belongs to the flavonoids. It is found quite often in medicinal plants and is considered to be anti-inflammatory, antibacterial, and antiviral, while also strengthening capillaries. Rutin is found in Self-heal, Greater Burnet, Chickweed, Biting

Stonecrop, Shepherd's Purse, Bogbean, Meadowsweet, Yarrow, and Heartsease.

Salicylic acid is found in many medicinal herbs and has well-known analgesic and anti-inflammatory properties. It also lowers fevers. Medicinal herbs that contain salicylic acid include Meadowsweet and Willow species.

Saponins are a big group of glycosides that are divided into three subgroups: triterpene glycosides, steroid glycosides, and steroid alkaloid glycosides. Saponins are widely found in more than 100 families of plants, including many vegetables, and the groups have three things in common: they are bitter, they produce foam when mixed with water, and they have a decaying effect on the cell membranes of red blood cells. Saponins have many actions; *in vitro* and *in vivo* tests show that saponins are anti-inflammatory, vulnerary, expectorant, diuretic, antibacterial, antifungal, and anthelmintic, besides lowering cholesterol. Herbs that contain saponins include Yarrow, Northern Dock, Stinging Nettle, Downy Birch, Horsetail, Purple Marshlocks, Daisy, and Dandelion.

Sesquiterpene lactones are substances that can be found in many herbs of the Asteraceae family (e.g., Dandelion). It is known that certain types of sesquiterpene lactones can cause allergic reactions on contact. They can lower cholesterol in the blood and may possibly also have antibacterial, antifungal, and vermifugal effects. Some types of sesquiterpene lactones are toxic (e.g., proto-anemonin, which is found in Marsh Marigold).

Sesquiterpenes are a group of active substances found in essential oils that have a variety of actions. One of these substances is chamazulene, which has anti-inflammatory effects and lowers fevers and is present in Yarrow.

Silicic acid is reputed to strengthen connective tissue, hair, nails, bones, and tendons, together with preventing osteoporosis and hastening the healing of broken bones. Horsetail contains a high level of silicic acid and the strengthening effect of this on connective tissue has also been said to be the reason why Horsetail has long been considered effective for rheumatoid arthritis, osteoarthritis, and lung diseases such as emphysema.

Stomachic: stimulating, strengthening, or toning the stomach.

Tannins have long been used for tanning skins for leather. They belong to the polyphenols and are very common constituents of Icelandic medicinal herbs. Medicinal herbs that contain tannins shrink or constrict bodily tissue. When an astringent herb is placed over wounds, it forms a thin, protective surface that inhibits fluid formation and protects against irritation. Tannins also have antibiotic properties and constrict veins, thereby reducing bleeding. Tannins protect inflamed mucous membranes, have a drying effect on mucous membranes, and reduce fluid formation, as well as reducing inflammation caused by infection. They also balance menstrual bleeding and diarrhea and are useful for external use in vaginal douches, nose powders, and eyewashes. Icelandic medicinal herbs that contain tannins include Meadowsweet, Eyebright, Wood Cranesbill, Knotgrass, Greater Burnet, Purple Marshlocks, Water Avens, Mountain Avens, Lady's Mantle, and Bearberry.

Terpenes are a big group of substances and are divided into many subgroups. They are found in essential oils and resins, among other things.

Triterpenes are a subgroup of terpenes and are divided into three main types: saponins, phytosterols, and steroids.

Ursolic acid belongs to the triterpenes. *In vitro* research has shown that it has antibacterial and anti-inflammatory properties as well as an inhibiting effect on the growth of cancer cells. Herbs that contain ursolic acid include Heather, Self-heal, Greater Burnet, and Greater Plantain.

Vitamins can be found in most medicinal herbs, but some herbs contain high quantities of vitamins. Examples of such herbs are Bilberry, Stinging Nettle, Crowberry, and Dandelion.

Vulnerary: promotes wound healing.

Bibliography

- Allen, David E., and G. Hatfield. 2004. *Medicinal Plants in Folk Tradition: An Ethnobotany of Britain & Ireland.* Timber Press, Portland.

- Barker, Julian. 2001. *The Medicinal Flora of Britain and Northwestern Europe.* Winter Press, West Wickham.

- Bartram, Thomas. 1998. *Bartram's Encyclopedia of Herbal Medicine.* Robinson Publishing, London.

- Bensky, Dan, S. Clavey, and E. Stöger. 2004. *Chinese Herbal Medicine Materia Medica.* 3rd Edition. Eastland Press, Seattle.

- BHMA (British Herbal Medicine Association). 1983. *British Herbal Pharmacopoeia.* British Herbal Medicine Association, Cowling.

- BHMA (British Herbal Medicine Association). 1996. *British Herbal Pharmacopoeia 1996.* British Herbal Medicine Association, Cowling.

- Bjarnason, Ágúst H. 1983. *Íslensk flóra með litmyndum.* Iðunn, Reykjavík.

- Bjarnason, Alexander. 1860. *Um íslenzkar drykkurtir, söfnun þeirra, geymslu, nytsemi, verkanir and tilreiðslu.* 2nd Edition. Ljósbrá, Reykjavík 1982.

- Blumenthal, Mark. 2003. *The ABC Clinical Guide to Herbs.* American Botanical Council, Austin.

- Blumenthal, Mark, A. Goldberg and J. Brinckmann. 2000. *Herbal Medicine.* Expanded Commission E Monographs. Integrative Medicine Communications, Newton.

- Bone, Kerry. 2003. *A Clinical Guide to Blending Liquid Herbs.* Churchill Livingstone, St. Louis.

- Bradley, Peter. 1992. *British Herbal Compendium Volume 1.* British Herbal Medicine Association, Bournemouth.

- Bradley, Peter. 2006. *British Herbal Compendium Volume 2.* British Herbal Medicine Association, Bournemouth.

- Chang, Hson-Mou, and Paul Pui-Hay But. 1986. *Pharmacology and Application of Chinese Materia Medica (Vol. 1).* World Scientific Publishing, Singapore.

- Chang, Hson-Mou, and Paul Pui-Hay But. 1987. *Pharmacology and Application of Chinese Materia Medica (Vol. 2).* World Scientific Publishing, Singapore.

- Chevallier, Andrew. 1996. *The Encyclopedia of Medicinal Plants.* Dorling Kindersley, London.

- Chiej, Roberto. 1984. *The Macdonald Encyclopedia of Medicinal Plants.* Macdonald & Co. Publishers, London.

- Chopra, R.N., I.C. Chopra, and B.S. Verma. 2005. *Supplement to Glossary of Indian Medicinal Plants.* National Institute of Science Communication and Information Resources, New Delhi.

- Crawford, Amanda McQuade. 2009. *The Natural Menopause Handbook.* Crossing Press, New York.

- Curtin, L.S.M. 1997. *Healing Herbs of the Upper Rio Grande.* Edited by Michael Moore. Western Edge Press, Santa Fe.

- Duke, James A., 1997. *The Green Pharmacy.* Rodale, New York.

- Duke, James A., and E.S. Ayensu. 1985. *Medicinal Plants of China, Volume One.* Reference Publications, Algonac.

- Duke, James A. and E.S. Ayensu. 1985. *Medicinal Plants of China, Volume Two.* Reference Publications, Algonac.

- Einarsdóttir, Ásdís Ragna. 2005. *Rhodiola rosea and its Indications for Some Psychiatric and Neurolandical Disorders.* Unpublished BSc thesis.

- Filippusson, Erlingu. 1963. *Íslenzkar nytjajurtir, læknaðu þig sjálfur.* Prents-miðjan Hólar, Reykjavík.

- European Scientific Cooperative on Phytotherapy. 2003. *ESCOP Monographs.* 2nd Edition. Georg Thieme Verlag, Stuttgart.

- Fluck, Hans. 1971. *Medicinal Plants.* W. Foulsham & Co., London.

- Foster, Steven, and J.A. Duke. 2000. *A Field Guide to Medicinal Plants and Herbs of Eastern and Central North America.* Houghton Mifflin Company, Boston.

- Grieve, M. 1980. *A Modern Herbal.* Penguin Books, London.

- Hákonardóttir, Hildur. 2005. *Ætigarðurinn: Handbók grasnytjungsins.* Salka, Reykjavík.

- Hedley, Christopher and Non Shaw. 1996. *Herbal Remedies: A Practical Beginner's Guide to Making Effective Remedies in the Kitchen.* Parragon Book Service, Bristol.

- Halldórsson, Björn. 1783. *Grasnytjar. Búnaðarfélag Íslands,* Reykjavík 1983.

- Hjaltalín, Oddur Jónsson. 1830. *Íslenzk grasafræði:* Hið Íslenzka bókmentafélag, Reykjavík. Found on http://baekur.is/is/bok/000295567/Islenzk_grasafraedi.

- Hoffmann, David. 2003. *Medical Herbalism: The Science and Practice of Herbal Medicine.* Healing Arts Press, Rochester.

- Holtom, Josie A. and W.H. Hylton. 1979. *The Complete Guide to Herbs.* Rodale Press, Aylesbury.

- Hörður Kristinsson. 2010. *Íslenska plöntuhandbókin—Blómplöntur and byrkingar.* Mál and menning, Reykjavík.

- Ísberg, Jón Ólafur and Örn Hrafnkelsson. 1996. *"Fyrst skal maður byrja að telja tungl...".* Læknafélag Íslands, Kópavandur.

- Jóhannsdóttir, Arnbjörg L. 1992. *Íslenskar lækningajurtir.* Örn and Örlygur, Reykjavík.

- Jóhannsson, Símon Jón. 1999. *Stóra hjátrúarbókin: Aðgengilegt uppflettirit um margvíslega hjátrú Íslendinga í hinu daglega lífi fyrr and nú.* Vaka-Helgafell, Reykjavík.

- Joshi, Kamal K. and S. D. Joshi. 2006. *Medicinal and Aromatic Plants Used in Nepal, Tibet and Trans-Himalayan Region.* Author House, Bloomington.

- Jónsson, Björn L. 1973. *Íslenzkar lækninga- and drykkjarjurtir.* Náttúrul-ækningafélag Íslands, Reykjavík.

- Jónsson, Jón. 1880. *Lítil ritgjörð um nytsemi nokkurra íslenzkra jurta eptir ýmsa höfunda.* Einar Þórðarson, Reykjavík.

- Kletter, Christa, and Monika Kriechbaum. 2001. *Tibetan Medicinal Plants.* Medpharm Scientific Publishers, Stuttgart.

- Launert, Edmund. 1989. *The Hamlyn Guide to Edible & Medicinal Plants of Britain and Northern Europe.* 4th Edition. Hamlyn Publishing Group, London.

- Lust, John. 1986. *The Herb Book.* Bantam Books, London.

- Manandhar, Narayan P. 2002. *Plants and People of Nepal.* Timber Press, Portland.

- McIntyre, Anne. 1994. *The Complete Woman's Herbal.* Gaia Books Limited, London.

- Mills, Simon and K. Bone. 2000. *Principles and Practice of Phytotherapy.* Churchill Livingstone, London.

- Mills, Simon and K. Bones. 2008. *The Essential Guide to Herbal Safety.* Churchill Livingstone, Philadelphia.

- Mills, Simon Y. 1985. *The Dictionary of Modern Herbalism.* Thorsons Publishing Group, Wellingborough.

- Moerman, Daniel E. 2009. *Native American Medicinal Plants.* Timber Press, Portland.

- Moore, Michael. 1989. *Medicinal Plants of the Desert and Canyon West.* Museum of New Mexico Press, Santa Fe.

- Moore, Michael. 2003. *Medicinal Plants of the Mountain West.* Museum of New Mexico Press, Santa Fe.

- Ólafsson, Eggert. 1943. *Ferðabók Eggerts Ólafssonar and Bjarna Pálssonar um ferðir þeirra á Íslandi árin 1752–1757 I-II.* Reykjavík.

- Rögnvaldardóttir, Nanna. 1998. *Matarást: Alfræðibók um mat and matargerð.* Iðunn, Reykjavík.

- Schofield, Janice I. 1998. *Discovering Wild Plants.* Alaska Northwest Books, Portland.

- Sigurðardóttir, Helga. 2009. *Matur and drykkur.* Bókaútgáfan Opna, Reykjavík.

- Stuart, Malcom. 1987. *The Encyclopedia of Herbs and Herbalism.* Black Cat, London.

- Tierra, Michael. 1998. *The Way of Herbs.* Pocket Books, New York.

- Treben, Maria. 1986. *Health from God's Garden.* Herbal remedies for Glowing Health and Well-being. Healing Arts Press, Rochester.

- Tsarong, Tsewang J. 1994. *Tibetan Medicinal Plants.* Tibetan Medical Publications, Kalimpong.

- Usher, George. 1974. *A Dictionary of Plants Used by Man.* Constable and Company, London.

- Weiss, Rudolf F. 1988. *Herbal Medicine.* AB Arcanum, Beaconsfield.

- Williamson, Elizabeth M. 2002. *Major Herbs of Ayurveda.* Elsevier Science, London.

- Williamson, Elizabeth M. 2003. *Potter's Herbal Cyclopaedia.* The C.W. Daniel Company, Essex.

- World Health Organization—Regional Office for the Western Pacific. 1998. *Medicinal Plants in the Republic of Korea.* Compiled by Natural Products Research Institute, Seoul National University. World Health Organization, Manila.

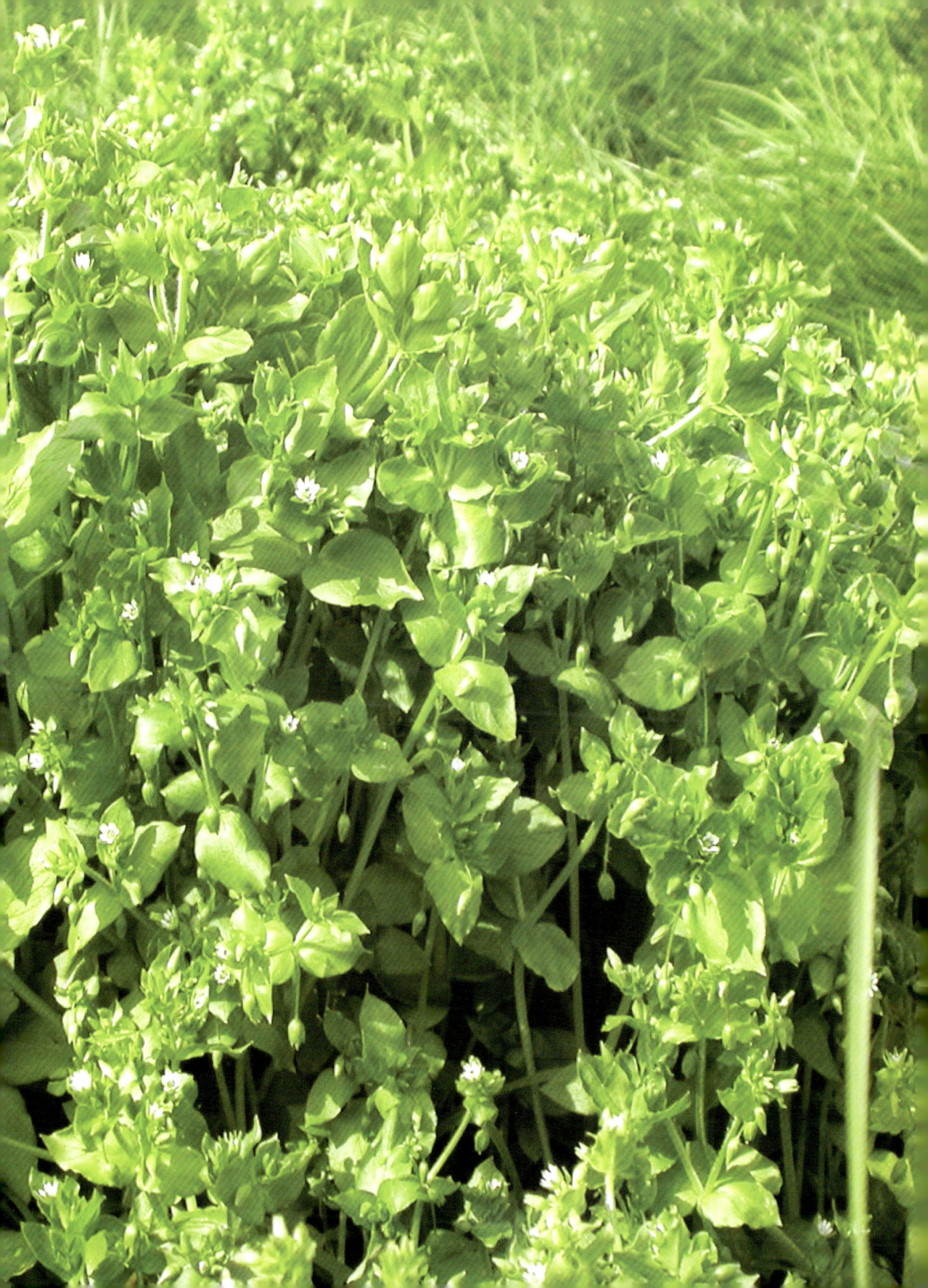

Research Bibliography

Most of the following research papers were found on open databases on the internet and are therefore easy to access. One particularly good website is the NCBI (National Center for Biotechnology Information) database, which has information on thousands of research papers on medicinal herbs. The website is: www.ncbi.nlm.nih.gov/guide/.

Alpine Bistort

1. Shen L, Yang L. [Identification of Yi nationality's secret recipe for treating snakebite] Zhongguo Zhong Yao Za Zhi. 1991 Jun; 16(6):328–9, 381. [Article in Chinese]

Angelica

1. Pathak S, Wanjari MM, Jain SK et al. Evaluation of Antiseizure Activity of Essential Oil from Roots of Angelica archangelica Linn. in Mice. Indian J Pharm Sci. 2010 May; 72(3):371–5.

2. Luszczki JJ, Wojda E et al. Anticonvulsant and acute neurotoxic effects of imperatorin, osthole and valproate in the maximal electroshock seizure and chimney tests in mice: a comparative study. Epilepsy Res. 2009 Aug; 85(2–3):293–9. Epub 2009 Apr 29.

3. Luszczki JJ, Glowniak K et al. Time-course and dose-response relationships of imperatorin in the mouse maximal electroshock seizure threshold model. Neurosci Res. 2007 Sep; 59(1):18–22. Epub 2007 May 25.

4. Sigurdsson S, Gudbjarnason S. Inhibition of acetylcholinesterase by extracts and constituents from Angelica archangelica and Geranium sylvaticum. Z Naturforsch C. 2007 Sep-Oct; 62(9–10):689–93.

5. Sigurdsson S, Ogmundsdottir HM et al. The cytotoxic effect of two chemotypes of essential oils from the fruits of Angelica archangelica L. Anticancer Res. 2005 May-Jun; 25(3B):1877–80.

6. Sigurdsson S, Ogmundsdottir HM et al. Antiproliferative effect of Angelica archangelica fruits. Z Naturforsch C. 2004 Jul-Aug; 59(7–8):523–7.

7. Sigurdsson S, Ogmundsdottir HM et al. Antitumor activity of Angelica archangelica leaf extract. In Vivo. 2005 Jan-Feb; 19(1):191–4.

8. Hensel A, Deters AM et al. Occurrence of N-phenylpropenoyl-L-amino acid amides in different herbal drugs and their influence on human keratinocytes, on human liver cells and on adhesion of Helicobacter pylori to the human stomach. Planta Med. 2007 Feb; 73(2):142–50. Epub 2007 Feb 13.

9. Yeh ML, Liu CF et al. Hepatoprotective effect of Angelica archangelica in chronically ethanol-treated mice. Pharmacology. 2003 Jun; 68(2):70–3.

10. Khayyal MT, el-Ghazaly MA et al. Antiulcerogenic effect of some gastrointestinally acting plant extracts and their combination. Arzneimittelforschung. 2001; 51(7):545–53.

11. Blumenthal M, Goldberg A, Brinckmann J. 2000. Herbal Medicine. Expanded Commission E Monographs. Integrative Medicine Communications, Newton.

12. Bradley P. 2006. *British Herbal Compendium Volume 2.* British Herbal Medicine Association, Bournemouth.

Bearberry

1. European Scientific Cooperative on Phytotherapy. 2003. *ESCOP Monographs.* 2nd Edition. Georg Thieme Verlag, Stuttgart.

2. Shimizu M, Shiota S et al. Marked potentiation of activity of beta-lactams against methicillin-resistant Staphylococcus aureus by corilagin. Antimicrob Agents Chemother. 2001 Nov; 45(11):3198–201.

3. Türi M, Türi E et al. Influence of aqueous extracts of medicinal plants on surface hydrophobicity of Escherichia coli strains of different origin. APMIS. 1997 Dec; 105(12):956–62.

4. WHO. 2004. WHO Monographs on selected medicinal plants, Volume 2. World Health Organization, Geneva.

5. Bol'shakova IV, Lozovskaia EL et al. [Antioxidant properties of plant extracts] Biofizika. 1998 Mar-Apr; 43(2):186–8. [Article in Russian]

6. Matsuda H, Nakamura S et al. [Pharmacological studies on leaf of Arctostaphylos uva-ursi (L.) Spreng. V. Effect of water extract from Arctostaphylos uva-ursi (L.) Spreng. (bearberry leaf) on the antiallergic and antiinflammatory activities of dexamethasone ointment] Yakugaku Zasshi. 1992 Sep; 112(9):673–7. [Article in Japanese]

7. Matsuda H, Nakata H et al. [Pharmacological study on Arctostaphylos uva-ursi (L.) Spreng. II. Combined effects of arbutin and prednisolone or dexamethazone on immuno-inflammation] Yakugaku Zasshi. 1990 Jan; 110(1):68–76. [Article in Japanese]

8. Beaux D, Fleurentin J et al. Effect of extracts of Orthosiphon stamineus Benth, Hieracium pilosella L., Sambucus nigra L. and Arctostaphylos uva-ursi (L.) Spreng. in rats. Phytother Res. 1999 May; 13(3):222–5.

9. Grases F, Melero G et al. Urolithiasis and phytotherapy. Int Urol Nephrol. 1994; 26(5):507–11.

10. Matsuda H, Higashino M et al. Studies of cuticle drugs from natural sources. IV. Inhibitory effects of some Arctostaphylos plants on melanin biosynthesis. Biol Pharm Bull. 1996 Jan; 19(1):153–6.

Bilberry

1. WHO. 2009. WHO monographs on selected medicinal plants. Vol. 4. World Health Organization, Geneva.

2. Perossini M, Guidi G et al. Diabetic and hypertensive retinopathy therapy with Vaccinium myrtillus anthocyanosides (Tegens TM). Double-blind placebo-controlled trial. Ann Ophthalmol Clin Ocul 1987; 113:1173–90.

3. Repossi P, Malagola R et al. The role of anthocyanosides on vascular permeability in diabetic retinopathy. Ann Ophthalmol Clin Ocul 1987; 113(4):357–361.

4. Vannini L, Samuelly R et al. Study of the pupillary reflex after anthocyanoside administration. Boll Ocul 1986; 65:11–2.

5. Orsucci P, Rossi M, Sabbatini G et al. Treatment of diabetic retinopathy with anthocyanosides: a preliminary report. Clin Ocul 1983; 4:377.

6. Scharrer A, Ober M. Anthocyanosides in treatment of retinopathies. Klin Monatsbl Augenheilkd 1981; 42:221–31. [Article in German]

7. Canter PH, Ernst E. Anthocyanosides of Vaccinium myrtillus (bilberry) for night vision—a systematic review of placebo-controlled trials. Surv. Ophthalmol. 2004 Jan-Feb; 49(1):38–50.

8. Muth ER, Laurent JM et al. The effect of bilberry nutritional supplementation on night visual acuity and contrast sensitivity. Altern Med Rev 2000; 5(2):164–73.

9. Yao N, Lan F et al. Protective effects of bilberry (Vaccinium myrtillus L.) extract against endotoxin-induced uveitis in mice. J Agric Food Chem. 2010 Apr 28; 58(8):4731–6.

10. Song J, Li Y et al. Protective effect of bilberry (Vaccinium myrtillus L.) extracts on cultured human corneal limbal epithelial cells (HCLEC). Phytother Res. 2010 Apr; 24(4):520–4.

11. Matsunaga N, Imai S et al. Bilberry and its main constituents have neuroprotective effects against retinal neuronal damage in vitro and in vivo. Mol Nutr Food Res. 2009 Jul; 53(7):869–77.

12. Matsunaga N, Chikaraishi Y et al. Vaccinium myrtillus (Bilberry) Extracts Reduce Angiogenesis In Vitro and In Vivo. Evid Based Complement Alternat Med. 2007 Oct 27.

13. Milbury PE, Graf B et al. Bilberry (Vaccinium myrtillus) anthocyanins modulate heme oxygenase-1 and glutathione S-transferase-pi expression in ARPE-19 cells. Invest Ophthalmol Vis Sci. 2007 May; 48(5):2343–9.

14. Chung HK, Choi SM et al. Efficacy of troxerutin on streptozotocin-induced rat model in the early stage of diabetic retinopathy. Arzneimittelforschung 2005; 55(10):573–80.

15. Fursova AZh, Gesarevich OG et al. [Dietary supplementation with bilberry extract prevents macular degeneration and cataracts in senesce-accelerated OXYS rats] Adv. Gerontol. 2005; 16:76–9.

16. Gatta L et al. Vaccinium myrtillus anthocyanosides in the treatment of venous stasis: controlled clinical study on sixty patients. Fitoterapia 1988; 59:19–26.

17. Teglio L, Mazzanti C et al. Vaccinium myrtillus anthocyanosides (Tegens™) in the treatment of venous insufficiency of lower limbs and acute piles in pregnancy. Quad Clin Ostet Ginecol 1987; 42:221–31.

18. Allegra C, Pollari G et al. Antocianosidi e sistema micro-vasculotessutale. Minerva Angiol. 1982; 7:39–44.

19. Grismondi G. Treatment of phlebopathies caused by statis in pregnancy. Minerva Ginecol. 1980; 32:221–30. [Article in Italian]

20. Ghiringhelli C, Gregoratti L et al. Capillarotropic action of anthocyanoides in high dosage in phlebopathic stasis. Minerva Cardioangiol. 1978; 26(4):255–76. [Article in Italian]

21. Mian E, Curri S et al. Anthocyanosides and the walls of the microvessels: further aspects of the mechanism of action of their protective effect in syndromes due to abnormal capillary fragility. Minerva MEd 1977; 68:3565–81.

22. Blumenthal, M. 2003. The ABC Clinical Guide to Herbs. American Botanical Council, Austin.

23. Gentile A. The use of anthocyanidins in bilberry (Tegens™—Inverni della Beffa) to prevent hemorrhaging. 1987. Unpublished: quotes in article, see Morazzoni P, Bombardelli E. Vaccinium myrtillus L. Fitoterapia 1996; 67(1):3–29. [Article in Italian]

24. Choi EH, Park JH et al. Alleviation of doxorubicin-induced toxicities by anthocyanin-rich bilberry (Vaccinium myrtillus L.) extract in rats and mice. Biofactors. 2010 Jul 7.

25. Mauray A, Milenkovic D et al. Atheroprotective effects of bilberry extracts in apo E-deficient mice. J Agric Food Chem. 2009 Dec 9; 57(23):11106–11.

26. Persson IA, Persson K et al. Effect of Vaccinium myrtillus and its polyphenols on angiotensin-converting enzyme activity in human endothelial cells. J Agric Food Chem. 2009 Jun 10; 57(11):4626–9.

27. Bell DR, Gochenaur K. Direct vasoactive and vasoprotective properties of anthocyanin-rich extracts. J. Appl. Physiol. 2006 Apr; 100(4):1164–70. Epub 2005 Dec 8.

28. Bertuglia S, Malandrino S et al. Effect of Vaccinium myrtillus anthocyanosides on ischaemia reperfusion injury in hamster cheek pouch microcirculation. Pharmacol Res. 1995 Mar-Apr; 31(3–4):183–7.

29. Detre Z, Jellinek H et al. Studies on vascular permeability in hypertension: action of anthocyanosides. Clin Physiol Biochem. 1986; 4(2):143–9.

30. Lietti A, Cristoni A et al. Studies on Vaccinium myrtillus anthocyanosides. I. Vasoprotective and antiinflammatory activity. Arzneimittelforschung. 1976; 26(5):829–32.

31. Piljac-Zegarac J, Belscak A et al. Antioxidant capacity and polyphenolic content of blueberry (Vaccinium corymbosum L.) leaf infusions. J Med Food. 2009 Jun; 12(3):608–14.

32. Savikin K, Zdunić G et al. Phenolic content and radical scavenging capacity of berries and related jams from certificated area in Serbia. Plant Foods Hum Nutr. 2009 Sep; 64(3):212–7.

33. Bao L, Yao XS et al. Protective effects of bilberry (Vaccinium myrtillus L.) extract on restraint stress-induced liver damage in mice. J Agric Food Chem. 2008 Sep 10; 56(17):7803–7. Epub 2008 Aug 9.

34. Rahman MM, Ichiyanagi T et al. Effects of anthocyanins on psychological stress-induced oxidative stress and neurotransmitter status. J Agric Food Chem. 2008 Aug 27; 56(16):7545–50. Epub 2008 Jul 29.

35. Bao L, Yao XS et al. Protective effects of bilberry (Vaccinium myrtillus L.) extract on KBrO3-induced kidney damage in mice. J Agric Food Chem. 2008 Jan 23; 56(2):420–5. Epub 2007 Dec 20.

36. Ryzhikov MA, Ryzhikova VO. [Application of chemiluminescent methods for analysis of the antioxidant activity of herbal extracts] Vopr Pitan. 2006; 75(2):22–6.

37. Sinitsyna O, Krysanova Z et al. Age-associated changes in oxidative damage and the activity of antioxidant enzymes in rats with inherited overgeneration of free radicals. J Cell Mol Med. 2006 Jan-Mar; 10(1):206–15.

38. Faria A, Oliveira J et al. Antioxidant properties of prepared blueberry (Vaccinium myrtillus) extracts. J Agric Food Chem. 2005 Aug 24; 53(17):6896–902.

39. Ehala S, Vaher M et al. Characterization of phenolic profiles of Northern European berries by capillary electrophoresis and determination of their antioxidant activity. J Agric Food Chem. 2005 Aug 10; 53(16):6484–90.

40. Nakajima JI, Tanaka I et al. LC/PDA/ESI-MS Profiling and Radical Scavenging Activity of Anthocyanins in Various Berries. J Biomed Biotechnol. 2004; 2004(5):241–247.

41. Viljanen K, Kylli P et al. Inhibition of protein and lipid oxidation in liposomes by berry phenolics. J Agric Food Chem. 2004 Dec 1; 52(24):7419–24.

42. Shabalina IG, Shalbueva NI et al. [Use of mirtilene forte and adrusen zinco for correction of oxidative lesions in mitochondria in rats OXYS with inherited hyperproduction of free radicals] Eksp Klin Farmakol. 2001 Jul-Aug; 64(4):34–6.

43. Laplaud PM, Lelubre A et al. Antioxidant action of Vaccinium myrtillus extract on human low density lipoproteins in vitro: initial observations. Fundam Clin Pharmacol. 1997; 11(1):35–40.

44. Nguyen V, Tang J et al. Cytotoxic effects of bilberry extract on MCF7-GFP-tubulin breast cancer cells. J Med Food. 2010 Apr; 13(2):278–85.

45. Thomasset S, Berry DP et al. Pilot study of oral anthocyanins for colorectal cancer chemoprevention. Cancer Prev Res (Phila Pa). 2009 Jul; 2(7):625–33.

46. Matsunaga N, Tsuruma K et al. Inhibitory actions of bilberry anthocyanidins on angiogenesis. Phytother Res. 2010 Jan; 24 Suppl 1:S42-7.

47. Teller N, Thiele W et al. Suppression of the kinase activity of receptor tyrosine kinases by anthocyanin-rich mixtures extracted from bilberries and grapes. J Agric Food Chem. 2009 Apr 22; 57(8):3094–101.

48. Mutanen M, Pajari AM et al. Berries as chemopreventive dietary constituents—a mechanistic approach with the ApcMin/+ mouse. Asia Pac J Clin Nutr. 2008; 17 Suppl 1:123–5.

49. Ozgurtas T, Aydin I et al. Bilberry inhibits angiogenesis in chick chorioallontoic membrane. Biofactors. 2008; 33(3):161–4.

50. Choi EH, Ok HE et al. Protective effect of anthocyanin-rich extract from bilberry (Vaccinium myrtillus L.) against myelotoxicity induced by 5-fluorouracil. Biofactors. 2007; 29(1):55–65.

51. Cooke D, Schwarz M et al. Effect of cyanidin-3-glucoside and an anthocyanin mixture from bilberry on adenoma development in the ApcMin mouse model of intestinal carcinogenesis—relationship with tissue anthocyanin levels. Int J Cancer. 2006 Nov 1; 119(9):2213–20.

52. Ichiyanagi T, Shida Y et al. Bioavailability and tissue distribution of anthocyanins in bilberry (Vaccinium myrtillus L.) extract in rats. J Agric Food Chem. 2006 Sep 6; 54(18):6578–87.

53. Zhao C, Giusti MM et al. Effects of commercial anthocyanin-rich extracts on colonic cancer and nontumorigenic colonic cell growth. J Agric Food Chem. 2004 Oct 6; 52(20):6122–8.

54. Katsube N, Iwashita K et al. Induction of apoptosis in cancer cells by Bilberry (Vaccinium myrtillus) and the anthocyanins. J Agric Food Chem. 2003 Jan 1; 51(1):68–75.

55. Burdulis D, Sarkinas A et al. Comparative study of anthocyanin composition, antimicrobial and antioxidant activity in bilberry (Vaccinium myrtillus L.) and blueberry (Vaccinium corymbosum L.) fruits. Acta Pol Pharm. 2009 Jul-Aug; 66(4):399–408.

56. Gordien AY, Gray AI et al. Activity of Scottish plant, lichen and fungal endophyte extracts against Mycobacterium aurum and Mycobacterium tuberculosis. Phytother Res. 2010 May; 24(5):692–8.

57. Huttunen S, Toivanen M et al. Inhibition Activity of Wild Berry Juice Fractions against Streptococcus pneumonia Binding to Human Bronchial Cells. Phytother Res. 2010 Jul 12.

58. Nohynek LJ, Alakomi HL et al. Berry phenolics: antimicrobial properties and mechanisms of action against severe human pathogens. Nutr Cancer. 2006; 54(1):18–32.

59. Chatterjee A, Yasmin T et al. Inhibition of Helicobacter pylori in vitro by various berry extracts, with enhanced susceptibility to clarithromycin. Mol Cell Biochem. 2004 Oct; 265(1–2):19–26.

60. Anthony JP, Fyfe L et al. The effect of blueberry extracts on Giardia duodenalis viability and spontaneous excystation of Cryptosporidium parvum oocysts, in vitro. Methods. 2007 Aug; 42(4):339–48.

61. Takikawa M, Inoue S et al. Dietary anthocyanin-rich bilberry extract ameliorates hyperglycemia and insulin sensitivity via activation of AMP-activated protein kinase in diabetic mice. J Nutr. 2010 Mar; 140(3):527–33. Epub 2010 Jan 20.

62. Cignarella A, Nastasi M et al. Novel lipid-lowering properties of Vaccinium myrtillus L. leaves, a traditional antidiabetic treatment, in several models of rat dyslipidaemia: a comparison with ciprofibrate. Thromb Res. 1996 Dec 1; 84(5):311–22.

63. Helmstädter A, Schuster N. Vaccinium myrtillus as an antidiabetic medicinal plant—research through the ages. Pharmazie. 2010 May; 65(5):315–21.

64. Svobodová A, Zdarilová A et al. Lonicera caerulea and Vaccinium myrtillus fruit polyphenols protect HaCaT keratinocytes against UVB-induced phototoxic stress and DNA damage. J Dermatol Sci. 2009 Dec; 56(3):196–204. Epub 2009 Sep 10.

65. Svobodová A, Rambousková J et al. Bilberry extract reduces UVA-induced oxidative stress in HaCaT keratinocytes: a pilot study. Biofactors. 2008; 33(4):249–66.

66. Colombo D, Vescovini R. Studio clinico controllato sull'efficacia degli antocianosidi del mirtillo cel trattamento della dismenorrea essenziale. Giorn It Ost Gin. 1985; 7:1033–8.

67. Liu J, Zhang W et al. Bog bilberry (Vaccinium uliginosum L.) extract reduces cultured Hep-G2, Caco-2, and 3T3-L1 cell viability, affects cell cycle progression, and has variable effects on membrane permeability. J Food Sci. 2010 Apr; 75(3):H103-7.

68. Zu XY, Zhang ZY et al. Anthocyanins extracted from Chinese blueberry (Vaccinium uliginosum L.) and its anticancer effects on DLD-1 and COLO205 cells. Chin Med J (Engl). 2010 Oct; 123(19):2714–9.

69. Kobayashi K, Baba E et al. Screening of Mongolian plants for influence on amylase activity in mouse plasma and gastrointestinal tube. Biol Pharm Bull. 2003 Jul; 26(7):1045–8.

70. Bae JY, Lim SS et al. Bog blueberry anthocyanins alleviate photoaging in ultraviolet-B irradiation-induced human dermal fibroblasts. Mol Nutr Food Res. 2009 Jun; 53(6):726–38.

71. Kim YH, Bang CY et al. Antioxidant activities of Vaccinium uliginosum L. extract and its active components. J Med Food. 2009 Aug; 12(4):885–92.

72. Yin L, Pi YL et al. [The effect of Vaccinium uliginosum to the electroretinogram and retina of rabbits before and after light-induced damage]. Zhonghua Yan Ke Za Zhi. 2010 May; 46(5):446–51. [Article in Chinese]

Bladderwrack

1. Kwak KW, Cho KS et al. Biological effects of fucoidan isolated from Fucus vesiculosus on thrombosis and vascular cells. Korean J Hematol. 2010 Mar; 45(1):51–7. Epub. 2010 Mar 31.

2. de Azevedo TC, Bezerra ME et al. Heparinoids algal and their anticoagulant, hemorrhagic activities and platelet aggregation. Biomed Pharmacother. 2009 Aug; 63(7):477–83. Epub. 2008 Oct 26.

3. Medeiros VP, Queiroz KC et al. Sulfated galactofucan from Lobophora variegata: anticoagulant and anti-inflammatory properties. Biochemistry (Mosc). 2008 Sep; 73(9):1018–24.

4. Cumashi A, Ushakova NA et al. Consorzio Interuniversitario Nazionale per la Bio-Oncologia, Italy. A comparative study of the anti-inflammatory, anticoagulant, antiangiogenic, and antiadhesive activities of nine different fucoidans from brown seaweeds. Glycobiology. 2007 May; 17(5):541–52. Epub 2007 Feb 12.

5. Dürig J, Bruhn T et al. Anticoagulant fucoidan fractions from Fucus vesiculosus induce platelet activation in vitro. Thromb Res. 1997 Mar 15; 85(6):479–91.

6. Parys S, Kehraus S et al. In vitro chemopreventive potential of fucophlorethols from the brown alga Fucus vesiculosus L. by anti-oxidant activity and inhibition of selected cytochrome P450 enzymes. Phytochemistry. 2010 Feb; 71(2–3):221–9. Epub 2009 Dec 1.

7. Wang T, Jónsdóttir R et al. Total phenolic compounds, radical scavenging and metal chelation of extracts from Icelandic seaweeds. Food Chemistry. 2009 Sep 1; 116 (1): 240–8.

8. Díaz-Rubio ME, Pérez-Jiménez J et al. Dietary fiber and antioxidant capacity in Fucus vesiculosus products. Int J Food Sci Nutr. 2009; 60 Suppl 2:23–34. Epub 2008 Oct 25.

9. Zaragozá MC, López D et al. Toxicity and antioxidant activity in vitro and in vivo of two Fucus vesiculosus extracts. J Agric Food Chem. 2008 Sep 10; 56(17):7773–80. Epub 2008 Aug 7.

10. Rocha de Souza MC, Marques CT et al. Antioxidant activities of sulfated polysaccharides from brown and red seaweeds. J Appl Phycol. 2007 Apr; 19(2):153–160. Epub 2006 Nov 30.

11. Rupérez P, Ahrazem O et al. Potential antioxidant capacity of sulfated polysaccharides from the edible marine brown seaweed Fucus vesiculosus. J Agric Food Chem. 2002 Feb 13; 50(4):840–5.

12. Skibola CF. The effect of Fucus vesiculosus, an edible brown seaweed, upon menstrual cycle length and hormonal status in three pre-menopausal women: a case report. BMC Complement Altern Med. 2004 Aug 4; 4:10.

13. Lamela M, Anca J et al. Hypoglycemic activity of several seaweed extracts. J Ethnopharmacol. 1989 Nov; 27(1–2):35–43.

14. Fujimura T, Tsukahara K et al. Effects of natural product extracts on contraction and mechanical properties of fibroblast populated collagen gel. Biol Pharm Bull. 2000 Mar; 23(3):291–7.

15. Fujimura T, Tsukahara K et al. Treatment of human skin with an extract of Fucus vesiculosus changes its thickness and mechanical properties. J Cosmet Sci. 2002 Jan-Feb; 53(1):1–9.

16. Kim MH, Joo HG. Immunostimulatory effects of fucoidan on bone marrow-derived dendritic cells. Immunol Lett. 2008 Jan 29; 115(2):138–43. Epub 2007 Nov 26.

17. Hirayasu H, Yoshikawa Y et al. Sulfated polysaccharides derived from dietary seaweeds increase the esterase activity of a lymphocyte tryptase, granzyme A. J Nutr Sci Vitaminol (Tokyo). 2005 Dec; 51(6):475–7.

18. Williamson, EM. 2003. Potter's Herbal Cyclopaedia. The C. W. Daniel Company, Essex.

19. Byon YY, Kim MH et al. Radioprotective effects of fucoidan on bone marrow cells: improvement of the cell survival and immunoreactivity. J Vet Sci. 2008 Dec; 9(4):359–65.

20. Béress A, Wassermann O et al. A new procedure for the isolation of anti-HIV compounds (polysaccharides and polyphenols) from the marine alga Fucus vesiculosus. J Nat Prod. 1993 Apr; 56(4):478–88.

21. Hyun JH, Kim SC et al. Apoptosis inducing activity of fucoidan in HCT-15 colon carcinoma cells. Biol Pharm Bull. 2009 Oct; 32(10):1760–4.

22. Veena CK, Josephine A et al. Mitochondrial dysfunction in an animal model of hyperoxaluria: a prophylactic approach with fucoidan. Eur J Pharmacol. 2008 Jan 28; 579(1–3):330–6. Epub 2007 Oct 16.

Bogbean

1. Jónsdóttir, G. Áhrif vatnsútdrátta af horblöðku og vallhumli á þroska angafrumna og getu þeirra til að ræsa ósamgena CD4+ T frumur in vitro. University of Iceland, Doctor's thesis, 2010. Found on 1.02.2011 at http://hdl.handle.net/1946/6959. [In Icelandic

2. Lindholm P, Gullbo J et al. Selective cytotoxicity evaluation in anticancer drug screening of fractionated plant extracts. J Biomol Screen. 2002 Aug; 7(4):333–40.

3. Kuduk-Jaworska J, Szpunar J et al. Immunomodulating polysaccharide fractions of Menyanthes trifoliata L. Z Naturforsch C. 2004 Jul-Aug; 59(7–8):485–93.

4. Heck AM, DeWitt BA et al. Potential interactions between alternative therapies and warfarin. Am J Health Syst Pharm. 2000 Jul 1; 57(13):1221–7; 1228–30.

Caraway

1. De Martino L, De Feo V et al. Chemistry, antioxidant, antibacterial and antifungal activities of volatile oils and their components. Nat Prod Commun. 2009 Dec; 4(12):1741–50.

2. Fazlara A, Najafzadeh H et al. The potential application of plant essential oils as natural preservatives against Escherichia coli O157:H7. Pak J Biol Sci. 2008 Sep 1; 11(17):2054–61.

3. Mohsenzadeh M. Evaluation of antibacterial activity of selected Iranian essential oils against Staphylococcus aureus and Escherichia coli in nutrient broth medium. Pak J Biol Sci. 2007 Oct 15; 10(20):3693–7.

4. Iacobellis NS, Lo Cantore P et al. Antibacterial activity of Cuminum cyminum L. and Carum carvi L. essential oils. J Agric Food Chem. 2005 Jan 12; 53(1):57–61.

5. Mahady GB, Pendland SL et al. In vitro susceptibility of Helicobacter pylori to botanical extracts used traditionally for the treatment of gastrointestinal disorders. Phytother Res. 2005 Nov; 19(11):988–91.

6. Hawrelak JA, Cattley T et al. Essential oils in the treatment of intestinal dysbiosis: A preliminary in vitro study. Altern Med Rev. 2009 Dec; 14(4):380–4.

7. Zare M, Shams-Ghahfarokhi M et al. Comparative study of the major Iranian cereal cultivars and some selected spices in relation to support Aspergillus parasiticus growth and aflatoxin production. Iran Biomed J. 2008 Oct; 12(4):229–36.

8. Park IK, Kim JN et al. Toxicity of plant essential oils and their components against Lycoriella ingenua (Diptera: Sciaridae). J Econ Entomol. 2008 Feb; 101(1):139–44.

9. Seo SM, Kim J et al. Fumigant antitermitic activity of plant essential oils and components from Ajowan (Trachyspermum ammi), Allspice (Pimenta dioica), caraway (Carum carvi), dill (Anethum graveolens), Geranium (Pelargonium graveolens), and Litsea (Litsea cubeba) oils against Japanese termite (Reticulitermes speratus Kolbe). J Agric Food Chem. 2009 Aug 12; 57(15):6596–602.

10. Pitasawat B, Champakaew D et al. Aromatic plant-derived essential oil: an alternative larvicide for mosquito control. Fitoterapia. 2007 Apr; 78(3):205–10. Epub 2007 Feb 6.

11. Chaiyasit D, Choochote W et al. Essential oils as potential adulticides against two populations of Aedes aegypti, the laboratory and natural field strains, in Chiang Mai province, northern Thailand. Parasitol Res. 2006 Nov; 99(6):715–21.

12. Sachin BS, Monica P et al. Pharmacokinetic interaction of some antitubercular drugs with caraway: implications in the enhancement of drug bioavailability. Hum Exp Toxicol. 2009 Apr; 28(4):175–84.

13. Lahlou S, Tahraoui A et al. Diuretic activity of the aqueous extracts of Carum carvi and Tanacetum vulgare in normal rats. J Ethnopharmacol. 2007 Apr 4; 110(3):458–63. Epub 2006 Oct 19.

14. Lemhadri A, Hajji L et al. Cholesterol and triglycerides lowering activities of caraway fruits in normal and streptozotocin diabetic rats. J Ethnopharmacol. 2006 Jul 19; 106(3):321–6. Epub 2006 Mar 6.

15. Eddouks M, Lemhadri A et al. Caraway and caper: potential antihyperglycaemic plants in diabetic rats. J Ethnopharmacol. 2004 Sep; 94(1):143–8.

16. Khayyal MT, el-Ghazaly MA et al. Antiulcerogenic effect of some gastrointestinally acting plant extracts and their combination. Arzneimittelforschung. 2001; 51(7):545–53.

17. Kapoor IP, Singh B et al. Chemistry and antioxidant activity of essential oil and oleoresins of black caraway (Carum bulbocastanum) fruits: Part 69. J Sci Food Agric. 2010 Feb; 90(3):385–90.

18. Rodov V, Vinokur Y et al. Hydrophilic and lipophilic antioxidant capacities of Georgian spices for meat and their possible health implications. Georgian Med News. 2010 Feb; (179):61–6.

19. Kamaleeswari M, Nalini N. Dose-response efficacy of caraway (Carum carvi L.) on tissue lipid peroxidation and antioxidant profile in rat colon carcinogenesis. J Pharm Pharmacol. 2006 Aug; 58(8):1121–30.

20. Satyanarayana S, Sushruta K et al. Antioxidant activity of the aqueous extracts of spicy food additives—evaluation and comparison with ascorbic acid in in-vitro systems. J Herb Pharmacother. 2004; 4(2):1–10.

21. Bogucka-Kocka A, Smolarz HD et al. Apoptotic activities of ethanol extracts from some Apiaceae on human leukaemia cell lines. Fitoterapia. 2008 Dec; 79(7–8):487–97. Epub 2008 Jul 10.

22. Naderi-Kalali B, Allameh A et al. Suppressive effects of caraway (Carum carvi) extracts on 2, 3, 7, 8-tetrachloro-dibenzo-p-dioxin-dependent gene expression of cytochrome P450 1A1 in the rat H4IIE cells. Toxicol In Vitro. 2005 Apr; 19(3):373–7. Epub 2005 Jan 26.

23. Zheng GQ, Kenney PM et al. Anethofuran, carvone, and limonene: potential cancer chemopreventive agents from dill weed oil and caraway oil. Planta Med. 1992 Aug; 58(4):338–41.

24. Deeptha K, Kamaleeswari M et al. Dose dependent inhibitory effect of dietary caraway on 1,2-dimethylhydrazine induced colonic aberrant crypt foci and bacterial enzyme activity in rats. Invest New Drugs. 2006 Nov; 24(6):479–88.

25. Kamaleeswari M, Deeptha K et al. Effect of dietary caraway (Carum carvi L.) on aberrant crypt foci development, fecal steroids, and intestinal alkaline phosphatase activities in 1,2-dimethylhydrazine-induced colon carcinogenesis. Toxicol Appl Pharmacol. 2006 Aug 1; 214(3):290–6. Epub 2006 Feb 17.

Chickweed

1. Chon SU, Heo BG et al. Total phenolics level, antioxidant activities and cytotoxicity of young sprouts of some traditional Korean salad plants. Plant Foods Hum Nutr. 2009 Mar; 64(1):25–31.

2. Pieroni A, Janiak V et al. In vitro antioxidant activity of non-cultivated vegetables of ethnic Albanians in southern Italy. Phytother Res. 2002 Aug; 16(5):467–73.

3. Budzianowski J, Pakulski G et al. Studies on antioxidative activity of some C-glycosylflavones. Pol J Pharmacol Pharm. 1991 Sep-Oct; 43(5):395–401.

Cold-weather Eyebright

1. Stoss M, Michels C et al. Prospective cohort trial of Euphrasia single-dose eye drops in conjunctivitis. J Altern Complement Med. 2000 Dec; 6(6):499–508.

2. Williamson, EM. 2003. Potter's Herbal Cyclopaedia. The C. W. Daniel Company, Essex.

3. Trovato A, Monforte MT et al. In vitro anti-mycotic activity of some medicinal plants containing flavonoids. Boll Chim Farm. 2000 Sep-Oct; 139(5):225–7.

4. Porchezhian E, Ansari SH et al. Antihyperglycemic activity of Euphrasia officinale leaves. Fitoterapia. 2000 Sep; 71(5):522–6.

Coltsfoot

1. Hwangbo C, Lee HS et al. The anti-inflammatory effect of tussilagone, from Tussilago farfara, is mediated by the induction of heme oxygenase-1 in murine macrophages. Int Immunopharmacol. 2009 Dec; 9(13–14):1578–84. Epub 2009 Oct 1.

2. Williamson, EM. 2003. Potter's Herbal Cyclopaedia. The C. W. Daniel Company, Essex.

3. Hwang SB, Chang MN et al. L-652,469—a dual receptor antagonist of platelet activating factor and dihydropyridines from Tussilago farfara L. Eur J Pharmacol. 1987 Sep 11; 141(2):269–81.

4. Turker AU, Usta C. Biological screening of some Turkish medicinal plant extracts for antimicrobial and toxicity activities. Nat Prod Res. 2008 Jan 20; 22(2):136–46.

5. Kokoska L, Polesny Z et al. Screening of some Siberian medicinal plants for antimicrobial activity. J Ethnopharmacol. 2002 Sep; 82(1):51–3.

6. Kim MR, Lee JY et al. Antioxidative effects of quercetin-glycosides isolated from the flower buds of Tussilago farfara L. Food Chem Toxicol. 2006 Aug; 44(8):1299–307. Epub 2006 Mar 6.

7. Cho J, Kim HM et al. Neuroprotective and antioxidant effects of the ethyl acetate fraction prepared from Tussilago farfara L. Biol Pharm Bull. 2005 Mar; 28(3):455–60.

8. Lim HJ, Lee HS et al. Suppression of inducible nitric oxide synthase and cyclooxygenase-2 expression by tussilagone from Farfarae flos in BV-2 microglial cells. Arch Pharm Res. 2008 May; 31(5):645–52. Epub 2008 May 15.

9. Park HR, Yoo MY et al. Sesquiterpenoids isolated from the flower buds of Tussilago farfara L. inhibit diacylglycerol acyltransferase. J Agric Food Chem. 2008 Nov 26; 56(22):10493–7.

10. Hirono I, Mori H, Culvenor CC. Carcinogenic activity of coltsfoot, Tussilago farfara l. Gann. 1976 Feb; 67(1):125–9.

Couch Grass

1. Hautmann, C, Scheithe, K. Fluid extract of Agropyron repens for the treatment of urinary tract infections or irritable bladder. Results of multicentric post-marketing surveillance. Zeitschrift für Phytotherapie 2000; 21(5):252–5

2. Bradley, P. 2006. British Herbal Compendium Volume 2. British Herbal Medicine Association, Bournemouth.

3. Grases F, Ramis M et al. Effect of Herniaria hirsuta and Agropyron repens on calcium oxalate urolithiasis risk in rats. J Ethnopharmacol. 1995 Mar; 45(3):211–4.

Cow Parsley

1. Lee SK, Kim Y et al. Inhibitory effects of Deoxypodophyllotoxin from Anthriscus sylvestris on human CYP2C9 and CYP3A4. Planta Med. 2010 May; 76(7):701–4. Epub 2009 Dec 3.

2. Yong Y, Shin SY et al. Antitumor activity of deoxypodophyllotoxin isolated from Anthriscus sylvestris: Induction of G2/M cell cycle arrest and caspase-dependent apoptosis. Bioorg Med Chem Lett. 2009 Aug 1; 19(15):4367–71. Epub 2009 May 28.

3. Jeong GS, Kwon OK et al. Lignans and coumarins from the roots of Anthriscus sylvestris and their increase of caspase-3 activity in HL-60 cells. Biol Pharm Bull. 2007 Jul; 30(7):1340–3.

4. Dall'Acqua S, Giorgetti M et al. Deoxypodophyllotoxin content and antioxidant activity of aerial parts of Anthriscus sylvestris Hoffm. Z Naturforsch C. 2006 Sep-Oct; 61(9–10):658–62.

5. Lin CX, Lee E et al. Deoxypodophyllotoxin (DPT) inhibits eosinophil recruitment into the airway and Th2 cytokine expression in an OVA-induced lung inflammation. Planta Med. 2006 Jul; 72(9):786–91. Epub 2006 May 29.

6. Lee SH, Son MJ et al. Dual inhibition of cyclooxygenases-2 and 5-lipoxygenase by deoxypodophyllotoxin in mouse bone marrow-derived mast cells. Biol Pharm Bull. 2004 Jun; 27(6):786–8.

7. Lim YH, Leem MJ et al. Cytotoxic constituents from the roots of Anthriscus sylvestris. Arch Pharm Res. 1999 Apr; 22(2):208–12.

8. Ikeda R, Nagao T et al. Antiproliferative constituents in umbelliferae plants. IV. Constituents in the fruits of Anthriscus sylvestris Hoffm. Chem Pharm Bull (Tokyo). 1998 May; 46(5):875–8.

9. Ikeda R, Nagao T et al. Antiproliferative constituents in umbelliferae plants. III. Constituents in the root and the ground part of Anthriscus sylvestris Hoffm. Chem Pharm Bull (Tokyo). 1998 May; 46(5):871–4.

10. Lin CX, Son MJ et al. Deoxypodophyllotoxin, a naturally occurring lignan, inhibits the passive cutaneous anaphylaxis reaction. Planta Med. 2004 May; 70(5):474–6.

Creeping Thyme

1. Komes D, Belščak-Cvitanović A et al. Phenolic composition and antioxidant properties of some traditionally used medicinal plants affected by the extraction time and hydrolysis. Phytochem Anal. 2010 Sep 16. [Previous Epub.]

2. Orhan I, Senol FS et al. Acetylcholinesterase inhibitory and antioxidant properties of Cyclotrichium niveum, Thymus praecox subsp. caucasicus var. caucasicus, Echinacea purpurea and E. pallida. Food Chem Toxicol. 2009 Jun; 47(6):1304–10. Epub 2009 Mar 12.

3. Topal U, Sasaki M et al. Chemical compositions and antioxidant properties of essential oils from nine species of Turkish plants obtained by supercritical carbon dioxide extraction and steam distillation. Int J Food Sci Nutr. 2008 Nov-Dec; 59(7–8):619–34.

4. Kulisić T, Krisko A et al. The effects of essential oils and aqueous tea infusions of oregano (Origanum vulgare L. spp. hirtum), thyme (Thymus vulgaris L.) and wild thyme (Thymus serpyllum L.) on the copper-induced oxidation of human low-density lipoproteins. Int J Food Sci Nutr. 2007 Mar; 58(2):87–93.

5. Alzoreky NS, Nakahara K. Antibacterial activity of extracts from some edible plants commonly consumed in Asia. Int J Food Microbiol. 2003 Feb 15; 80(3):223–30.

6. Rasooli I, Mirmostafa SA. Antibacterial properties of Thymus pubescens and Thymus serpyllum essential oils. Fitoterapia. 2002 Jun; 73(3):244–50.

7. Isman MB, Wan AJ, Passreiter CM. Insecticidal activity of essential oils to the tobacco cutworm, Spodoptera litura. Fitoterapia. 2001 Jan; 72(1):65–8.

8. Oral N, Gülmez M, Vatansever L et al. Application of antimicrobial ice for extending shelf life of fish. J Food Prot. 2008 Jan; 71(1):218–22.

Crowberry

1. Kim KC, Kang KA et al. Risk reduction of ethyl acetate fraction of Empetrum nigrum var. japonicum via antioxidant properties against hydrogen peroxide-induced cell damage. J Toxicol Environ Health A. 2009; 72(21–22):1499–508.

2. Ogawa K, Sakakibara H et al. Anthocyanin composition and antioxidant activity of the Crowberry (Empetrum nigrum) and other berries. J Agric Food Chem. 2008 Jun 25; 56(12):4457–62. Epub 2008 Jun 4.

3. Gordien AY, Gray AI et al. Activity of Scottish plant, lichen and fungal endophyte extracts against Mycobacterium aurum and Mycobacterium tuberculosis. Phytother Res. 2010 May; 24(5):692–8.

4. McCutcheon AR, Ellis SM et al. Antifungal screening of medicinal plants of British Columbian native peoples. J Ethnopharmacol. 1994 Dec; 44(3):157–69.

5. Huttunen S, Toivanen M et al. Inhibition Activity of Wild Berry Juice Fractions against Streptococcus pneumoniae Binding to Human Bronchial Cells. Phytother Res. 2010 Jul 12.

6. McCutcheon R, RW Stokes et al. Towers Anti-Mycobacterial Screening of British Columbian Medicinal Plants Pharmaceutical Biology. 1997 Apr; 35(2):77–83.

7. Gunnarsdóttir R, Hilmarsdóttir I et al. Bakt"eríuhemjandi efni úr krækilyngi. Tólfta ráðstefna um rannsóknir í líf- og heilbrigðisvísindum í Háskóla Íslands. Reykjavík, 4.-5. January 2005. Læknablaðið 90 (suppl 50, p. 98) 2004.

Daisy

1. Siatka T, Kašparová M. Seasonal variation in total phenolic and flavonoid contents and DPPH scavenging activity of Bellis perennis L. flowers. Molecules. 2010 Dec 21; 15(12):9450–61.

2. Kavalcioğlu N, Açik L et al. Biological activities of Bellis perennis volatiles and extracts. Nat Prod Commun. 2010 Jan; 5(1):147–50.

3. Avato P, Vitali C et al. Antimicrobial activity of polyacetylenes from Bellis perennis and their synthetic derivatives. Planta Med. 1997 Dec; 63(6):503–7.

4. Bader G, Kulhanek Y et al. [The antifungal action of polygalacic acid glycosides]. Pharmazie. 1990 Jul;45(8):618–20. [Article in German]

5. Morikawa T, Muraoka O et al. [Pharmaceutical food science: search for anti-obese constituents from medicinal foods-anti-hyperlipidemic saponin constituents from the flowers of Bellis perennis]. Yakugaku Zasshi. 2010 May; 130(5):673–8. [Article in Japanese]

6. Morikawa T, Li X et al. Perennisosides I-VII, acylated triterpene saponins with antihyperlipidemic activities from the flowers of Bellis perennis. J Nat Prod. 2008 May; 71(5):828–35. Epub 2008 Mar 26.

Dandelion

1. Bradley, P. 2006. *British Herbal Compendium Volume 2.* British Herbal Medicine Association, Bournemouth.

2. European Scientific Cooperative on Phytotherapy. 2003. *ESCOP Monographs.* 2nd Edition. Georg Thieme Verlag, Stuttgart.

3. Sengul M, Yildiz H et al. Total phenolic content, antioxidant and antimicrobial activities of some medicinal plants. Pak J Pharm Sci. 2009 Jan; 22(1):102–6.

4. Williamson, EM. 2003. Potter's Herbal Cyclopaedia. The C. W. Daniel Company, Essex.

5. WHO. 2010. *WHO Monographs on medicinal plants commonly used in the Newly Independent states (NIS).* World Health Organization, Geneva.

Downy Birch

1. European Scientific Cooperative on Phytotherapy. 2003. *ESCOP Monographs.* 2nd Edition. Georg Thieme Verlag, Stuttgart.

2. Weckesser S, Laszczyk MN et al. Topical treatment of necrotising herpes zoster with betulin from birch bark. Forsch Komplementmed. 2010 Oct; 17(5):271–3. Epub 2010 Sep 9.

3. Gong Y, Raj KM et al. The synergistic effects of betulin with acyclovir against herpes simplex viruses. Antiviral Res. 2004 Nov; 64(2):127–30.

4. Reuter J, Wölfle U et al. Which plant for which skin disease? Part 2: Dermatophytes, chronic venous insufficiency, photoprotection, actinic keratoses, vitiligo, hair loss, cosmetic indications. J Dtsch Dermatol Ges. 2010 Aug 5. [Epub before print]

5. Kim EC, Lee HS et al. The bark of Betula platyphylla var. japonica inhibits the development of atopic dermatitis-like skin lesions in NC/Nga mice. J Ethnopharmacol. 2008 Mar 5; 116(2):270–8. Epub 2007 Dec

6. Huyke C, Laszczyk M et al. [Treatment of actinic keratoses with birch bark extract: a pilot study]. J Dtsch Dermatol Ges. 2006 Feb; 4(2):132–6. [Article in German]

7. Nozdrin VI, Belousova TA et al. [Morphogenetic aspect of the influence of purified birch tar on skin]. Morfologiia. 2004; 126(5):56–60. [Article in Russian]

8. Drag M, Surowiak P et al. Comparison of the cytotoxic effects of birch bark extract, betulin and betulinic acid towards human gastric carcinoma and pancreatic carcinoma drug-sensitive and drug-resistant cell lines. Molecules. 2009 Apr 24; 14(4):1639–51.

9. Chen Z, Wu QL et al. [Effect of betulinic acid on proliferation and apoptosis in Jurkat cells and its mechanism]. Zhonghua Zhong Liu Za Zhi. 2008 Aug; 30(8):588–92. [Article in Chinese]

10. Pyo JS, Roh SH et al. Anti-cancer effect of Betulin on a human lung cancer cell line: a pharmacoproteomic approach using 2 D SDS PAGE coupled with nano-HPLC tandem Mass Spectrometry. Planta Med. 2009 Feb; 75(2):127–31. Epub 2008 Dec 12.

11. Zhang XJ, Han L et al. [Studies of betuionic acid on cell cycle and related protein expressions on mice of bearing H22 tumor cells]. Zhongguo Zhong Yao Za Zhi. 2008 Jul; 33(14):1739–43. [Article in Chinese]

12. Mshvildadze V, Legault J et al. Anticancer diarylheptanoid glycosides from the inner bark of Betula papyrifera. Phytochemistry. 2007 Oct; 68(20):2531–6. Epub 2007 Jun 27.

13. Rzeski W, Stepulak A et al. Betulinic acid decreases expression of bcl-2 and cyclin D1, inhibits proliferation, migration and induces apoptosis in cancer cells. Naunyn Schmiedebergs Arch Pharmacol. 2006 Oct; 374(1):11–20. Epub 2006 Sep 9.

14. Ju EM, Lee SE et al. Antioxidant and anticancer activity of extract from Betula platyphylla var. japonica. Life Sci. 2004 Jan 9; 74(8):1013–26.

15. Calliste CA, Trouillas P et al. Free radical scavenging activities measured by electron spin resonance spectroscopy and B16 cell antiproliferative behaviors of seven plants. J Agric Food Chem. 2001 Jul; 49(7):3321–7.

16. Han S, Li Z et al. [Antitumor effect of the extract of birch bark and its influence to the immune function]. Zhong Yao Cai. 2000 Jun; 23(6):343–5. [Article in Chinese]

17. Kim SH, Park JH et al. Inhibition of antigen-induced degranulation by aryl compounds isolated from the bark of Betula platyphylla in RBL-2H3 cells. Bioorg Med Chem Lett. 2010 May 1; 20(9):2824–7. Epub 2010 Mar 15.

18. Huh JE, Baek YH et al. Protective effects of butanol fraction from Betula platyphylla var. japonica on cartilage alterations in a rabbit collagenase-induced osteoarthritis. J Ethnopharmacol. 2009 Jun 25; 123(3):515–21. Epub 2008 Sep 4.

19. Cho YJ, Huh JE et al. Effect of Betula platyphylla var. japonica on proteoglycan release, type II collagen degradation, and matrix metalloproteinase expression in rabbit articular cartilage explants. Biol Pharm Bull. 2006 Jul; 29(7):1408–13.

20. Matsuda H, Ishikado A et al. Hepatoprotective, superoxide scavenging, and antioxidative activities of aromatic constituents from the bark of Betula platyphylla var. japonica. Bioorg Med Chem Lett. 1998 Nov 3; 8(21):2939–44.

21. Shimizu I, Isshiki Y et al. The antibacterial activity of fragrance ingredients against Legionella pneumophila. Biol Pharm Bull. 2009 Jun; 32(6):1114–7.

22. Demikhova OV, Balakshin VV et al. [Antimycobacterial activity of a dry birch bark extract on a model of experimental pulmonary tuberculosis]. Probl Tuberk Bolezn Legk. 2006; (1):55–7. [Article in Russian]

23. Rauha JP, Remes S et al. Antimicrobial effects of Finnish plant extracts containing flavonoids and other phenolic compounds. Int J Food Microbiol. 2000 May 25; 56(1):3–12.

24. Webster D, Taschereau P et al. Antifungal activity of medicinal plant extracts; preliminary screening studies. J Ethnopharmacol. 2008 Jan 4; 115(1):140–6. Epub 2007 Sep 25.

25. Buruk K, Sokmen A et al. Antimicrobial activity of some endemic plants growing in the Eastern Black Sea Region, Turkey. Fitoterapia. 2006 Jul; 77(5):388–91. Epub 2006 Apr 18.

26. Sur TK, Pandit S et al. Studies on the antiinflammatory activity of Betula alnoides bark. Phytother Res. 2002 Nov; 16(7):669–71.

27. Havlik J, Gonzalez de la Huebra R et al. Xanthine oxidase inhibitory properties of Czech medicinal plants. J Ethnopharmacol. 2010 Nov 11; 132(2):461–5. Epub 2010 Aug 26.

. . . .

Dulse

1. McGrath BM, Harmon JP et al. Palmaria palmata (Dulse) as an unusual maritime aetiology of hyperkalemia in a patient with chronic renal failure: a case report. J Med Case Reports. 2010 Sep 8; 4:301.

2. Yuan YV, Walsh NA. Antioxidant and antiproliferative activities of extracts from a variety of edible seaweeds. Food Chem Toxicol. 2006 Jul; 44(7):1144–50. Epub 2006 Mar 22.

3. Yuan YV, Carrington MF et al. Extracts from dulse (Palmaria palmata) are effective antioxidants and inhibitors of cell proliferation in vitro. Food Chem Toxicol. 2005 Jul; 43(7):1073–81.

. . . .

Fir Clubmoss

1. Felgenhauer N, Zilker T et al. Intoxication with huperzine A, a potent anticholinesterase found in the fir club moss. J Toxicol Clin Toxicol. 2000;38(7):803–8.

2. Halldorsdottir ES, Jaroszewski JW et al. Acetylcholinesterase inhibitory activity of lycopodane-type alkaloids from the Icelandic Lycopodium annotinum ssp. alpestre. Phytochemistry. 2010 Feb; 1(2–3):149–57. Epub 2009 Nov 24.

3. Pálmadóttir RH. Lýkópódium alkalóíðar í litunarjafna (Diphasiastrum alpinum). Einangrun, efnabyggingar og asetýlkólinesterasavirkni. University of Iceland. MSc thesis, 2010. Found on 30.03.2011 at http://hdl.handle.net/1946/4905. [In Icelandic]

4. Ingibjörg Sigurðardóttir. Áhrif lýkópódíum alkalóíða úr lyngjafna og skollafingri á angafrumur in vitro. University of Iceland. M.Sc. thesis, 2009. Found on 30.03.2011 at http://hdl.handle.net/1946/4030. In Icelandic.

. . . .

Grass of Parnassus

1. Sunil Kumar KCa, Müller K. Medicinal plants from Nepal; II. Evaluation as inhibitors of lipid peroxidation in biological membranes. Journal of Ethnopharmacology, 1999 Feb 1; 64(2): 135–9.

2. Müller K. Antiproliferative activity of selected Nepalese medicinal plants against the growth of human keratinocytes. Pharm. Pharmacol. Lett. 1997; 7(2/3):63–65.

. . . .

Greater Burnet

1. Chang HM, But PPH. 1986. *Pharmacology and Application of Chinese Materia Medica (Vol. 1)*. World Scientific Publishing, Singapore.

2. Kim TG, Kang SY et al. Antiviral activities of extracts isolated from Terminalis chebula Retz., Sanguisorba officinalis L., Rubus coreanus Miq. and Rheum palmatum L. against hepatitis B virus. Phytother Res. 2001 Dec; 15(8):718–20.

3. Kokoska L, Polesny Z et al. Screening of some Siberian medicinal plants for antimicrobial activity. J Ethnopharmacol. 2002 Sep; 82(1):51–3.

4. Cho JY, Yoo ES et al. The inhibitory effect of triterpenoid glycosides originating from Sanguisorba officinalis on tissue factor activity and

the production of TNF-alpha. Planta Med. 2006 Nov; 72(14):1279–84. Epub. 2006 Oct 4.

5. Liao H, Banbury LK et al. Antioxidant activity of 45 Chinese herbs and the relationship with their TCM characteristics. Evid Based Complement Alternat Med. 2008 Dec; 5(4):429–34. Epub 2007 Jun 11.

6. Ferreira A, Proença C et al. The in vitro screening for acetylcholinesterase inhibition and antioxidant activity of medicinal plants from Portugal. J Ethnopharmacol. 2006 Nov 3; 108(1):31–7. Epub 2006 Apr 28.

7. Masaki H, Sakaki S et al. Active-oxygen scavenging activity of plant extracts. Biol Pharm Bull. 1995 Jan; 18(1):162–6.

8. Kim YH, Chung CB et al. Anti-wrinkle activity of ziyuglycoside I isolated from a Sanguisorba officinalis root extract and its application as a cosmeceutical ingredient. Biosci Biotechnol Biochem. 2008 Feb; 72(2):303–11. Epub 2008 Feb 7.

9. Tsukahara K, Moriwaki S et al. Inhibitory effect of an extract of Sanguisorba officinalis L. on ultraviolet-B-induced photodamage of rat skin. Biol Pharm Bull. 2001 Sep; 24(9):998–1003.

10. Hachiya A, Kobayashi A et al. The inhibitory effect of an extract of Sanguisorba officinalis L. on ultraviolet B-induced pigmentation via the suppression of endothelin-converting enzyme-1alpha. Biol Pharm Bull. 2001 Jun; 24(6):688–92.

11. Konishi K, Urada M et al. Inhibitory effect of sanguiin H-11 on chemotaxis of neutrophil. Biol Pharm Bull. 2000 Feb; 23(2):213–8.

12. Park KH, Koh D et al. Antiallergic activity of a disaccharide isolated from Sanguisorba officinalis. Phytother Res. 2004 Aug; 18(8):658–62.

13. Shin TY, Lee KB et al. Anti-allergic effects of Sanguisorba officinalis on animal models of allergic reactions. Immunopharmacol Immunotoxicol. 2002 Aug; 24(3):455–68.

14. Liu X, Cui Y et al. Triterpenoids from Sanguisorba officinalis. Phytochemistry. 2005 Jul; 66(14):1671–9.

15. Goun EA, Petrichenko VM et al. Anticancer and antithrombin activity of Russian plants. J Ethnopharmacol. 2002 Aug; 81(3):337–42.

16. Nguyen TT, Cho SO et al. Neuroprotective effect of Sanguisorbae radix against oxidative stress-induced brain damage: in vitro and in vivo. Biol Pharm Bull. 2008 Nov; 31(11):2028–35.

17. Ban JY, Nguyen HT et al. Neuroprotective properties of gallic acid from Sanguisorbae radix on amyloid beta protein (25–35)-induced toxicity in cultured rat cortical neurons. Biol Pharm Bull. 2008 Jan; 31(1):149–53.

. . . .

Greater Plantain

1. Chang, HM, But PPH. 1986. *Pharmacology and Application of Chinese Materia Medica (Vol. 1)*. World Scientific Publishing, Singapore.

2. Hetland G, Samuelsen AB et al. Protective effect of Plantago major L. Pectin polysaccharide against systemic Streptococcus pneumoniae infection in mice. Scand J Immunol. 2000 Oct; 52(4):348–55.

3. Velasco-Lezama R, Tapia-Aguilar R et al. Effect of Plantago major on cell proliferation in vitro. J Ethnopharmacol. 2006 Jan 3; 103(1):36–42. Epub 2005 Oct 14.

4. Chiang LC, Chiang W et al. In vitro cytotoxic, antiviral and immunomodulatory effects of Plantago major and Plantago asiatica. Am J Chin Med. 2003; 31(2):225–34.

5. Holetz FB, Pessini GL et al. Screening of some plants used in the Brazilian folk medicine for the treatment of infectious diseases. Mem Inst Oswaldo Cruz. 2002 Oct; 97(7):1027–31.

6. Bol'shakova IV, Lozovskaia EL et al. [Antioxidant properties of plant extracts] Biofizika. 1998 Mar-Apr; 43(2):186–8. [Article in Russian]

7. Hriscu A, Stănescu U et al. [A pharmacodynamic investigation of the effect of polyholozidic substances extracted from Plantago sp. on the digestive tract] Rev Med Chir Soc Med Nat Iasi. 1990 Jan-Mar; 94(1):165–70. [Article in Rumanian]

8. Atta AH, Mouneir SM. Evaluation of some medicinal plant extracts for antidiarrheal activity. Phytother Res. 2005 Jun; 19(6):481–5.

9. Ponce-Macotela M, Navarro-Alegría I et al. [In vitro effect against Giardia of 14 plant extracts] Rev Invest Clin. 1994 Sep-Oct; 46(5):343–7. [Article in Spanish]

10. Türel I, Ozbek H et al. Hepatoprotective and anti-inflammatory activities of Plantago major L. Indian J Pharmacol. 2009 Jun; 41(3):120–4.

11. Beara IN, Orčić DZ et al. Liquid chromatography/tandem mass spectrometry study of anti-inflammatory activity of plantain (Plantago L.) species. J Pharm Biomed Anal. 2010 Sep 5; 52(5):701–6. Epub 2010 Feb 18.

12. Ringbom T, Huss U et al. Cox-2 inhibitory effects of naturally occurring and modified fatty acids. J Nat Prod. 2001 Jun; 64(6):745–9.

13. Ringbom T, Segura L et al. Ursolic acid from Plantago major, a selective inhibitor of cyclooxygenase-2 catalyzed prostaglandin biosynthesis. J Nat Prod. 1998 Oct; 61(10):1212–5.

14. Chiang LC, Chiang W et al. Antiviral activity of Plantago major extracts and related compounds in vitro. Antiviral Res. 2002 Jul; 55(1):53–62.

15. Gomez-Flores R, Calderon CL et al. Immunoenhancing properties of Plantago major leaf extract. Phytother Res. 2000 Dec; 14(8):617–22.

16. Atta AH, Abo EL-Sooud K. The antinociceptive effect of some Egyptian medicinal plant extracts. J Ethnopharmacol. 2004 Dec; 95(2–3):235–8.

17. Karpilovskaia ED, Gorban' GP et al. [Inhibiting effect of the polyphenolic complex from Plantago major (plantastine) on the carcinogenic effect of endogenously synthesized nitro-sodimethylamine] Farmakol Toksikol. 1989 Jul-Aug; 52(4):64–7. [Article in Russian]

18. Shipochliev T. [Uterotonic action of extracts from a group of medicinal plants] Vet Med Nauki. 1981; 18(4):94–8. [Article in Bulgarian]

19. Ikawati Z, Wahyuono S et al. Screening of several Indonesian medicinal plants for their inhibitory effect on histamine release from RBL-2H3 cells. J Ethnopharmacol. 2001 May; 75(2–3):249–56.

20. Beara IN, Lesjak MM et al. Plantain (Plantago L.) species as novel sources of flavonoid antioxidants. J Agric Food Chem. 2009 Oct 14; 57(19):9268–73.

21. Chiang LC, Ng LT et al. Immunomodulatory activities of flavonoids, monoterpenoids, triterpenoids, iridoid glycosides and phenolic compounds of Plantago species. Planta Med. 2003 Jul; 69(7):600–4.

22. Ozaslan M, Didem Karagöz I et al. In vivo antitumoral effect of Plantago major L. extract on Balb/C mouse with Ehrlich ascites tumor. Am J Chin Med. 2007; 35(5):841–51.

23. Gálvez M, Martín-Cordero C et al. Cytotoxic effect of Plantago spp. on cancer cell lines. J Ethnopharmacol. 2003 Oct; 88(2–3):125–30.

24. Lithander A. Intracellular fluid of waybread (Plantago major) as a prophylactic for mammary cancer in mice. Tumor Biol. 1992; 13(3):138–41.

25. Ruffa MJ, Ferraro G et al. Cytotoxic effect of Argentine medicinal plant extracts on human hepatocellular carcinoma cell line. J Ethnopharmacol. 2002 Mar; 79(3):335–9.

26. Doan DD, Nguyen NH et al. Studies on the individual and combined diuretic effects of four Vietnamese traditional herbal remedies (Zea mays, Imperata cylindrica, Plantago major and Orthosiphon stamineus). J Ethnopharmacol. 1992 Jun; 36(3):225–31.

Groundsel

1. Vilar JH, Garcia M et al. [Veno-occlusive liver disease induced by Senecio vulgaris toxicity] Gastroenterol Hepatol. 2000 Jun-Jul; 23(6):285–6. [Article in Spanish]

2. Ortiz Cansado A, Crespo Valadés E et al. [Veno-occlusive liver disease due to intake of Senecio vulgaris tea]. Gastroenterol Hepatol. 1995 Oct; 18(8):413–6. [Article in Spanish]

3. Uzun E, Sariyar G, Adsersen A et al. Traditional medicine in Sakarya province (Turkey) and antimicrobial activities of selected species. J Ethnopharmacol. 2004 Dec; 95(2–3):287–96.

4. Loizzo MR, Statti GA et al. Antibacterial and antifungal activity of Senecio inaequidens DC. and Senecio vulgaris L. Phytother Res. 2004 Sep; 18(9):777–9.

Hawkweed

1. Williamson, EM. 2003. *Potter's Herbal Cyclopaedia*. The C. W. Daniel Company, Essex.

Heartsease

1. Toiu A, Pârvu AE et al. Evaluation of anti-inflammatory activity of alcoholic extract from Viola tricolor. Rev Med Chir Soc Med Nat Iasi. 2007 Apr-Jun; 111(2):525–9.

2. Bradley, P. 2006. British Herbal Compendium Volume 2. British Herbal Medicine Association, Bournemouth.

3. Vukics V, Kery A et al. Analysis of polar antioxidants in Heartsease (Viola tricolor L.) and Garden pansy (Viola x wittrockiana Gams.). J Chromatogr Sci. 2008 Oct; 46(9):823–7.

4. Vukics V, Kery A et al. Major flavonoid components of heartsease (Viola tricolor L.) and their antioxidant activities. Anal Bioanal Chem. 2008 Apr; 390(7):1917–25. Epub 2008 Feb 8.

5. Svangård E, Göransson U et al. Cytotoxic cyclotides from Viola tricolor. J Nat Prod. 2004 Feb; 67(2):144–7.

Heather

1. Williamson, EM. 2003. Potter's Herbal Cyclopaedia. The C. W. Daniel Company, Essex.

2. Gordien AY, Gray AI et al. Activity of Scottish plant, lichen and fungal endophyte extracts against Mycobacterium aurum and

Mycobacterium tuberculosis. Phytother Res. 2010 May; 24(5):692–8.

3. Tunón H, Olavsdotter C et al. Evaluation of anti-inflammatory activity of some Swedish medicinal plants. Inhibition of prostaglandin biosynthesis and PAF-induced exocytosis. J Ethnopharmacol. 1995 Oct; 48(2):61–76.

4. Najid A, Simon A et al. Characterization of ursolic acid as a lipoxygenase and cyclooxygenase inhibitor using macrophages, platelets and differentiated HL60 leukemic cells. FEBS Lett. 1992 Mar 16; 299(3):213–7.

5. Orhan I, Küpeli E et al. Bioassay-guided isolation of kaempferol-3-O-beta-D-galactoside with anti-inflammatory and antinociceptive activity from the aerial part of Calluna vulgaris L. J Ethnopharmacol. 2007 Oct 8; 114(1):32–7. Epub 2007 Jul 3.

6. Simon A, Najid A et al. Inhibition of lipoxygenase activity and HL60 leukemic cell proliferation by ursolic acid isolated from heather flowers (Calluna vulgaris). Biochim Biophys Acta. 1992 Apr 8; 1125(1):68–72.

7. Najid A, Simon A et al. A Calluna vulgaris extract 5-lipoxygenase inhibitor shows potent antiproliferative effects on human leukemia HL-60 cells. Eicosanoids. 1992; 5(1):45–51.

8. Pavlović RD, Lakusić B et al. Arbutin content and antioxidant activity of some Ericaceae species. Pharmazie. 2009 Oct; 64(10):656–9.

9. Saaby L, Rasmussen HB et al. MAO-A inhibitory activity of quercetin from Calluna vulgaris (L.) Hull. J Ethnopharmacol. 2009 Jan 12; 121(1):178–81. Epub 2008 Nov 1.

Hemp-nettle

1. Matkowski, A, Tasarz, P et al. Antioxidant activity of herb extracts from five medicinal plants from Lamiaceae, subfamily Lamioideae. Journal of Medicinal Plants Research. 2008 Nov; 2(11):321–30

Horsetail

1. Williamson, EM. 2003. Potter's Herbal Cyclopaedia. The C. W. Daniel Company, Essex.

2. WHO. 2010. WHO monographs on medicinal plants commonly used in the Newly Independent States (NIS). World Health Organization, Geneva.

3. Cetojević-Simin DD, Canadanović-Brunet JM et al. Antioxidative and antiproliferative activities of different horsetail (Equisetum arvense L.) extracts. J Med Food. 2010 Apr; 13(2):452–9.

4. Stajner D, Popović BM et al. Exploring Equisetum arvense L., Equisetum ramosissimum L. and Equisetum telmateia L. as sources of natural antioxidants. Phytother Res. 2009 Apr; 23(4):546–50.

5. Mimica-Dukic N, Simin N et al. Phenolic compounds in field horsetail (Equisetum arvense L.) as natural antioxidants. Molecules. 2008 Jul 17; 13(7):1455–64.

6. Milovanović V, Radulović N et al. Antioxidant, antimicrobial and genotoxicity screening of hydro-alcoholic extracts of five serbian Equisetum species. Plant Foods Hum Nutr. 2007 Sep; 62(3):113–9. Epub 2007 Aug 4.

7. Guilherme dos Santos J Jr, Hoffmann Martins do Monte F et al. Cognitive enhancement in aged rats after chronic administration of Equisetum arvense L. with demonstrated antioxidant properties in vitro. Pharmacol Biochem Behav. 2005 Jul; 81(3):593–600.

8. Myagmar BE, Aniya Y. Free radical scavenging action of medicinal herbs from Mongolia. Phytomedicine. 2000 Jun; 7(3):221–9.

9. Stajner D, Popović BM et al. Free radical scavenging activity of three Equisetum species from Fruska gora mountain. Fitoterapia. 2006 Dec; 77(7–8):601–4. Epub 2006 Jul 6.

10. Radulović N, Stojanović G et al. Composition and antimicrobial activity of Equisetum arvense L. essential oil. Phytother Res. 2006 Jan; 20(1):85–8.

11. Dos Santos JG Jr, Blanco MM et al. Sedative and anticonvulsant effects of hydroalcoholic extract of Equisetum arvense. Fitoterapia. 2005 Sep; 76(6):508–13.

12. Do Monte FH, dos Santos JG Jr et al. Antinociceptive and anti-inflammatory properties of the hydroalcoholic extract of stems from Equisetum arvense L. in mice. Pharmacol Res. 2004 Mar; 49(3):239–43.

13. Tamaki M, Nakashima M et al. [Assessment of clinical usefulness of Eviprostat for benign prostatic hyperplasia—comparison of Eviprostat tablet with a formulation containing two-times more active ingredients] Hinyokika Kiyo. 2008 Jun; 54(6):435–45. [Article in Japanese]

14. Oka M, Tachibana M et al. Relevance of anti-reactive oxygen species activity to anti-inflammatory activity of components of eviprostat, a phytotherapeutic agent for benign prostatic hyperplasia. Phytomedicine. 2007 Aug; 14(7–8):465–72. Epub 2007 Jun 20.

15. Soleimani S, Azarbaizani FF et al. The effect of Equisetum arvense L. (Equisetaceae) in histological changes of pancreatic beta-cells in streptozotocin-induced diabetic in rats. Pak J Biol Sci. 2007 Dec 1; 10(23):4236–40.

16. Safiyeh S, Fathallah FB et al. Antidiabetic effect of Equisetum arvense L. (Equisetaceae) in streptozotocin-induced diabetes in male rats. Pak J Biol Sci. 2007 May 15; 10(10):1661–6.

17. Blumenthal, M, A, Goldberg J. Brinckmann. 2000. Herbal Medicine. Expanded Commission E Monographs. Integrative Medicine Communications, Newton.

18. Grases F, Melero G et al. Urolithiasis and phytotherapy. Int Urol Nephrol. 1994; 26(5):507–11.

19. Baracho NC, Vicente BB et al. Study of acute hepatotoxicity of Equisetum arvense L. in rats. Acta Cir Bras. 2009 Nov-Dec; 24(6):449–53.

20. Oh H, Kim DH et al. Hepatoprotective and free radical scavenging activities of phenolic petrosins and flavonoids isolated from Equisetum arvense. J Ethnopharmacol. 2004 Dec; 95(2–3):421–4.

21. Tepkeeva II, Aushev VN et al. Cytostatic activity of peptide extracts of medicinal plants on transformed A549, H1299, and HeLa Cells. Bull Exp Biol Med. 2009 Jan; 147(1):48–51.

22. Chaadaeva AV, Tenkeeva II et al. [Antitumor activity of the plant remedy peptide extract PE-PM in a new mouse T-lymphoma/eukemia model] Biomed Khim. 2009 Jan-Feb; 55(1):81–8. [Article in Russian]

23. Tepkeeva II, Moiseeva EV et al. Evaluation of antitumor activity of peptide extracts from medicinal plants on the model of transplanted breast cancer in CBRB-Rb(8.17)1Iem mice. Bull Exp Biol Med. 2008 Apr; 145(4):464–6.

Iceland Moss

1. Kempe C, Grüning H et al. [Icelandic moss lozenges in the prevention or treatment of oral mucosa irritation and dried out throat mucosa] Laryngorhinootologie. 1997 Mar; 76(3):186–8. [Article in German]

2. European Scientific Cooperative on Phytotherapy. 2003. *ESCOP Monographs*. 2nd Edition. Georg Thieme Verlag, Stuttgart.

3. Freysdottir J, Omarsdottir S et al. In vitro and in vivo immunomodulating effects of traditionally prepared extract and purified compounds from Cetraria islandica. Int Immunopharmacol. 2008 Mar; 8(3):423–30. Epub 2007 Dec 7.

4. Ogmundsdóttir HM, Zoëga GM et al. Anti-proliferative effects of lichen-derived inhibitors of 5-lipoxygenase on malignant cell-lines and mitogen-stimulated lymphocytes. J Pharm Pharmacol. 1998 Jan; 50(1):107–15.

5. Gülçin I, Oktay M et al. Determination of antioxidant activity of lichen Cetraria islandica (L) Ach. J Ethnopharmacol. 2002 Mar; 79(3):325–9.

6. Krämer P, Wincierz U et al. Rational approach to fractionation, isolation, and characterization of polysaccharides from the lichen Cetraria islandica. Arzneimittelforschung. 1995 Jun; 45(6):726–31.

7. Ingolfsdottir K, Hjalmarsdottir MA et al. In vitro susceptibility of Helicobacter pylori to protolichesterinic acid from the lichen Cetraria islandica. Antimicrob Agents Chemother. 1997 Jan; 41(1):215–7.

8. Ingólfsdóttir K, Chung GA et al. Antimycobacterial activity of lichen metabolites in vitro. Eur J Pharm Sci. 1998 Apr; 6(2):141–4.

9. Pengsuparp T, Cai L et al. Mechanistic evaluation of new plant-derived compounds that inhibit HIV-1 reverse transcriptase. J Nat Prod. 1995 Jul; 58(7):1024–31.

10. Ingolfsdottir K. Bioactive compounds from Iceland moss. Proceedings of the Phytochemistry Society of Europe, 2000, 44:25–36.

11. Olafsdottir ES, Ingolfsdottir K et al. Immunologically active (1->3)-(1->4)-alpha-D-glucan from Cetraria islandica. Phytomedicine. 1999 Mar; 6(1):33–9.

12. Ingolfsdottir K, Jurcic K et al. Immunologically active polysaccharide from Cetraria islandica. Planta Med. 1994 Dec; 60(6):527–31.

13. Ágústsdóttir, H. Áhrif prótólichesterínsýru á frumufjölgun og tjáningu STAT3 próteins í frumulínum úr mergæxli. University of Iceland, MSc. thesis, 2009. Found on 22.03.2011 at http://hdl.handle.net/1946/3025. [In Icelandic].

14. Kristmundsdóttir T, Jónsdóttir E et al. Solubilization of poorly soluble lichen metabolites for biological testing on cell lines. Eur J Pharm Sci. 2005 Apr; 24(5):539–43.

15. Pang Z, Otaka K et al. Structure of beta-glucan oligomer from laminarin and its effect on human monocytes to inhibit the proliferation of U937 cells. Biosci Biotechnol Biochem. 2005 Mar; 69(3):553–8.

Irish Moss

1. Williamson, EM. 2003. *Potter's Herbal Cyclopaedia*. The C. W. Daniel Company, Essex.

Juniper

1. Wanner J, Schmidt E et al. Chemical composition and antibacterial activity of selected essential oils and some of their main compounds. Nat Prod Commun. 2010 Sep; 5(9):1359–64.

2. Lawrence HA, Palombo EA. Activity of essential oils against Bacillus subtilis spores. J Microbiol Biotechnol. 2009 Dec; 19(12):1590–5.

3. Cavaleiro C, Pinto E et al. Antifungal activity of Juniperus essential oils against dermatophyte, Aspergillus and Candida strains. J Appl Microbiol. 2006 Jun; 100(6):1333–8.

4. Pepeljnjak S, Kosalec I et al. Antimicrobial activity of juniper berry essential oil (Juniperus communis L., Cupressaceae). Acta Pharm. 2005 Dec; 55(4):417–22.

5. Marino A, Bellinghieri V et al. In vitro effect of branch extracts of Juniperus species from Turkey on Staphylococcus aureus biofilm. FEMS Immunol Med Microbiol. 2010 Aug; 59(3):470–6. Epub 2010 May 28.

6. Martz F, Peltola R et al. Effect of latitude and altitude on the terpenoid and soluble phenolic composition of juniper (Juniperus communis) needles and evaluation of their antibacterial activity in the boreal zone. J Agric Food Chem. 2009 Oct 28; 57(20):9575–84.

7. Miceli N, Trovato A et al. Comparative analysis of flavonoid profile, antioxidant and antimicrobial activity of the berries of Juniperus communis L. var. communis and Juniperus communis L. var. saxatilis Pall. from Turkey. Agric Food Chem. 2009 Aug 12; 57(15):6570–7.

8. Gordien AY, Gray AI et al. Activity of Scottish plant, lichen and fungal endophyte extracts against Mycobacterium aurum and Mycobacterium tuberculosis. Phytother Res. 2010 May; 24(5):692–8.

9. Gordien AY, Gray AI et al. Antimycobacterial terpenoids from Juniperus communis L. (Cuppressaceae). J Ethnopharmacol. 2009 Dec 10; 126(3):500–5. Epub 2009 Sep 13.

10. Jimenez-Arellanes A, Meckes M et al. Activity against multidrug-resistant Mycobacterium tuberculosis in Mexican plants used to treat respiratory diseases. Phytother Res. 2003 Sep; 17(8):903–8.

11. Al-Mustafa AH, Al-Thunibat OY. Antioxidant activity of some Jordanian medicinal plants used traditionally for treatment of diabetes. Pak J Biol Sci. 2008 Feb 1; 11(3):351–8.

12. Emami SA, Asili J et al. Antioxidant activity of leaves and fruits of Iranian conifers. Evid Based Complement Alternat Med. 2007 Sep; 4(3):313–9.

13. Van Slambrouck S, Daniels AL et al. Effects of crude aqueous medicinal plant extracts on growth and invasion of breast cancer cells. Oncol Rep. 2007 Jun; 17(6):1487–92.

14. Sánchez de Medina F, Gámez MJ et al. Hypoglycemic activity of juniper "berries." Planta Med. 1994 Jun; 60(3):197–200.

15. Swanston-Flatt SK, Day C, Bailey CJ et al. Traditional plant treatments for diabetes. Studies in normal and streptozotocin diabetic mice. Diabetologia. 1990 Aug; 33(8):462–4.

Kidney Vetch

1. Suganda AG, Amoros M et al. [Inhibitory effects of some crude and semi-purified extracts of indigenous French plants on the multiplication of human herpesvirus 1 and poliovirus 2 in cell culture] J Nat Prod. 1983 Sep-Oct; 46(5):626–32. [Article in French]

2. Godevac D, Zdunić G, et al. Antioxidant activity of nine Fabaceae species growing in Serbia and Montenegro. 2008 Apr; 79(3): 185–7.

Knotgrass

1. González Begné M et al. Clinical effect of a Mexican sanguinaria extract (Polygonum aviculare L.) on gingivitis. J Ethnopharmacol. 2001 Jan; 74(1):45–51.

2. Chevallier, A. 1996. The Encyclopedia of Medicinal Plants. Dorling Kindersley, London.

3. Salama H, Marraiki N. Antimicrobial Activity and Phytochemical Analysis of Polygonum Aviculare L.(Polygonaceae), Naturally Growing in Egypt, Australian Journal of Basic and Applied Sciences. 2009; 3(3):2008–15.

4. Williamson, Elizabeth M. 2002. Major Herbs of Ayurveda. Elsevier Science, London.

5. Hsu CY. Antioxidant activity of extract from Polygonum aviculare L. Biol Res. 2006; 39(2):281–8. Epub 2006 Jul 25.

6. Yin MH, Kang DG et al. Screening of vasorelaxant activity of some medicinal plants used in Oriental medicines. J Ethnopharmacol. 2005 May 13; 99(1):113–7.

7. Tunón H, Olavsdotter C et al. Evaluation of anti-inflammatory activity of some Swedish medicinal plants. Inhibition of prostaglandin biosynthesis and PAF-induced exocytosis. J Ethnopharmacol. 1995 Oct; 48(2):61–76.

8. Nan JX, Park EJ et al. Antifibrotic effects of the methanol extract of Polygonum aviculare in fibrotic rats induced by bile duct ligation and scission. Biol Pharm Bull. 2000 Feb; 23(2):240–3.

Lady's Bedstraw

1. Mavi A, Terzi Z, Ozgen U et al. Antioxidant properties of some medicinal plants: Prangos ferulacea (Apiaceae), Sedum sempervivoides (Crassulaceae), Malva neglecta (Malvaceae), Cruciata taurica (Rubiaceae), Rosa pimpinellifolia (Rosaceae), Galium verum subsp. verum (Rubiaceae), Urtica dioica (Urticaceae). Biol Pharm Bull. 2004 May; 27(5):702–5.

Lady's Mantle

1. Bradley, P. 2006. British Herbal Compendium Volume 2. British Herbal Medicine Association, Bournemouth.

2. Shrivastava R, John GW. Treatment of Aphthous Stomatitis with topical Alchemilla vulgaris in glycerine. Clin Drug Investig. 2006; 26(10):567–73.

3. Shrivastava R, Cucuat N et al. Effects of Alchemilla vulgaris and glycerine on epithelial and myofibroblast cell growth and cutaneous lesion healing in rats. Phytother Res. 2007 Apr; 21(4):369–73.

4. Oktyabrsky O, Vysochina G et al. Assessment of anti-oxidant activity of plant extracts using microbial test systems. J Appl Microbiol. 2009 Apr; 106(4):1175–83. Epub 2009 Jan 30.

5. Kiselova Y, Ivanova D et al. Correlation between the in vitro antioxidant activity and polyphenol content of aqueous extracts from Bulgarian herbs. Phytother Res. 2006 Nov; 20(11):961–5.

6. Williamson, EM. 2003. Potter's Herbal Cyclopaedia. The C. W. Daniel Company, Essex.

7. Jonadet M, Meunier MT et al. [Flavonoids extracted from Ribes nigrum L. and Alchemilla vulgaris L.: 1. In vitro inhibitory activities on elastase, trypsin and chymotrypsin. 2. Angioprotective activities compared in vivo] J Pharmacol. 1986 Jan-Mar; 17(1):21–7. [Article in French]

8. Said O, Saad B et al. Weight Loss in Animals and Humans Treated with "Weighlevel," a Combination of Four Medicinal Plants Used in Traditional Arabic and Islamic Medicine. Evid Based Complement Alternat Med. 2008 Oct 24. [Previous Epub.]

Large-flowered Wintergreen

1. Chang, HM, But PPH . 1987. Pharmacology and Application of Chinese Materia Medica (Vol. 2). World Scientific Publishing, Singapore.

2. Chang J, Inui T. Novel phenolic glycoside dimer and trimer from the whole herb of Pyrola rotundifolia. Chem Pharm Bull (Tokyo). 2005 Aug; 53(8):1051–3.

3. Xuan W, Dong M et al. Effects of compound injection of Pyrola rotundifolia L and Astragalus membranaceus Bge on experimental guinea pigs' gentamicin ototoxicity. Ann Otol Rhinol Laryngol. 1995 May; 104(5):374–80.

4. Wang CH, Wu CG. [Clinical observation on the treatment of 101 hypertension patients with Pyrola rotundifolia preparation] Zhong Xi Yi Jie He Za Zhi. 1986 Oct; 6(10):604–5, 581. [Article in Chinese]

Male Fern

1. Williamson, Elizabeth M. 2003. Potter's Herbal Cyclopaedia. The C. W. Daniel Company, Essex.

2. Magalhães LG, Kapadia GJ et al. In vitro schistosomicidal effects of some phloroglucinol derivatives from Dryopteris species against Schistosoma mansoni adult worms. Parasitol Res. 2010 Jan; 106(2):395–401. Epub 2009 Nov 7.

3. Kantemir I, Akder G et al. [Preliminary report on an unexpected effect of an extract from Dryopteris filix mas]. Arzneimittelforschung. 1976 Feb; 26(2):261–2. [Article in German]

Marsh Marigold

1. Duke, JA, and Ayensu ES. 1985. Medicinal Plants of China, Volume Two. Reference Publications, Algonac.

Meadowsweet

1. Peresun'ko AP, Bespalov VG et al. [Clinico-experimental study of using plant preparations from the flowers of Filipendula ulmaria (L.) Maxim for the treatment of precancerous changes and prevention of uterine cervical cancer] Vopr Onkol. 1993; 39(7–12):291–5. [Article in Russian]

2. Spiridonov NA, Konovalov DA et al. Cytotoxicity of some Russian ethnomedicinal plants and plant compounds. Phytother Res. 2005 May; 19(5):428–32.

3. Cwikla C, Schmidt K et al. Investigations into the antibacterial activities of phytotherapeutics against Helicobacter pylori and Campylobacter jejuni. Phytother Res. 2010 May; 24(5):649–56.

4. Nesterova IuV, Povet'eva TN et al. [Evaluation of anti-inflammatory activity of extracts from Siberian plants] Vestn Ross Akad Med Nauk. 2009; (11):30–4. [Article in Russian]

5. Churin AA, Masnaia NV et al. [Effect of Filipendula ulmaria extract on immune system of CBA/CaLac and C57Bl/6 mice] Eksp Klin Farmakol. 2008 Sep-Oct; 71(5):32–6. [Article in Russian]

6. Rauha JP, Remes S et al. Antimicrobial effects of Finnish plant extracts containing flavonoids and other phenolic compounds. Int J Food Microbiol. 2000 May 25; 56(1):3–12.

7. Ryzhikov MA, Ryzhikova VO. [Application of chemiluminescent methods for analysis of the antioxidant activity of herbal extracts] Vopr Pitan. 2006; 75(2):22–6. [Article in Russian]

8. Calliste CA, Trouillas P et al. Free radical scavenging activities measured by electron spin resonance spectroscopy and B16 cell antiproliferative behaviors of seven plants. J Agric Food Chem. 2001 Jul; 49(7):3321–7.

9. Liapina LA, Koval'chuk GA. [A comparative study of the action on the hemostatic system of extracts from the flowers and seeds of the meadowsweet (Filipendula ulmaria (L.) Maxim.] Izv Akad Nauk Ser Biol. 1993 Jul-Aug; (4):625–8. [Article in Russian]

10. Barnaulov OD, Denisenko PP. [Anti-ulcer action of a decoction of the flowers of the dropwort, Filipendula ulmaria (L.) Maxim] Farmakol Toksikol. 1980 Nov-Dec; 43(6):700–5. [Article in Russian]

Nootka Lupine

1. Research on Ævar Jóhannesson's decoction. Lecture given by the biochemist Steinþór Sigurðsson at the autumn meeting of Heilsuhringurinn magazine, 1997.

Northern Dock

1. Suh HJ, Lee KS et al. Determination of singlet oxygen quenching and protection of biological systems by various extracts from seed of Rumex crispus L. J Photochem Photobiol B. 2010 Dec 22. [Previous Epub.]

2. Maksimović Z, Kovacević N et al. Antioxidant activity of yellow dock (Rumex crispus L., Polygonaceae) fruit extract. Phytother Res. 2011 Jan; 25(1):101–5. doi: 10.1002/ptr.3234.

3. Yildirim A, Mavi A et al. Determination of antioxidant and antimicrobial activities of Rumex crispus L. extracts. J Agric Food Chem. 2001 Aug; 49(8):4083–9.

4. Reig R, Sanz P et al. Fatal poisoning by Rumex crispus (curled dock): pathological findings and application of scanning electron microscopy. Vet Hum Toxicol. 1990 Oct; 32(5):468–70.

5. Panciera RJ, Martin T et al. Acute oxalate poisoning attributable to ingestion of curly dock (Rumex crispus) in sheep. J Am Vet Med Assoc. 1990 Jun 15;196(12):1981–4.

Purple Marshlocks

1. Yerschik OA, Lovkova MY et al. Antiinflammatory activity of proanthocyanidins of rhizomes with roots of Comarum palustre L. Dokl Biol Sci. 2009 Nov-Dec; 429:535–7.

2. Popov SV, Popova GY et al. Antiinflammatory activity of the pectic polysaccharide from Comarum palustre. Fitoterapia. 2005 Jun; 76(3–4):281–7.

3. Popov SV, Ovodova RG et al. Adhesion of human neutrophils to fibronectin is inhibited by comaruman, pectin of marsh cinquefoil Comarum palustre L., and by its fragments. Biochemistry (Mosc). 2005 Jan; 70(1):108–12.

4. Popov SV, Ovodova RG et al. Protective effect of comaruman, a pectin of cinquefoil Comarum palustre L., on acetic acid-induced colitis in mice. Dig Dis Sci. 2006 Sep; 51(9):1532–7. Epub 2006 Aug 22.

5. Mondodoev AG, Bikmulina GA et al. [Nefroprotective influence of the Comarum palustre L. on chronic experimental glomerulonephritis] Patol Fiziol Eksp Ter. 2010 Jan-Mar; (1):24–7. [Article in Russian]

6. Buzuk GN, Lovkova MY et al. A new source of proanthocyanidins with antiarthritic activity: purple marshlocks (Comarum palustre L.) rhizome and roots. Dokl Biochem Biophys. 2008 Jul-Aug; 421:211–3.

Red Clover

1. WHO. 2009. WHO Monographs on selected medicinal plants. Vol. 4. World Health Organization, Geneva.

2. Hidalgo LA, Chedraui PA et al. The effect of red clover isoflavones on menopausal symptoms, lipids and vaginal cytology in menopausal women: a randomized, double-blind, placebo-controlled study. Gynecol Endocrinol. 2005 Nov; 21(5):257–64.

3. Tice JA, Ettinger B et al. Phytoestrogen supplements for the treatment of hot flashes: the Isoflavone Clover Extract (ICE) Study: a randomized controlled trial. JAMA. 2003 Jul 9; 290(2):207–14.

4. Geller SE, Shulman LP et al. Safety and efficacy of black cohosh and red clover for the management of vasomotor symptoms: a randomized controlled trial. Menopause. 2009 Nov-Dec; 16(6):1156–66.

5. Maki PM, Rubin LH et al. Effects of botanicals and combined hormone therapy on cognition in postmenopausal women. Menopause. 2009 Nov-Dec; 16(6):1167–77.

6. Lipovac M, Chedraui P et al. Improvement of postmenopausal depressive and anxiety symptoms after treatment with isoflavones derived from red clover extracts. Maturitas. 2010 Mar; 65(3):258–61. Epub 2009 Nov 30.

7. Vishali N, Kamakshi K et al. Red clover Trifolium pratense (Linn.) isoflavones extract on the pain threshold of normal and ovariectomized rats—a long-term study. Phytother Res. 2010 Jul 7. [Previous Epub.]

8. Pakalapati G, Li L et al. Influence of red clover (Trifolium pratense) isoflavones on gene and protein expression profiles in liver of ovariectomized rats. Phytomedicine. 2009 Sep; 16(9):845–55. Epub 2009 May 5.

9. Alves DL, Lima SM et al. Effects of Trifolium pratense and Cimicifuga racemosa on the endometrium of Wistar rats. Maturitas. 2008 Dec 20; 61(4):364–70. Epub 2008 Dec 17.

10. Adaikan PG, Srilatha B et al. Efficacy of red clover isoflavones in the menopausal rabbit model. Fertil Steril. 2009 Dec; 92(6):2008–13. Epub 2008 Oct 29.

11. Mu H, Bai YH et al. Research on antioxidant effects and estrogenic effect of formononetin from Trifolium pratense (red clover). Phytomedicine. 2009 Apr; 16(4):314–9. Epub 2008 Aug 30.

12. Occhiuto F, Zangla G et al. The phytoestrogenic isoflavones from Trifolium pratense L. (Red clover) protects human cortical neurons from glutamate toxicity. Phytomedicine. 2008 Sep; 15(9):676–82. Epub 2008 Jun 6.

13. Nissan HP, Lu J et al. A red clover (Trifolium pratense) phase II clinical extract possesses opiate activity. J Ethnopharmacol. 2007 May 30; 112(1):207–10. Epub 2007 Feb 11.

14. Overk CR, Yao P et al. Comparison of the in vitro estrogenic activities of compounds from hops (Humulus lupulus) and red clover (Trifolium pratense). J Agric Food Chem. 2005 Aug 10; 53(16):6246–53.

15. Burdette JE, Liu J et al. Trifolium pratense (red clover) exhibits estrogenic effects in vivo in ovariectomized Sprague-Dawley rats. J Nutr. 2002 Jan; 132(1):27–30.

16. Overk CR, Guo J et al. In vivo estrogenic comparisons of Trifolium pratense (red clover) Humulus lupulus (hops), and the pure compounds isoxanthohumol and 8-prenylnaringenin. Chem Biol Interact. 2008 Oct 22; 176(1):30–9. Epub 2008 Jun 20.

17. Circosta C, De Pasquale R et al. Effects of isoflavones from red clover (Trifolium pratense) on skin changes induced by ovariectomy in rats. Phytother Res. 2006 Dec; 20(12):1096–9.

18. Terzic MM, Dotlic J et al. Influence of red clover-derived isoflavones on serum lipid profile in postmenopausal women. J Obstet Gynaecol Res. 2009 Dec; 35(6):1091–5.

19. Chedraui P, San Miguel G et al. Effect of Trifolium pratense-derived isoflavones on the lipid profile of postmenopausal women with increased body mass index. Gynecol Endocrinol. 2008 Nov; 24(11):620–4.

20. Atkinson C, Oosthuizen W et al. Modest protective effects of isoflavones from a red clover-derived dietary supplement on cardiovascular disease risk factors in perimenopausal women, and evidence of an interaction with ApoE genotype in 49–65 year-old women. J Nutr. 2004 Jul; 134(7):1759–64.

21. Blakesmith SJ, Lyons-Wall PM et al. Effects of supplementation with purified red clover (Trifolium pratense) isoflavones on plasma lipids and insulin resistance in healthy premenopausal women. Br J Nutr. 2003 Apr; 89(4):467–74.

22. Simoncini T, Garibaldi S et al. Effects of phytoestrogens derived from red clover on atherogenic adhesion molecules in human endothelial cells. Menopause. 2008 May-Jun; 15(3):542–50.

23. Campbell MJ, Woodside JV et al. Effect of red clover-derived isoflavone supplementation on insulin-like growth factor, lipid and antioxidant status in healthy female volunteers: a pilot study. Eur J Clin Nutr. 2004 Jan; 58(1):173–9.

24. Haines C, James A et al. Comparison between phytoestrogens and estradiol in the prevention of atheroma in ovariectomized cholesterol-fed rabbits. Climacteric. 2006 Dec; 9(6):430–6.

25. Mueller M, Hobiger S et al. Red clover extract: a source for substances that activate peroxisome proliferator-activated receptor alpha and ameliorate the cytokine secretion profile of lipopolysaccharide-stimulated macrophages. Menopause. 2010 Mar; 17(2):379–87.

26. Mueller M, Jungbauer A. Red clover extract: a putative source for simultaneous treatment of menopausal disorders and the metabolic syndrome. Menopause. 2008 Nov-Dec; 15(6):1120–31.

27. García-Martínez MC, Hermenegildo C et al. Phytoestrogens increase the capacity of serum to stimulate prostacyclin release in human endothelial cells. Acta Obstet Gynecol Scand. 2003 Aug; 82(8):705–10.

28. Howes JB, Tran D et al. Effects of dietary supplementation with isoflavones from red clover on ambulatory blood pressure and endothelial function in postmenopausal type 2 diabetes. Diabetes Obes Metab. 2003 Sep; 5(5):325–32.

29. Weaver CM, Martin BR et al. Antiresorptive effects of phytoestrogen supplements compared with estradiol or risedronate in postmenopausal women using (41)Ca methodology. J Clin Endocrinol Metab. 2009 Oct; 94(10):3798–805. Epub 2009 Jul 7.

30. Kawakita S, Marotta F et al. Effect of an isoflavones-containing red clover preparation and alkaline supplementation on bone metabolism in ovariectomized rats. Clin Interv Aging. 2009; 4:91–100. Epub 2009 May 14.

31. Occhiuto F, Pasquale RD et al. Effects of phytoestrogenic isoflavones from red clover (Trifolium pratense L.) on experimental osteoporosis. Phytother Res. 2007 Feb; 21(2):130–4.

32. Chen MY, Yan SC et al. [Red clover isoflavones inhibit the proliferation and promote the apoptosis of benign prostatic hyperplasia stromal cells] Zhonghua Nan Ke Xue. 2010 Jan; 16(1):34–9. [Article in Chinese]

33. Wuttke W, Jarry H et al. Plant-derived alternative treatments for the aging male: facts and myths. Aging Male. 2010 Jun; 13(2):75–81.

34. Krenn L, Paper DH. Inhibition of angiogenesis and inflammation by an extract of red clover (Trifolium pratense L.). Phytomedicine. 2009 Dec; 16(12):1083–8. Epub 2009 Aug 7.

35. Medjakovic S, Jungbauer A. Red clover isoflavones biochanin A and formononetin are potent ligands of the human aryl hydrocarbon receptor. Steroid Biochem Mol Biol. 2008 Jan; 108(1–2):171–7. Epub 2007 Oct 22.

36. Roberts DW, Doerge DR et al. Inhibition of extrahepatic human cytochromes P450 1A1 and 1B1 by metabolism of isoflavones found in Trifolium pratense (red clover). J Agric Food Chem. 2004 Oct 20; 52(21):6623–32.

37. Lam AN, Demasi M et al. Effect of red clover isoflavones on cox-2 activity in murine and human monocyte/macrophage cells. Nutr Cancer. 2004; 49(1):89–93.

38. Slater M, Brown D et al. In the prostatic epithelium, dietary isoflavones from red clover significantly increase estrogen receptor beta and E-cadherin expression but decrease transforming growth factor beta1. Prostate Cancer Prostatic Dis. 2002; 5(1):16–21.

39. Cassady JM, Zennie TM et al. Use of a mammalian cell culture benzo(a)pyrene metabolism assay for the detection of potential anticarcinogens from natural products: inhibition of metabolism by biochanin A, an isoflavone from Trifolium pratense L. Cancer Res. 1988 Nov 15; 48(22):6257–61.

40. Engelhardt PF, Riedl CR. Effects of one-year treatment with isoflavone extract from red clover on prostate, liver function, sexual function, and quality of life in men with elevated PSA levels and negative prostate biopsy findings. Urology. 2008 Feb; 71(2):185–90; discussion 190.

41. Alleva LM, Cai C et al. Using Complementary and Alternative Medicines to Target the Host Response during Severe Influenza. Evid Based Complement Alternat Med. 2009 Sep 24. [Previous Epub.]

42. Yang Z, Huang XY et al. Effects of red clover extract on the activation and proliferation of mouse T lymphocytes and the NO secretion of mouse macrophages. Yao Xue Xue Bao. 2008 Oct; 43(10):1019–24.

43. Occhiuto F, Palumbo DR et al. The isoflavones mixture from Trifolium pratense L. protects HCN 1-A neurons from oxidative stress. Phytother Res. 2009 Feb; 23(2):192–6.

44. Danilets MG, Bel'skiĭ IuP et al. [Effect of plant polysaccharides on TH1-dependent immune response: screening investigation] Eksp Klin Farmakol. 2010 Jun; 73(6):19–22. [Article in Russian]

45. Powles TJ, Howell A et al. Red clover isoflavones are safe and well tolerated in women with a family history of breast cancer. Menopause Int. 2008 Mar; 14(1):6–12.

46. Imhof M, Gocan A et al. Effects of a red clover extract (MF11RCE) on endometrium and sex hormones in postmenopausal women. Maturitas. 2006 Aug 20; 55(1):76–81. Epub 2006 Mar 2.

47. Atkinson C, Warren RM et al. Red-clover-derived isoflavones and mammographic breast density: a double-blind, randomized,

placebo-controlled trial [ISRCTN42940165]. Breast Cancer Res. 2004; 6(3):R170-9. Epub 2004 Feb 24.

48. Powles T. Isoflavones and women's health. Breast Cancer Res. 2004; 6(3):140-2. Epub 2004 Apr 6.

Ribwort Plantain

1. Beara IN, Orčić DZ et al. Liquid chromatography/tandem mass spectrometry study of anti-inflammatory activity of plantain (Plantago L.) species. J Pharm Biomed Anal. 2010 Sep 5; 52(5):701-6. Epub 2010 Feb 18.

2. Vigo E, Cepeda A et al. In-vitro anti-inflammatory activity of Pinus sylvestris and Plantago lanceolata extracts: effect on inducible NOS, COX-1, COX-2 and their products in J774A.1 murine macrophages. J Pharm Pharmacol. 2005 Mar; 57(3):383-91.

3. Herold A, Cremer L et al. Antioxidant properties of some hydroalcoholic plant extracts with antiinflammatory activity. Roum Arch Microbiol Immunol. 2003 Jul-Dec; 62(3-4):217-27.

4. Herold A, Cremer L et al. Hydroalcoholic plant extracts with anti-inflammatory activity. Roum Arch Microbiol Immunol. 2003 Jan-Jun; 62(1-2):117-29.

5. Wegener T, Kraft K. [Plantain (Plantago lanceolata L.): anti-inflammatory action in upper respiratory tract infections] Wien Med Wochenschr. 1999; 149(8-10):211-6. [Article in German]

6. Murai M, Tamayama Y et al. Phenylethanoids in the herb of Plantago lanceolata and inhibitory effect on arachidonic acid-induced mouse ear edema. Planta Med. 1995 Oct; 61(5):479-80.

7. Shipochliev T, Dimitrov A et al. [Anti-inflammatory action of a group of plant extracts] Vet Med Nauki. 1981; 18(6):87-94. [Article in Bulgarian]

8. Hausmann M, Obermeier F et al. In vivo treatment with the herbal phenylethanoid acteoside ameliorates intestinal inflammation in dextran sulphate sodium-induced colitis. Clin Exp Immunol. 2007 May; 148(2):373-81.

9. Adam M, Dobiás P et al. Extraction of antioxidants from plants using ultrasonic methods and their antioxidant capacity. J Sep Sci. 2009 Jan; 32(2):288-94.

10. Kardosová A, Machová E. Antioxidant activity of medicinal plant polysaccharides. Fitoterapia. 2006 Jul; 77(5):367-73. Epub 2006 May 24.

11. Gálvez M, Martín-Cordero C et al. Antioxidant activity of methanol extracts obtained from Plantago species. J Agric Food Chem. 2005 Mar 23; 53(6):1927-33.

12. Yiğit D, Yiğit N et al. An investigation on the anticandidal activity of some traditional medicinal plants in Turkey. Mycoses. 2009 Mar; 52(2):135-40. Epub 2008 Jun 3.

13. Kozan E, Küpeli E et al. Evaluation of some plants used in Turkish folk medicine against parasitic infections for their in vivo anthelmintic activity. J Ethnopharmacol. 2006 Nov 24; 108(2):211-6. Epub 2006 May 16.

14. Fleer H, Verspohl EJ. Antispasmodic activity of an extract from Plantago lanceolata L. and some isolated compounds. Phytomedicine. 2007 Jun; 14(6):409-15. Epub 2007 Feb 12.

15. Hriscu A, Stănescu U et al. [A pharmacodynamic investigation of the effect of polyholozidic substances extracted from Plantago sp. on the digestive tract] Rev Med Chir Soc Med Nat Iasi. 1990 Jan-Mar; 94(1):165-70. [Article in Rumanian]

16. Shipochliev T. [Uterotonic action of extracts from a group of medicinal plants] Vet Med Nauki. 1981; 18(4):94-8. [Article in Bulgarian]

Rose Bay Willow Herb

1. Battinelli L, Tita B, Evandri MG et al. Antimicrobial activity of Epilobium spp. extracts. Farmaco. 2001 May-Jul; 56(5-7):345-8.

2. Rauha JP, Remes S et al. Antimicrobial effects of Finnish plant extracts containing flavonoids and other phenolic compounds. Int J Food Microbiol. 2000 May 25; 56(1):3-12.

3. Webster D, Taschereau P et al. Antifungal activity of medicinal plant extracts; preliminary screening studies. J Ethnopharmacol. 2008 Jan 4; 115(1):140-6. Epub 2007 Sep 25.

4. Schepetkin IA, Kirpotina LN et al. Immunomodulatory activity of oenothein B isolated from Epilobium angustifolium. J Immunol. 2009 Nov 15; 183(10):6754-66. Epub 2009 Oct 21.

5. Hevesi Tóth B, Blazics B et al. Polyphenol composition and antioxidant capacity of Epilobium species. J Pharm Biomed Anal. 2009 Jan 15; 49(1):26-31. Epub 2008 Oct 8.

6. Ryzhikov MA, Ryzhikova VO. [Application of chemiluminescent methods for analysis of the antioxidant activity of herbal extracts]. Vopr Pitan. 2006; 75(2):22-6. [Article in Russian]

7. Kiss A, Kowalski J et al. Induction of neutral endopeptidase activity in PC-3 cells by an aqueous extract of Epilobium angustifolium L. and oenothein B. Phytomedicine. 2006 Mar; 13(4):284-9. Epub 2005 Jun 27.

8. Kiss A, Kowalski J et al. Effect of Epilobium angustifolium L. extracts and polyphenols on cell proliferation and neutral endopeptidase activity in selected cell lines. Pharmazie. 2006 Jan; 61(1):66-9.

9. Kiss A, Kowalski J et al. Compounds from Epilobium angustifolium inhibit the specific metallopeptidases ACE, NEP and APN. Planta Med. 2004 Oct; 70(10):919-23.

10. Vitalone A, McColl J et al. Characterization of the effect of Epilobium extracts on human cell proliferation. Pharmacology. 2003 Oct; 69(2):79-87.

11. Hiermann A, Reidlinger M et al. [Isolation of the antiphlogistic principle from Epilobium angustifolium]. Planta Med. 1991 Aug; 57(4):357-60. [Article in German]

12. Hiermann A, Juan H et al. Influence of Epilobium extracts on prostaglandin biosynthesis and carrageenin induced edema of the rat paw. J Ethnopharmacol. 1986 Aug; 17(2):161-9.

13. Tita B, Abdel-Haq H et al. Analgesic properties of Epilobium angustifolium, evaluated by the hot plate test and the writhing test. Farmaco. 2001 May-Jul; 56(5-7):341-3.

14. Vitalone A, Bordi F et al. Anti-proliferative effect on a prostatic epithelial cell line (PZ-HPV-7) by Epilobium angustifolium L. Farmaco. 2001 May-Jul; 56(5-7):483-9.

Roseroot

1. Parisi A, Tranchita E et al. Effects of chronic Rhodiola Rosea supplementation on sport performance and antioxidant capacity in trained male: preliminary results. J Sports Med Phys Fitness. 2010 Mar; 50(1):57-63.

2. Evdokimov VG. [Effect of cryopowder Rhodiola rosae L. on cardiorespiratory parameters and physical performance of humans] Aviakosm Ekolog Med. 2009 Nov-Dec; 43(6):52-6. [Article in Russian]

3. Zhang ZJ, Tong Y et al. Dietary supplement with a combination of Rhodiola crenulata and Ginkgo biloba enhances the endurance performance in healthy volunteers. Chin J Integr Med. 2009 Jun; 15(3):177–83. Epub 2009 Jul 2.

4. Schutgens FW, Neogi P et al. The influence of adaptogens on ultraweak biophoton emission: a pilot-experiment. Phytother Res. 2009 Aug; 23(8):1103–8.

5. Abidov M, Grachev S et al. Extract of Rhodiola rosea radix reduces the level of C-reactive protein and creatinine kinase in the blood. Bull Exp Biol Med. 2004 Jul; 138(1):63–4.

6. De Bock K, Eijnde BO et al. Acute Rhodiola rosea intake can improve endurance exercise performance. Int J Sport Nutr Exerc Metab. 2004 Jun; 14(3):298–307.

7. Spasov AA, Wikman GK et al. A double-blind, placebo-controlled pilot study of the stimulating and adaptogenic effect of Rhodiola rosea SHR-5 extract on the fatigue of students caused by stress during an examination period with a repeated low-dose regimen. Phytomedicine. 2000 Apr; 7(2):85–9.

8. Huang SC, Lee FT et al. Attenuation of long-term Rhodiola rosea supplementation on exhaustive swimming-evoked oxidative stress in the rat. Chin J Physiol. 2009 Oct 31; 52(5):316–24.

9. Lee FT, Kuo TY et al. Chronic Rhodiola rosea extract supplementation enforces exhaustive swimming tolerance. J Chin Med. 2009; 37(3):557–72.

10. Wang Q, Wang J et al. [Salidroside protects the hypothalamic-pituitary-gonad axis of male rats undergoing negative psychological stress in experimental navigation and intensive exercise] Zhonghua Nan Ke Xue. 2009 Apr; 15(4):331–6. [Article in Chinese]

11. Tan CB, Gao M et al. Protective effects of salidroside on endothelial cell apoptosis induced by cobalt chloride. Biol Pharm Bull. 2009 Aug; 32(8):1359–63.

12. Panossian A, Nikoyan N et al. Comparative study of Rhodiola preparations on behavioral despair of rats. Phytomedicine. 2008 Jan; 15(1–2):84–91. Epub 2007 Dec 3.

13. Zhang WS, Zhu LQ et al. [Protective effects of salidroside on injury induced by hypoxia/hypoglycemia in cultured neurons] Zhongguo Zhong Yao Za Zhi. 2004 May; 29(5):459–62. [Article in Chinese]

14. Abidov M, Crendal F et al. Effect of extracts from Rhodiola rosea and Rhodiola crenulata (Crassulaceae) roots on ATP content in mitochondria of skeletal muscles. Bull Exp Biol Med. 2003 Dec; 136(6):585–7.

15. Azizov AP, Seĭfulla RD. [The effect of elton, leveton, fitoton and adapton on the work capacity of experimental animals] Eksp Klin Farmakol. 1998 May-Jun; 61(3):61–3. [Article in Russian]

16. Blomkvist J, Taube A et al. Perspective on Roseroot (Rhodiola rosea) studies. Planta Med. 2009 Sep; 75(11):1187–90. Epub 2009 May 25.

17. Walker TB, Altobelli SA et al. Failure of Rhodiola rosea to alter skeletal muscle phosphate kinetics in trained men. Metabolism. 2007 Aug; 56(8):1111–7.

18. Colson SN, Wyatt FB et al. Cordyceps sinensis- and Rhodiola rosea-based supplementation in male cyclists and its effect on muscle tissue oxygen saturation. J Strength Cond Res. 2005 May; 19(2):358–63.

19. Wing SL, Askew EW et al. Lack of effect of Rhodiola or oxygenated water supplementation on hypoxemia and oxidative stress. Wilderness Environ Med. 2003 Spring; 14(1):9–16.

20. Bystritsky A, Kerwin L et al. A pilot study of Rhodiola rosea (Rhodax) for generalized anxiety disorder (GAD). J Altern Complement Med. 2008 Mar; 14(2):175–80.

21. Darbinyan V, Aslanyan G et al. Clinical trial of Rhodiola rosea L. extract SHR-5 in the treatment of mild to moderate depression. Nord J Psychiatry. 2007; 61(5):343–8.

22. Olsson EM, von Schéele B et al. A randomised, double-blind, placebo-controlled, parallel-group study of the standardised extract SHR-5 of the roots of Rhodiola rosea in the treatment of subjects with stress-related fatigue. Planta Med. 2009 Feb; 75(2):105–12. Epub 2008 Nov 18.

23. Fintelmann V, Gruenwald J. Efficacy and tolerability of a Rhodiola rosea extract in adults with physical and cognitive deficiencies. Adv Ther. 2007 Jul-Aug; 24(4):929–39.

24. Shevtsov VA, Zholus BI et al. A randomized trial of two different doses of a SHR-5 Rhodiola rosea extract versus placebo and control of capacity for mental work. Phytomedicine. 2003 Mar; 10(2–3):95–105.

25. Darbinyan V, Kteyan A et al. Rhodiola rosea in stress induced fatigue—a double blind cross-over study of a standardized extract SHR-5 with a repeated low-dose regimen on the mental performance of healthy physicians during night duty. Phytomedicine. 2000 Oct; 7(5):365–71.

26. Spasov AA, Mandrikov VB et al. [The effect of the preparation rodakson on the psychophysiological and physical adaptation of students to an academic load] Eksp Klin Farmakol. 2000 Jan-Feb; 63(1):76–8. [Article in Russian]

27. Ha Z, Zhu Y et al. [The effect of rhodiola and acetazolamide on the sleep architecture and blood oxygen saturation in men living at high altitude] Zhonghua Jie He He Hu Xi Za Zhi. 2002 Sep; 25(9):527–30. [Article in Chinese]

28. Qin YJ, Zeng YS et al. [Effects of Rhodiola rosea on level of 5-hydroxytryptamine, cell proliferation and differentiation, and number of neuron in cerebral hippocampus of rats with depression induced by chronic mild stress] Zhongguo Zhong Yao Za Zhi. 2008 Dec; 33(23):2842–6. [Article in Chinese]

29. Panossian A, Hovhannisyan A et al. Pharmacokinetic and pharmacodynamic study of interaction of Rhodiola rosea SHR-5 extract with warfarin and theophylline in rats. Phytother Res. 2009 Mar; 23(3):351–7.

30. Chen TS, Liou SY et al. Antioxidant evaluation of three adaptogen extracts. Am J Chin Med. 2008; 36(6):1209–17.

31. Mattioli L, Funari C et al. Effects of Rhodiola rosea L. extract on behavioural and physiological alterations induced by chronic mild stress in female rats. J Psychopharmacol. 2009 Mar; 23(2):130–42. Epub 2008 May 30.

32. Jafari M, Felgner JS et al. Rhodiola: a promising anti-aging Chinese herb. Rejuvenation Res. 2007 Dec; 10(4):587–602.

33. Mattioli L, Perfumi M. Rhodiola rosea L. extract reduces stress- and CRF-induced anorexia in rats. J Psychopharmacol. 2007 Sep; 21(7):742–50. Epub 2007 Jan 26.

34. Perfumi M, Mattioli L. Adaptogenic and central nervous system effects of single doses of 3% rosavin and 1% salidroside Rhodiola rosea L. extract in mice. Phytother Res. 2007 Jan; 21(1):37–43.

35. Chen CH, Chan HC et al. Antioxidant activity of some plant extracts towards xanthine oxidase, lipoxygenase and tyrosinase. Molecules. 2009 Aug 10; 14(8):2947–58.

36. van Diermen D, Marston A et al. Monoamine oxidase inhibition by Rhodiola rosea L. roots. J Ethnopharmacol. 2009 Mar 18; 122(2):397–401. Epub 2009 Jan 9.

37. Arbuzov AG, Maslov LN et al. [Phytoadaptogens-induced phenomenon similar to ischemic preconditioning] Ross Fiziol Zh Im I M Sechenova. 2009 Apr; 95(4):398–404. [Article in Russian]

38. Maslov LN, Lishmanov YB et al. Antiarrhythmic activity of phytoadaptogens in short-term ischemia-reperfusion of the heart and postinfarction cardiosclerosis. Bull Exp Biol Med. 2009 Mar; 147(3):331–4.

39. Zhang J, Liu A et al. Salidroside protects cardiomyocyte against hypoxia-induced death: a HIF-1alpha-activated and VEGF-mediated pathway. J Pharmacol. 2009 Apr 1; 607(1–3):6–14.

40. Wu T, Zhou H et al. Cardioprotection of salidroside from ischemia/reperfusion injury by increasing N-acetylglucosamine linkage to cellular proteins. Eur J Pharmacol. 2009 Jun 24; 613(1–3):93–9. Epub 2009 Apr 17.

41. Kobayashi K, Yamada K et al. Constituents of Rhodiola rosea showing inhibitory effect on lipase activity in mouse plasma and alimentary canal. Planta Med. 2008 Nov; 74(14):1716–9. Epub 2008 Nov 3.

42. Shen W, Fan WH et al. [Effects of rhodiola on expression of vascular endothelial cell growth factor and angiogenesis in aortic atherosclerotic plaque of rabbits] Zhongguo Zhong Xi Yi Jie He Za Zhi. 2008 Nov; 28(11):1022–5. [Article in Chinese]

43. Maslov LN, Lishmanov IuB. [Cardioprotective and antiarrhythmic properties of Rhodiolae roseae preparations] Eksp Klin Farmakol. 2007 Sep-Oct; 70(5):59–67. [Article in Russian]

44. Kwon YI, Jang HD et al. Evaluation of Rhodiola crenulata and Rhodiola rosea for management of type II diabetes and hypertension. Asia Pac J Clin Nutr. 2006; 15(3):425–32.

45. Li J, Fan WH et al. [Effect of rhodiola on expressions of Flt-1, KDR and Tie-2 in rats with ischemic myocardium] Zhongguo Zhong Xi Yi Jie He Za Zhi. 2005 May; 25(5):445–8. [Article in Chinese]

46. Zhang Z, Liu J et al. [The effect of Rhodiola capsules on oxygen consumption of myocardium and coronary artery blood flow in dogs] Zhongguo Zhong Yao Za Zhi. 1998 Feb; 23(2):104–6. [Article in Chinese]

47. Maĭmeskulova LA, Maslov LN. [The anti-arrhythmia action of an extract of Rhodiola rosea and of n-tyrosol in models of experimental arrhythmias] Eksp Klin Farmakol. 1998 Mar-Apr; 61(2):37–40. [Article in Russian]

48. Lishmanov IuB, Naumova AV et al. [Contribution of the opioid system to realization of inotropic effects of Rhodiola rosea extracts in ischemic and reperfusion heart damage in vitro] Eksp Klin Farmakol. 1997 May-Jun; 60(3):34–6. [Article in Russian]

49. Maĭmeskulova LA, Maslov LN et al. [The participation of the mu-, delta- and kappa-opioid receptors in the realization of the anti-arrhythmia effect of Rhodiola rosea] Eksp Klin Farmakol. 1997 Jan-Feb; 60(1):38–9. [Article in Russian]

50. Maslova I.V, Kondrat'ev BIu et al. [The cardioprotective and antiadrenergic activity of an extract of Rhodiola rosea in stress] Eksp Klin Farmakol. 1994 Nov-Dec; 57(6):61–3. [Article in Russian]

51. Lishmanov IuB, Maslova LV et al. [The anti-arrhythmia effect of Rhodiola rosea and its possible mechanism] Biull Eksp Biol Med. 1993 Aug; 116(8):175–6. [Article in Russian]

52. Zhu J, Wan X et al. Evaluation of salidroside in vitro and in vivo genotoxicity. Drug Chem Toxicol. 2010 Apr; 33(2):220–6.

53. Wang H, Ding Y et al. The in vitro and in vivo antiviral effects of salidroside from Rhodiola rosea L. against coxsackievirus B3. Phytomedicine. 2009 Mar; 16(2–3):146–55. Epub 2008 Sep 24.

54. McGovern E, McDonnell TJ. Herbal medicine—sets the heart racing! Ir Med J. 2010 Jul-Aug; 103(7):219.

55. Pooja, Bawa AS et al. Anti-inflammatory activity of Rhodiola rosea—"a second-generation adaptogen." Phytother Res. 2009 Aug; 23(8):1099–102.

56. Xu KJ, Zhang SF et al. [Preventive and treatment effect of composite Rhodiolae on acute lung injury in patients with severe pulmonary hypertension during extracorporeal circulation] Zhongguo Zhong Xi Yi Jie He Za Zhi. 2003 Sep; 23(9):648–50. [Article in Chinese]

57. Zhang S, Gao W et al. [Early use of Chinese drug rhodiola compound for patients with post-trauma and inflammation in prevention of ALI/ARDS] Zhonghua Wai Ke Za Zhi. 1999 Apr; 37(4):238–40. [Article in Chinese]

58. Bocharova OA, Matveev BP et al. [The effect of a Rhodiola rosea extract on the incidence of recurrences of a superficial bladder cancer (experimental clinical research)] Urol Nefrol (Mosk). 1995 Mar-Apr; (2):46–7. [Article in Russian]

59. Hu X, Zhang X et al. Salidroside induces cell-cycle arrest and apoptosis in human breast cancer cells. Biochem Biophys Res Commun. 2010 Jul 16; 398(1):62–7. Epub 2010 Jun 10.

60. Hu X, Lin S et al. A preliminary study: the anti-proliferation effect of salidroside on different human cancer cell lines. Cell Biol Toxicol. 2010 Dec; 26(6):499–507. Epub 2010 Mar 23.

61. Majewska A, Hoser G et al. Antiproliferative and antimitotic effect, S phase accumulation and induction of apoptosis and necrosis after treatment of extract from Rhodiola rosea rhizomes on HL-60 cells. J Ethnopharmacol. 2006 Jan 3; 103(1):43–52. Epub 2005 Sep 19.

62. Ming DS, Hillhouse BJ et al. Bioactive compounds from Rhodiola rosea (Crassulaceae). Phytother Res. 2005 Sep; 19(9):740–3.

63. Salikhova RA, Aleksandrova IV et al. [Effect of Rhodiola rosea on the yield of mutation alterations and DNA repair in bone marrow cells] Patol Fiziol Eksp Ter. 1997 Oct-Dec; (4):22–4. [Article in Russian]

64. Udintsev SN, Krylova SG et al. [The enhancement of the efficacy of adriamycin by using hepatoprotectors of plant origin in metastases of Ehrlich's adenocarcinoma to the liver in mice] Vopr Onkol. 1992; 38(10):1217–22. [Article in Russian]

65. Udintsev SN, Shakhov VP. The role of humoral factors of regenerating liver in the development of experimental tumors and the effect of Rhodiola rosea extract on this process. Neoplasma. 1991; 38(3):323–31.

66. Udintsev SN, Shakhov VP. [Changes in clonogenic properties of bone marrow and transplantable mice tumor cells during combined use of cyclophosphane and biological response modifiers of adaptogenic origin] Eksp Onkol. 1990; 12(6):55–6. [Article in Russian]

67. Udintsev SN, Shakhov VP [Decrease in the growth rate of Ehrlich's tumor and Pliss' lymphosarcoma with partial hepatectomy] Vopr Onkol. 1989; 35(9):1072–5. [Article in Russian]

68. Dement'eva LA, Iaremenko KV. [Effect of a Rhodiola extract on the tumor process in an experiment] Vopr Onkol. 1987; 33(7):57–60. [Article in Russian]

69. Mattioli L, Perfumi M. Effects of a Rhodiola rosea L. extract on acquisition and expression of morphine tolerance and dependence in mice. J Psychopharmacol. 2010 Feb 8. [Previous Epub.]

70. Mattioli L, Perfumi M. Evaluation of Rhodiola rosea L. extract on affective and physical signs of nicotine withdrawal in mice. J Psychopharmacol. 2009 Nov 25. [Previous Epub.]

71. Blum K, Chen TJ et al. Manipulation of catechol-O-methyl-transferase (COMT) activity to influence the attenuation of substance seeking behavior, a subtype of Reward Deficiency Syndrome (RDS), is dependent upon gene polymorphisms: a

hypothesis. Med Hypotheses. 2007; 69(5):1054–60. Epub 2007 Apr 30.

72. Cifani C, Micioni Di Bonaventura MV et al. Effect of salidroside, active principle of Rhodiola rosea extract, on binge eating. Physiol Behav. 2010 Sep 16. [Previous Epub.]

73. Schriner SE, Abrahamyan A et al. Decreased mitochondrial superoxide levels and enhanced protection against paraquat in Drosophila melanogaster supplemented with Rhodiola rosea. Free Radic Res. 2009 Sep; 43(9):836–43. Epub 2009 Jul 24.

74. Yu S, Shen Y et al. Involvement of ERK1/2 pathway in neuroprotection by salidroside against hydrogen peroxide-induced apoptotic cell death. J Mol Neurosci. 2010 Mar; 40(3):321–31. Epub 2009 Sep 29.

75. Calcabrini C, De Bellis R et al. Rhodiola rosea ability to enrich cellular antioxidant defences of cultured human keratinocytes. Arch Dermatol Res. 2010 Apr; 302(3):191–200. Epub 2009 Aug 25.

76. Battistelli M, De Sanctis R et al. Rhodiola rosea as antioxidant in red blood cells: ultrastructural and hemolytic behaviour. Eur J Histochem. 2005 Jul-Sep; 49(3):243–54.

77. Boon-Niermeijer EK, van den Berg A et al. Phyto-adaptogens protect against environmental stress-induced death of embryos from the freshwater snail Lymnaea stagnalis. Phytomedicine. 2000 Oct; 7(5):389–99.

78. Zhang L, Yu H et al. Neuroprotective effects of salidroside against beta-amyloid-induced oxidative stress in SH-SY5Y human neuroblastoma cells. Neurochem Int. 2010 Nov; 57(5):547–55. Epub 2010 Jul 6.

79. Chen X, Zhang Q et al. Protective effect of salidroside against H2O2-induced cell apoptosis in primary culture of rat hippocampal neurons. Mol Cell Biochem. 2009 Dec; 332(1–2):85–93. Epub 2009 Jun 25.

80. Qu ZQ, Zhou Y et al. Pretreatment with Rhodiola rosea extract reduces cognitive impairment induced by intracerebroventricular streptozotocin in rats: implication of anti-oxidative and neuroprotective effects. Biomed Environ Sci. 2009 Aug; 22(4):318–26.

81. Bocharov EV, Kucherianu VG et al. [Neuroprotective features of phytoadaptogens] Vestn Ross Akad Med Nauk. 2008; (4):47–50. [Article in Russian]

82. Yu S, Liu M et al. Neuroprotective effects of salidroside in the PC12 cell model exposed to hypoglycemia and serum limitation. Cell Mol Neurobiol. 2008 Dec; 28(8):1067–78. Epub 2008 May 15.

83. Zhang L, Yu H et al. Protective effects of salidroside on hydrogen peroxide-induced apoptosis in SH-SY5Y human neuroblastoma cells. Eur J Pharmacol. 2007 Jun 14; 564(1–3):18–25. Epub 2007 Feb 15.

84. Yin D, Yao W et al. Salidroside, the main active compound of Rhodiola plants, inhibits high glucose-induced mesangial cell proliferation. Planta Med. 2009 Sep; 75(11):1191–5. Epub 2009 May 14.

85. Kim SH, Hyun SH et al. Antioxidative effects of Cinnamomi cassiae and Rhodiola rosea extracts in liver of diabetic mice. Biofactors. 2006; 26(3):209–19.

86. Molokovskiĭ DS, Davydov VV et al. [The action of adaptogenic plant preparations in experimental alloxan diabetes] Probl Endokrinol (Mosk). 1989 Nov-Dec; 35(6):82–7. [Article in Russian]

87. Dieamant Gde C, Velazquez Pereda Mdel C et al. Neuroimmunomodulatory compound for sensitive skin care: in vitro and clinical assessment. J Cosmet Dermatol. 2008 Jun; 7(2):112–9.

88. Zubeldia JX, Nabi HA et al. Exploring New Applications for Rhodiola rosea: Can We Improve the Quality of Life of Patients with Short-Term Hypothyroidism Induced by Hormone Withdrawal? J Med Food. 2010 Oct 14. [Previous Epub.]

89. Jeong HJ, Ryu YB et al. Neuraminidase inhibitory activities of flavonols isolated from Rhodiola rosea roots and their in vitro anti-influenza viral activities. Bioorg Med Chem. 2009 Oct 1; 17(19):6816–23. Epub 2009 Aug 21.

90. Pashkevich IA, Uspenskaia IuA et al. [Comparative evaluation of effects of p-tyrosol and Rhodiola rosea extract on bone marrow cells in vivo] Eksp Klin Farmakol. 2003 Jul-Aug; 66(4):50–2. [Article in Russian]

91. Zhang Y, Liu Y. [Study on effects of salidroside on lipid peroxidation on oxidative stress in rat hepatic stellate cells] Zhong Yao Cai. 2005 Sep; 28(9):794–6. [Article in Chinese]

92. Iaremiĭ IN, Grigor'eva NF. [Hepatoprotective properties of liquid extract of Rhodiola rosea] Eksp Klin Farmakol. 2002 Nov-Dec; 65(6):57–9. [Article in Russian]

Rowan

1. Olszewska MA, Michel P. Antioxidant activity of inflorescences, leaves and fruits of three Sorbus species in relation to their polyphenolic composition. Nat Prod Res. 2009; 23(16):1507–21.

2. Hukkanen AT, Pölönen SS et al. Antioxidant capacity and phenolic content of sweet rowanberries. J Agric Food Chem. 2006 Jan 11; 54(1):112–9.

Sea Mayweed

1. Suganda AG, Amoros M et al. [Inhibitory effects of some crude and semi-purified extracts of indigenous French plants on the multiplication of human herpesvirus 1 and poliovirus 2 in cell culture] J Nat Prod. 1983 Sep-Oct; 46(5):626–32. [Article in French]

Self-heal

1. Song YW, Lee EY et al. Assessment of comparative pain relief and tolerability of SKI306X compared with celecoxib in patients with rheumatoid arthritis: a 6-week, multicenter, randomized, double-blind, double-dummy, phase III, noninferiority clinical trial. Clin Ther. 2007 May; 29(5):862–73.

2. Jung YB, Roh KJ et al. Effect of SKI 306X, a new herbal anti-arthritic agent, in patients with osteoarthritis of the knee: a double-blind placebo controlled study. Am J Chin Med. 2001; 29(3–4):485–91.

3. Adámková H, Vicar J et al. Macleya cordata and Prunella vulgaris in oral hygiene products—their efficacy in the control of gingivitis. Biomed Pap Med Fac Univ Palacky Olomouc Czech. Epub. 2004 Jul; 148(1):103–5.

4. Zdarilová A, Svobodová A et al. Prunella vulgaris extract and rosmarinic acid suppress lipopolysaccharide-induced alteration in human gingival fibroblasts. Toxicol In Vitro. 2009 Apr; 23(3):386–92. Epub. 2008 Dec 30.

5. Fang X, Yu MM et al. Immune modulatory effects of Prunella vulgaris L. on monocytes/macrophages. Int J Mol Med. 2005 Dec; 16(6):1109–16.

6. Fang X, Chang RC et al. Immune modulatory effects of Prunella vulgaris L. Int J Mol Med. 2005 Mar; 15(3):491–6.

7. Psotová J, Kolár M et al. Biological activities of Prunella vulgaris extract. Phytother Res. 2003 Nov; 17(9):1082–7.

8. Zheng MS, Zhang YZ. [Anti-HBsAg herbs employing ELISA technique] Zhong Xi Yi Jie He Za Zhi. 1990 Sep; 10(9):560–2, 518. [Article in Chinese]

9. Reichling J, Nolkemper S et al. Impact of ethanolic lamiaceae extracts on herpesvirus infectivity in cell culture. Forsch Komplementmed. 2008 Dec; 15(6):313–20. Epub. 2008 Nov 3.

10. Zhang Y, But PP et al. Chemical properties, mode of action, and in vivo anti-herpes activities of a lignin-carbohydrate complex from Prunella vulgaris. Antiviral Res. 2007 Sep; 75(3):242–9. Epub. 2007 Apr 17.

11. Nolkemper S, Reichling J et al. Antiviral effect of aqueous extracts from species of the Lamiaceae family against Herpes simplex virus type 1 and type 2 in vitro. Planta Med. 2006 Dec; 72(15):1378–82. Epub. 2006 Nov 7.

12. Chiu LC, Zhu W et al. A polysaccharide fraction from medicinal herb Prunella vulgaris downregulates the expression of herpes simplex virus antigen in Vero cells. J Ethnopharmacol. 2004 Jul; 93(1):63–8.

13. Xu HX, Lee SH et al. Isolation and characterization of an anti-HSV polysaccharide from Prunella vulgaris. Antiviral Res. 1999 Nov; 44(1):43–54.

14. Zheng M. [Experimental study of 472 herbs with antiviral action against the herpes simplex virus] Zhong Xi Yi Jie He Za Zhi. 1990 Jan; 10(1):39–41, 6. [Article in Chinese]

15. Liu S, Jiang S et al. Identification of inhibitors of the HIV-1 gp41 six-helix bundle formation from extracts of Chinese medicinal herbs Prunella vulgaris and Rhizoma cibotte. Life Sci. 2002 Aug 30; 71(15):1779–91.

16. Au TK, Lam TL et al. A comparison of HIV-1 integrase inhibition by aqueous and methanol extracts of Chinese medicinal herbs. Life Sci. 2001 Feb 23; 68(14):1687–94.

17. Kageyama S, Kurokawa M et al. Extract of Prunella vulgaris spikes inhibits HIV replication at reverse transcription in vitro and can be absorbed from intestine in vivo. Antivir Chem Chemother. 2000 Mar; 11(2):157–64.

18. Lam TL, Lam ML et al. A comparison of human immunodeficiency virus type-1 protease inhibition activities by the aqueous and methanol extracts of Chinese medicinal herbs. Life Sci. 2000 Oct 27; 67(23):2889–96.

19. Yamasaki K, Nakano M et al. Anti-HIV-1 activity of herbs in Labiatae. Biol Pharm Bull. 1998 Aug; 21(8):829–33.

20. Yamasaki K, Otake T et al. [Screening test of crude drug extract on anti-HIV activity] Yakugaku Zasshi. 1993 Nov; 113(11):818–24. [Article in Japanese]

21. Yao XJ, Wainberg MA et al. Mechanism of inhibition of HIV-1 infection in vitro by purified extract of Prunella vulgaris. Virology. 1992 Mar; 187(1):56–62.

22. Brindley MA, Widrlechner MP et al. Inhibition of lentivirus replication by aqueous extracts of Prunella vulgaris. Virol J. 2009 Jan 20; 6:8.

23. Huang N, Hauck C et al. Rosmarinic acid in Prunella vulgaris ethanol extract inhibits lipopolysaccharide-induced prostaglandin E2 and nitric oxide in RAW 264.7 mouse macrophages. J Agric Food Chem. 2009 Nov 25; 57(22):10579–89.

24. Park SH, Oh HS et al. The structure-activity relationship of the series of non-peptide small antagonists for p56lck SH2 domain. Bioorg Med Chem. 2007 Jun 1; 15(11):3938–50. Epub 2007 Apr 5.

25. Harput US, Saracoglu I et al. Effects of two Prunella species on lymphocyte proliferation and nitric oxide production. Phytother Res. 2006 Feb; 20(2):157–9.

26. Ryu SY, Oak MH et al. Anti-allergic and anti-inflammatory triterpenes from the herb of Prunella vulgaris. Planta Med. 2000 May; 66(4):358–60.

27. Han EH, Choi JH et al. Immunostimulatory activity of aqueous extract isolated from Prunella vulgaris. Food Chem Toxicol. 2009 Jan; 47(1):62–9. Epub 2008 Oct 17.

28. Liu F, Ng TB. Antioxidative and free radical scavenging activities of selected medicinal herbs. Life Sci. 2000 Jan 14; 66(8):725–35.

29. Lamaison JL, Petitjean-Freytet C et al. [Medicinal Lamiaceae with antioxidant properties, a potential source of rosmarinic acid] Pharm Acta Helv. 1991; 66(7):185–8. [Article in French]

30. Psotova J, Chlopcíková S et al. Cytoprotectivity of Prunella vulgaris on doxorubicin-treated rat cardiomyocytes. Fitoterapia. 2005 Sep; 76(6):556–61.

31. Chang, HM, PPH. But. 1987. *Pharmacology and Application of Chinese Materia Medica (Vol. 2)*. World Scientific Publishing, Singapore.

32. Zheng J, He J et al. Antihyperglycemic activity of Prunella vulgaris L. in streptozotocin-induced diabetic mice. Asia Pac J Clin Nutr. 2007; 16 Suppl 1:427–31.

33. Valentová K, Truong NT et al. Induction of glucokinase mRNA by dietary phenolic compounds in rat liver cells in vitro. J Agric Food Chem. 2007 Sep 19; 55(19):7726–31. Epub 2007 Aug 23.

34. Skottová N, Kazdová L et al. Phenolics-rich extracts from Silybum marianum and Prunella vulgaris reduce a high-sucrose diet induced oxidative stress in hereditary hypertriglyceridemic rats. Pharmacol Res. 2004 Aug; 50(2):123–30.

35. Kim SY, Kim SH et al. Effects of Prunella vulgaris on mast cell-mediated allergic reaction and inflammatory cytokine production. Exp Biol Med (Maywood). 2007 Jul; 232(7):921–6.

36. Shin TY, Kim YK et al. Inhibition of immediate-type allergic reactions by Prunella vulgaris in a murine model. Immunopharmacol Immunotoxicol. 2001 Aug; 23(3):423–35.

37. Collins NH, Lessey EC et al. Characterization of antiestrogenic activity of the Chinese herb, prunella vulgaris, using in vitro and in vivo (Mouse Xenograft) models. Biol Reprod. 2009 Feb; 80(2):375–83. Epub 2008 Oct 15.

38. Huang JC, Ruan CH et al. Prunella stica inhibits the proliferation but not the prostaglandin production of Ishikawa cells. Life Sci. 2006 Jun 27; 79(5):436–41. Epub 2006 Feb 14.

39. Vostálová J, Zdarilová A et al. Prunella vulgaris extract and rosmarinic acid prevent UVB-induced DNA damage and oxidative stress in HaCaT keratinocytes. Arch Dermatol Res. 2010 Apr; 302(3):171–81. Epub 2009 Oct 28.

40. Psotova J, Svobodova A et al. Photoprotective properties of Prunella vulgaris and rosmarinic acid on human keratinocytes. J Photochem Photobiol B. 2006 Sep 1; 84(3):167–74. Epub 2006 Apr 21.

41. World Health Organization—Regional Office for the Western Pacific. 1998. Medicinal Plants in the Republic of Korea. Compiled by Natural Products Research Institute, Seoul National University. World Health Organization, Manila.

42. Choi JH, Kim DY et al. Effects of SKI 306X, a new herbal agent, on proteoglycan degradation in cartilage explant culture and collagenase-induced rabbit osteoarthritis model. Osteoarthritis Cartilage. 2002 Jun; 10(6):471–8.

43. Park SJ, Kim DH et al. The ameliorating effect of the extract of the flower of Prunella vulgaris var.lilacina on drug-induced memory impairments in mice. Food Chem Toxicol. 2010 Apr 1. [Epub Previous.]

44. Choi JH, Han EH et al. Suppression of PMA-induced tumor cell invasion and metastasis by aqueous extract isolated from Prunella vulgaris via the inhibition of NF-kappaB-dependent MMP-9 expression. Food Chem Toxicol. 2010 Feb; 48(2):564–71. Epub 2009 Nov 14.

45. Zhang MZ, Sun ZC et al. [Study on proteomics of Jurkat cells treated with the extracts from Prunella vulgaris] Zhong Yao Cai. 2009 Jun; 32(6):917–22. [Article in Chinese]

46. Zhang KJ, Zhang MZ et al. [The experimental research about the effect of Prunella vulgaris L. on Raji cells growth and expression of apoptosis related protein] Zhong Yao Cai. 2006 Nov; 29(11):1207–10. [Article in Chinese]

47. Sun HX, Qin F et al. In vitro and in vivo immunosuppressive activity of Spica Prunellae ethanol extract on the immune responses in mice. J Ethnopharmacol. 2005 Oct 3; 101(1–3):31–6.

48. Won J, Hur YG et al. Rosmarinic acid inhibits TCR-induced T cell activation and proliferation in an Lck-dependent manner. Eur J Immunol. 2003 Apr; 33(4):870–9.

49. Ahn SC, Oh WK et al. Inhibitory effects of rosmarinic acid on Lck SH2 domain binding to a synthetic phosphopeptide. Planta Med. 2003 Jul; 69(7):642–6.

50. Horikawa K, Mohri T et al. Moderate inhibition of mutagenicity and carcinogenicity of benzo[a]pyrene, 1,6-dinitropyrene and 3,9-dinitrofluoranthene by Chinese medicinal herbs. Mutagenesis. 1994 Nov; 9(6):523–6.

51. Lee H, Lin JY. Antimutagenic activity of extracts from anticancer drugs in Chinese medicine. Mutat Res. 1988 Feb; 204(2):229–34.

52. Lee SW, Chung WT et al. Clematis mandshurica protected to apoptosis of rat chondrocytes. J Ethnopharmacol. 2005 Oct 3; 101(1–3):294–8.

Sheep's Sorrel

1. Leonard SS, Keil D et al. Essiac tea: scavenging of reactive oxygen species and effects on DNA damage. J Ethnopharmacol. 2006 Jan 16; 103(2):288–96. Epub 2005 Oct 13.

2. Sardari S, Shokrgozar MA et al. Cheminformatics based selection and cytotoxic effects of herbal extracts. Toxicol In Vitro. 2009 Oct; 23(7):1412–21. Epub 2009 Jul 12.

Shepherd's Purse

1. Bradley, Peter. 2006. British Herbal Compendium Volume 2. British Herbal Medicine Association, Bournemouth.

2. El-Abyad MS, Morsi NM et al. Preliminary screening of some Egyptian weeds for antimicrobial activity. Microbios. 1990; 62(250):47–57.

3. Shipochliev T. [Uterotonic action of extracts from a group of medicinal plants] Vet Med Nauki. 1981; 18(4):94–8. [Article in Bulgarian]

4. Kuroda K, Akao M. Antitumor and anti-intoxication activities of fumaric acid in cultured cells. Gann. 1981 Oct; 72(5):777–82.

5. Kuroda K, Akao M et al. Inhibitory effect of Capsella bursa-pastoris extract on growth of Ehrlich solid tumor in mice. Cancer Res. 1976 Jun; 36(6):1900–3.

6. Hwang JH, Lee BM. et al. Inhibitory effects of plant extracts on tyrosinase, L-DOPA oxidation, and melanin synthesis. J Toxicol Environ Health A. 2007 Mar 1; 70(5):393–407.

Silverweed

1. Tomczyk M, Pleszczyńska M et al. Variation in total polyphenolics contents of aerial parts of Potentilla species and their anticariogenic activity. Molecules. 2010 Jun 29; 15(7):4639–51.

2. Tomczyk M, Leszczyńska K et al. Antimicrobial activity of Potentilla species. Fitoterapia. 2008 Dec; 79(7–8):592–4. Epub 2008 Jul 10.

3. Zhao YL, Cai GM et al. Anti-hepatitis B virus activities of triterpenoid saponin compound from Potentilla anserine L. Phytomedicine. 2008 Apr; 15(4):253–8. Epub 2008 Mar 11.

4. Chen JR, Yang ZQ et al. Immunomodulatory activity in vitro and in vivo of polysaccharide from Potentilla anserina. Fitoterapia. 2010 Dec; 81(8):1117–24. Epub 2010 Jul 17.

5. Huber R, Ditfurth AV et al. Tormentil for active ulcerative colitis: an open-label, dose-escalating study. J Clin Gastroenterol. 2007 Oct; 41(9):834–8.

6. Tunón H, Olavsdotter C et al. Evaluation of anti-inflammatory activity of some Swedish medicinal plants. Inhibition of prostaglandin biosynthesis and PAF-induced exocytosis. J Ethnopharmacol. 1995 Oct; 48(2):61–76.

7. Nikitina VS, Kuz'mina LIu et al. [Antibacterial activity of polyphenolic compounds isolated from plants of Geraniaceae and Rosaceae families] Prikl Biokhim Mikrobiol. 2007 Nov-Dec; 43(6):705–12. [Article in Russian]

8. Spiridonov NA, Konovalov DA et al. Cytotoxicity of some Russian ethnomedicinal plants and plant compounds. Phytother Res. 2005 May; 19(5):428–32.

Sorrel

1. Lee NJ, Choi JH et al. Antimutagenicity and cytotoxicity of the constituents from the aerial parts of Rumex acetosa. Biol Pharm Bull. 2005 Nov; 28(11):2158–61.

2. Ito H. Effects of the antitumor agents from various natural sources on drug-metabolizing system, phagocytic activity and complement system in sarcoma 180-bearing mice. Jpn J Pharmacol. 1986 Mar; 40(3):435–43.

Speedwell

1. Crişan G, Tămaş M et al. A comparative study of some Veronica species. Rev Med Chir Soc Med Nat Iasi. 2007 Jan-Mar; 111(1):280–4.

2. Scarlat M, Sandor V et al. Experimental anti-ulcer activity of Veronica officinalis L. extracts. J Ethnopharmacol. 1985 May; 13(2):157–63.

Stinging Nettle

1. Safarinejad MR. Urtica dioica for treatment of benign prostatic hyperplasia: a prospective, randomized, double-blind, placebo-controlled, crossover study. J Herb Pharmacother. 2005; 5(4):1–11.

2. Schneider T, Rübben H. [Stinging nettle root extract (Bazoton-uno) in long term treatment of benign prostatic syndrome (BPS). Results of a randomized, double-blind, placebo controlled multicenter

study after 12 months] Urologe A. 2004 Mar; 43(3):302–6. [Article in German]

3. WHO. 2004. WHO monographs on selected medicinal plants. Vol. 2. World Health Organization, Geneva.

4. European Scientific Cooperative on Phytotherapy. 2003. *ESCOP Monographs.* 2nd Edition. Georg Thieme Verlag, Stuttgart.

5. Lopatkin N, Sivkov A et al. Efficacy and safety of a combination of Sabal and Urtica extract in lower urinary tract symptoms—long-term follow-up of a placebo-controlled, double-blind, multicenter trial. Int Urol Nephrol. 2007; 39(4):1137–46. Epub 2007 Feb 15.

6. Lopatkin NA, Sivkov AV et al. Combined extract of Sabal palm and nettle in the treatment of patients with lower urinary tract symptoms in double blind, placebo-controlled trial] Urologiia. 2006 Mar-Apr; (2):12, 14–9. [Article in Russian]

7. Lopatkin N, Sivkov A et al. Long-term efficacy and safety of a combination of sabal and urtica extract for lower urinary tract symptoms—a placebo-controlled, double-blind, multicenter trial. World J Urol. 2005 Jun; 23(2):139–46. Epub. 2005 Jun 1.

8. Popa G, Hägele-Kaddour H et al. [Efficacy of a combined Sabal-urtica preparation in the symptomatic treatment of benign prostatic hyperplasia. Results of a placebo-controlled double-blind study] MMW Fortschr Med. 2005 Oct 6; 147 Suppl 3:103–8. [Article in German]

9. Sökeland J. Combined sabal and urtica extract compared with finasteride in men with benign prostatic hyperplasia: analysis of prostate volume and therapeutic outcome. BJU Int. 2000 Sep; 86(4):439–42.

10. Bercovich E, Saccomanni M. [Analysis of the results obtained with a new phytotherapeutic association for benign prostatic hyperplasia versus controls.] Urologia. 2010 Oct 2; 77(3):180–186. [Article in Italian]

11. Pavone C, Abbadessa D et al. [Associating Serenoa repens, Urtica dioica and Pinus pinaster. Safety and efficacy in the treatment of lower urinary tract symptoms. Prospective study on 320 patients] Urologia. 2010 Sep 23; 77(1):43–51. [Article in Italian]

12. Schöttner M, Gansser D et al. Lignans from the roots of Urtica dioica and their metabolites bind to human sex hormone binding globulin (SHBG). Planta Med. 1997 Dec; 63(6):529–32.

13. Lichius JJ, Muth C. The inhibiting effects of Urtica dioica root extracts on experimentally induced prostatic hyperplasia in the mouse. Planta Med. 1997 Aug; 63(4):307–10.

14. Cai T, Mazzoli S et al. Serenoa repens associated with Urtica dioica (ProstaMEV) and curcumin and quercitin (FlogMEV) extracts are able to improve the efficacy of prulifloxacin in bacterial prostatitis patients: results from a prospective randomised study. Int J Antimicrob Agents. 2009 Jun; 33(6):549–53. Epub 2009 Jan 31.

15. Durak I, Biri H et al. Aqueous extract of Urtica dioica makes significant inhibition on adenosine deaminase activity in prostate tissue from patients with prostate cancer. Cancer Biol Ther. 2004 Sep; 3(9):855–7. Epub 2004 Sep 18.

16. Konrad L, Müller HH et al. Antiproliferative effect on human prostate cancer cells by a stinging nettle root (Urtica dioica) extract. Planta Med. 2000 Feb; 66(1):44–7.

17. Kayser K, Bubenzer J et al. Expression of lectin, interleukin-2 and histopathologic blood group binding sites in prostate cancer and its correlation with integrated optical density and syntactic structure analysis. Anal Quant Cytol Histol. 1995 Apr; 17(2):135–42.

18. Hirano T, Homma M et al. Effects of stinging nettle root extracts and their steroidal components on the Na+,K(+)-ATPase of the benign prostatic hyperplasia. Planta Med. 1994 Feb; 60(1):30–3.

19. Schulze-Tanzil G, de SP et al. Effects of the antirheumatic remedy hox alpha—a new stinging nettle leaf extract—on matrix metalloproteinases in human chondrocytes in vitro. Histol Histopathol. 2002 Apr; 17(2):477–85.

20. Broer J, Behnke B. Immunosuppressant effect of IDS 30, a stinging nettle leaf extract, on myeloid dendritic cells in vitro. J Rheumatol. 2002 Apr; 29(4):659–66.

21. Obertreis B, Ruttkowski T et al. Ex-vivo in-vitro inhibition of lipopolysaccharide stimulated tumor necrosis factor-alpha and interleukin-1 beta secretion in human whole blood by extractum urticae dioicae foliorum. Arzneimittelforschung. 1996 Apr; 46(4):389–94.

22. Obertreis B, Giller K et al. [Anti-inflammatory effect of Urtica dioica folia extract in comparison to caffeic malic acid] Arzneimittelforschung. 1996 Jan; 46(1):52–6. [Article in German]

23. Christensen R, Bliddal H. Is Phytalgic(R) a goldmine for osteoarthritis patients or is there something fishy about this nutraceutical? A summary of findings and risk-of-bias assessment. Arthritis Res Ther. 2010; 12(1):105. Epub 2010 Feb 8.

24. Jacquet A, Girodet PO et al. Phytalgic, a food supplement, vs placebo in patients with osteoarthritis of the knee or hip: a randomised double-blind placebo-controlled clinical trial. Arthritis Res Ther. 2009; 11(6):R192. Epub. 2009 Dec 16.

25. Tahri A, Yamani S et al. Acute diuretic, natriuretic and hypotensive effects of a continuous perfusion of aqueous extract of Urtica dioica in the rat. J Ethnopharmacol. 2000 Nov; 73(1–2):95–100.

26. Randall C, Dickens A et al. Nettle sting for chronic knee pain: a randomised controlled pilot study. Complement Ther Med. 2008 Apr; 16(2):66–72. Epub 2007 Apr 17.

27. Randall C, Randall H et al. Randomized controlled trial of nettle sting for treatment of base-of-thumb pain. J R Soc Med. 2000 Jun; 93(6):305–9.

28. Randall C, Meethan K et al. Nettle sting of Urtica dioica for joint pain—an exploratory study of this complementary therapy. Complement Ther Med. 1999 Sep; 7(3):126–31.

29. Komes D, Belščak-Cvitanović A et al. Phenolic composition and antioxidant properties of some traditionally used medicinal plants affected by the extraction time and hydrolysis. Phytochem Anal. 2010 Sep 16. [Previous Epub.]

30. Yener Z, Celik I et al. Effects of Urtica dioica L. seed on lipid peroxidation, antioxidants and liver pathology in aflatoxin-induced tissue injury in rats. Food Chem Toxicol. 2009 Feb; 47(2):418–24. Epub 2008 Dec 3.

31. Toldy A, Atalay M et al. The beneficial effects of nettle supplementation and exercise on brain lesion and memory in rat. J Nutr Biochem. 2009 Dec; 20(12):974–81. Epub 2008 Dec 13.

32. Yildiz L, Başkan KS et al. Combined HPLC-CUPRAC (cupric ion reducing antioxidant capacity) assay of parsley, celery leaves, and nettle. Talanta. 2008 Oct 19; 77(1):304–13. Epub 2008 Jun 27.

33. Celik I, Tuluce Y. Elevation protective role of Camellia sinensis and Urtica dioica infusion against trichloroacetic acid-exposed in rats. Phytother Res. 2007 Nov; 21(11):1039–44.

34. Hudec J, Burdová M et al. Antioxidant capacity changes and phenolic profile of Echinacea purpurea, nettle (Urtica dioica L.), and dandelion (Taraxacum officinale) after application of polyamine and phenolic biosynthesis regulators. J Agric Food Chem. 2007 Jul 11; 55(14):5689–96. Epub 2007 Jun 19.

35. Ozyurt D, Demirata B et al. Determination of total antioxidant capacity by a new spectrophotometric method based on Ce(IV)

reducing capacity measurement. Talanta. 2007 Feb 28; 71(3):1155–65. Epub. 2006 Jul 17.

36. Kanter M, Coskun O et al. Hepatoprotective effects of Nigella sativa L and Urtica dioica L on lipid peroxidation, antioxidant enzyme systems and liver enzymes in carbon tetrachloride-treated rats. World J Gastroenterol. 2005 Nov 14; 11(42):6684–8.

37. Ozen T, Korkmaz H. Modulatory effect of Urtica dioica L. (Urticaceae) leaf extract on biotransformation enzyme systems, antioxidant enzymes, lactate dehydrogenase and lipid peroxidation in mice. Phytomedicine. 2003; 10(5):405–15.

38. Pieroni A, Janiak V et al. In vitro antioxidant activity of non-cultivated vegetables of ethnic Albanians in southern Italy. Phytother Res. 2002 Aug; 16(5):467–73.

39. Exarchou V, Fiamegos YC et al. Hyphenated chromatographic techniques for the rapid screening and identification of antioxidants in methanolic extracts of pharmaceutically used plants. J Chromatogr A. 2006 Apr 21; 1112(1–2):293–302. Epub 2005 Dec 15.

40. Toldy A, Stadler K et al. The effect of exercise and nettle supplementation on oxidative stress markers in the rat brain. Brain Res Bull. 2005 May 30; 65(6):487–93. Epub 2005 Mar 31.

41. Cetinus E, Kilinc M et al. The role of urtica dioica (urticaceae) in the prevention of oxidative stress caused by tourniquet application in rats. Tohoku J Exp Med. 2005 Mar; 205(3):215–21.

42. Gülçin I, Küfrevioglu OI et al. Antioxidant, antimicrobial, antiulcer and analgesic activities of nettle (Urtica dioica L.). J Ethnopharmacol. 2004 Feb; 90(2–3):205–15.

43. Mavi A, Terzi Z et al. Antioxidant properties of some medicinal plants: Prangos ferulacea (Apiaceae), Sedum sempervivoides (Crassulaceae), Malva neglecta (Malvaceae), Cruciata taurica (Rubiaceae), Rosa pimpinellifolia (Rosaceae), Galium verum subsp. verum (Rubiaceae), Urtica dioica (Urticaceae). Biol Pharm Bull. 2004 May; 27(5):702–5.

44. Kanter M, Meral I et al. Effects of Nigella sativa L. and Urtica dioica L. on lipid peroxidation, antioxidant enzyme systems and some liver enzymes in CCl4-treated rats. J Vet Med A Physiol Pathol Clin Med. 2003 Jun; 50(5):264–8.

45. Turker AU, Usta C. Biological screening of some Turkish medicinal plant extracts for antimicrobial and toxicity activities. Nat Prod Res. 2008 Jan 20; 22(2):136–46.

46. van der Meer FJ, de Haan CA et al. The carbohydrate-binding plant lectins and the non-peptidic antibiotic pradimicin A target the glycans of the coronavirus envelope glycoproteins. J Antimicrob Chemother. 2007 Oct; 60(4):741–9. Epub 2007 Aug 18.

47. van der Meer FJ, de Haan CA et al. Antiviral activity of carbohydrate-binding agents against Nidovirales in cell culture. Antiviral Res. 2007 Oct; 76(1):21–9. Epub 2007 May 21.

48. Balzarini J, Van Herrewege Y et al. Carbohydrate-binding agents efficiently prevent dendritic cell-specific intercellular adhesion molecule-3-grabbing nonintegrin (DC-SIGN)-directed HIV-1 transmission to T lymphocytes. Mol Pharmacol. 2007 Jan; 71(1):3–11. Epub 2006 Oct 20.

49. Balzarini J, Neyts J et al. The mannose-specific plant lectins from Cymbidium hybrid and Epipactis helleborine and the (N-acetylglucosamine)n-specific plant lectin from Urtica dioica are potent and selective inhibitors of human immunodeficiency virus and cytomegalovirus replication in vitro. Antiviral Res. 1992 Jun; 18(2):191–207.

50. Turville SG, Vermeire K et al. Sugar-binding proteins potently inhibit dendritic cell human immunodeficiency virus type 1 (HIV-1) infection and dendritic-cell-directed HIV-1 transfer. J Virol. 2005 Nov; 79(21):13519–27.

51. Uncini Manganelli RE, Zaccaro L et al. Antiviral activity in vitro of Urtica dioica L., Parietaria diffusa M. et K. and Sambucus nigra L. J Ethnopharmacol. 2005 Apr 26; 98(3):323–7.

52. De Clercq E. Current lead natural products for the chemotherapy of human immunodeficiency virus (HIV) infection. Med Res Rev. 2000 Sep; 20(5):323–49.

53. Hadizadeh I, Peivastegan B et al. Antifungal activity of nettle (Urtica dioica L.), colocynth (Citrullus colocynthis L. Schrad), oleander (Nerium oleander L.) and koнar (Ziziphus spina-christi L.) extracts on plants pathogenic fungi. Pak J Biol Sci. 2009 Jan 1; 12(1):58–63.

54. Bnouham M, Merhfour FZ et al. Antidiabetic effect of some medicinal plants of Oriental Morocco in neonatal non-insulin-dependent diabetes mellitus rats. Hum Exp Toxicol. 2010 Oct; 29(10):865–71. Epub 2010 Feb 12.

55. Fazeli SA, Gharravi AM et al. The granule cell density of the dentate gyrus following administration of Urtica dioica extract to young diabetic rats. Folia Morphol (Warsz). 2008 Aug; 67(3):196–204.

56. Jahanshahi M, Golalipour MJ et al. The effect of Urtica dioica extract on the number of astrocytes in the dentate gyrus of diabetic rats. Folia Morphol (Warsz). 2009 May; 68(2):93–7.

57. Golalipour MJ, Khori V. The protective activity of Urtica dioica leaves on blood glucose concentration and beta-cells in streptozotocin-diabetic rats. Pak J Biol Sci. 2007 Apr 15; 10(8):1200–4.

58. Rau O, Wurglics M et al. Screening of herbal extracts for activation of the human peroxisome proliferator-activated receptor. Pharmazie. 2006 Nov; 61(11):952–6.

59. Onal S, Timur S et al. Inhibition of alpha-glucosidase by aqueous extracts of some potent antidiabetic medicinal herbs. Prep Biochem Biotechnol. 2005; 35(1):29–36.

60. Bnouham M, Merhfour FZ et al. Antihyperglycemic activity of the aqueous extract of Urtica dioica. Fitoterapia. 2003 Dec; 74(7–8):677–81.

61. Farzami B, Ahmadvand D et al. Induction of insulin secretion by a component of Urtica dioica leave extract in perifused Islets of Langerhans and its in vivo effects in normal and streptozotocin diabetic rats. Ethnopharmacol. 2003 Nov; 89(1):47–53.

62. Mekhfi H, El Haouari M et al. Platelet anti-aggregant property of some Moroccan medicinal plants. J Ethnopharmacol. 2004 Oct; 94(2–3):317–22.

63. Legssyer A, Ziyyat A et al. Cardiovascular effects of Urtica dioica L. in isolated rat heart and aorta. Phytother Res. 2002 Sep; 16(6):503–7.

64. Testai L, Chericoni S et al. Cardiovascular effects of Urtica dioica L. (Urticaceae) roots extracts: in vitro and in vivo pharmacological studies. J Ethnopharmacol. 2002 Jun; 81(1):105–9.

65. Nassiri-Asl M, Zamansoltani F et al. Effects of Urtica dioica extract on lipid profile in hypercholesterolemic rats. Zhong Xi Yi Jie He Xue Bao. 2009 May; 7(5):428–33.

66. Daher CF, Baroody KG et al. Effect of Urtica dioica extract intake upon blood lipid profile in the rats. Fitoterapia. 2006 Apr; 77(3):183–8. Epub 2006 Feb 23.

67. Avci G, Kupeli E et al. Antihypercholesterolaemic and antioxidant activity assessment of some plants used as remedy in Turkish folk medicine. J Ethnopharmacol. 2006 Oct 11; 107(3):418–23. Epub 2006 Apr 15.

68. Harput US, Saracoglu I et al. Stimulation of lymphocyte proliferation and inhibition of nitric oxide production by aqueous Urtica dioica extract. Phytother Res. 2005 Apr; 19(4):346–8.

69. Riehemann K, Behnke B et al. Plant extracts from stinging nettle (Urtica dioica), an antirheumatic remedy, inhibit the proinflammatory transcription factor NF-kappaB. FEBS Lett. 1999 Jan 8; 442(1):89–94.

70. Konrad A, Mähler M et al. Ameliorative effect of IDS 30, a stinging nettle leaf extract, on chronic colitis. Int J Colorectal Dis. 2005 Jan; 20(1):9–17. Epub 2004 Aug 25.

71. Akbay P, Basaran AA et al. In vitro immunomodulatory activity of flavonoid glycosides from Urtica dioica L. Phytother Res. 2003 Jan; 17(1):34–7.

72. Roschek B Jr, Fink RC et al. Nettle extract (Urtica dioica) affects key receptors and enzymes associated with allergic rhinitis. Phytother Res. 2009 Jul; 23(7):920–6.

73. Mittman P. Randomized, double-blind study of freeze-dried Urtica dioica in the treatment of allergic rhinitis. Planta Med. 1990 Feb; 56(1):44–7.

74. El Haouari M, Bnouham M et al. Inhibition of rat platelet aggregation by Urtica dioica leaves extracts. Phytother Res. 2006 Jul; 20(7):568–72.

75. Golalipour MJ, Ghafari S et al. Protective role of Urtica dioica L. (Urticaceae) extract on hepatocytes morphometric changes in STZ diabetic Wistar rats. Turk J Gastroenterol. 2010 Sep; 21(3):262–9.

Sundew

1. Williamson, EM. 2003. *Potter's Herbal Cyclopaedia*. The C. W. Daniel Company, Essex.

2. Fukushima K, Nagai K et al. Drosera rotundifolia and Drosera tokaiensis suppress the activation of HMC-1 human mast cells. J Ethnopharmacol. 2009 Aug 17; 125(1):90–6. Epub 2009 Jun 18.

3. Paper DH, Karall E et al. Comparison of the antiinflammatory effects of Drosera rotundifolia and Drosera madagascariensis in the HET-CAM assay. Phytother Res. 2005 Apr; 19(4):323–6.

4. Krenn L, Beyer G et al. In vitro antispasmodic and anti-inflammatory effects of Drosera rotundifolia. Arzneimittelforschung. 2004; 54(7):402–5.

Sweet Grass

1. Nemeikaite-Ceniene A, Maroziene A et al. Redox properties of novel antioxidant 5,8-Dihydroxycoumarin: implications for its prooxidant cytotoxicity. Z Naturforsch C. 2005 Nov-Dec; 60(11–12):849–54.

2. Pukalskas A, van Beek TA et al. Identification of radical scavengers in sweet grass (Hierochloe odorata). J Agric Food Chem. 2002 May 8; 50(10):2914–9.

3. Zainuddin A, Pokorný J et al. Antioxidant activity of sweetgrass (Hierochloë odorata Wahlnb.) extract in lard and rapeseed oil emulsions. Nahrung. 2002 Feb; 46(1):15–7.

Sweet Vernal Grass

1. Dwyer CJ, Downing GM et al. Dicoumarol toxicity in neonatal calves associated with the feeding of sweet vernal (Anthoxanthum odoratum) hay. Aust Vet J. 2003 Jun; 81(6):332–5.

2. Pritchard DG, Markson LM et al. Haemorrhagic syndrome of cattle associated with the feeding of sweet vernal (Anthoxanthum

odoratum) hay containing dicoumarol. Vet Rec. 1983 Jul 23; 113(4):78–84.

Valerian

1. Fernández-San-Martín MI, Masa-Font R et al. Effectiveness of Valerian on insomnia: a meta-analysis of randomized placebo-controlled trials. Sleep Med. 2010 Jun; 11(6):505–11. Epub 2010 Mar 26.

2. Oxman AD, Flottorp S et al. A televised, web-based randomised trial of an herbal remedy (valerian) for insomnia. PLoS One. 2007 Oct 17; 2(10):e1040.

3. Dimpfel W, Brattström A et al. Central action of a fixed Valerian-hops extract combination (Ze 91019) in freely moving rats. Eur J Med Res. 2006 Nov 30; 11(11):496–500.

4. Bent S, Padula A et al. Valerian for sleep: a systematic review and meta-analysis. Am J Med. 2006 Dec; 119(12):1005–12.

5. Lacher SK, Mayer R et al. Interaction of valerian extracts of different polarity with adenosine receptors: identification of isovaltrate as an inverse agonist at A1 receptors. Biochem Pharmacol. 2007 Jan 15; 73(2):248–58. Epub 2006 Oct 6.

6. Komori T, Matsumoto T et al. The sleep-enhancing effect of valerian inhalation and sleep-shortening effect of lemon inhalation. Chem Senses. 2006 Oct; 31(8):731–7. Epub 2006 Jul 20.

7. Shinomiya K, Fujimura K et al. Effects of valerian extract on the sleep-wake cycle in sleep-disturbed rats. Acta Med Okayama. 2005 Jun; 59(3):89–92.

8. Wheatley D. Medicinal plants for insomnia: a review of their pharmacology, efficacy and tolerability. J Psychopharmacol. 2005 Jul; 19(4):414–21.

9. Dietz BM, Mahady GB et al. Valerian extract and valerenic acid are partial agonists of the 5-HT5a receptor in vitro. Brain Res Mol Brain Res. 2005 Aug 18; 138(2):191–7.

10. Fernández S, Wasowski C et al. Sedative and sleep-enhancing properties of linarin, a flavonoid-isolated from Valeriana officinalis. Pharmacol Biochem Behav. 2004 Feb; 77(2):399–404.

11. Yuan CS, Mehendale S et al. The gamma-aminobutyric acidergic effects of valerian and valerenic acid on rat brainstem neuronal activity. Anesth Analg. 2004 Feb; 98(2):353–8.

12. Hadley S, Petry JJ. Valerian. Am Fam Physician. 2003 Apr 15; 67(8):1755–8.

13. Blumenthal, M. 2003. The ABC Clinical Guide to Herbs. American Botanical Council, Austin.

14. Pallesen S, Bjorvatn B et al. [Valerian as a sleeping aid?] Tidsskr Nor Laegeforen. 2002 Dec 10; 122(30):2857–9. [Article in Norwegian]

15. Ziegler G, Ploch M et al. Efficacy and tolerability of valerian extract LI 156 compared with oxazepam in the treatment of non-organic insomnia--a randomized, double-blind, comparative clinical study. Eur J Med Res. 2002 Nov 25; 7(11):480–6.

16. Wheatley D. Stress-induced insomnia treated with kava and valerian: singly and in combination. Hum Psychopharmacol. 2001 Jun; 16(4):353–356.

17. Wheatley D. Kava and valerian in the treatment of stress-induced insomnia. Phytother Res. 2001 Sep; 15(6):549–51.

18. Poyares DR, Guilleminault C et al. Can valerian improve the sleep of insomniacs after benzodiazepine withdrawal? Prog Neuro-psychopharmacol Biol Psychiatry. 2002 Apr; 26(3):539–45.

19. Dominguez RA, Bravo-Valverde RL et al. Valerian as a hypnotic for Hispanic patients. Cultur Divers Ethnic Minor Psychol. 2000 Feb; 6(1):84–92.

20. Dorn M. [Efficacy and tolerability of Baldrian versus oxazepam in non-organic and non-psychiatric insomniacs: a randomised, double-blind, clinical, comparative study] Forsch Komplementarmed Klass Naturheilkd. 2000 Apr; 7(2):79–84. [Article in German]

21. Donath F, Quispe S et al. Critical evaluation of the effect of valerian extract on sleep structure and sleep quality. Pharmacopsychiatry. 2000 Mar; 33(2):47–53.

22. Ammer K, Melnizky P. [Medicinal baths for treatment of generalized fibromyalgia] Forsch Komplementarmed. 1999 Apr; 6(2):80–5. [Article in German]

23. WHO. 1999. WHO monographs on selected medicinal plants. Vol. 1. World Health Organization, Geneva.

24. Schulz H, Stolz C et al. The effect of valerian extract on sleep polygraphy in poor sleepers: a pilot study. Pharmacopsychiatry. 1994 Jul; 27(4):147–51.

25. Leuschner J, Müller J et al. Characterisation of the central nervous depressant activity of a commercially available valerian root extract. Arzneimittelforschung. 1993 Jun; 43(6):638–41.

26. Lindahl O, Lindwall L. Double blind study of a valerian preparation. Pharmacol Biochem Behav. 1989 Apr; 32(4):1065–6.

27. Balderer G, Borbély AA. Effect of valerian on human sleep. Psychopharmacology (Berl). 1985; 87(4):406–9.

28. Leathwood PD, Chauffard F et al. Aqueous extract of valerian root (Valeriana officinalis L.) improves sleep quality in man. Pharmacol Biochem Behav. 1982 Jul; 17(1):65–71.

29. Taibi DM, Bourguignon C et al. A feasibility study of valerian extract for sleep disturbance in person with arthritis. Biol Res Nurs. 2009 Apr; 10(4):409–17. Epub 2008 Dec 28.

30. Taibi DM, Vitiello MV et al. A randomized clinical trial of valerian fails to improve self-reported, polysomnographic, and actigraphic sleep in older women with insomnia. Sleep Med. 2009 Mar; 10(3):319–28. Epub 2008 May 14.

31. Hattesohl M, Feistel B et al. Extracts of Valeriana officinalis L. s.l. show anxiolytic and antidepressant effects but neither sedative nor myorelaxant properties. Phytomedicine. 2008 Jan; 15(1–2):2–15.

32. Diaper A, Hindmarch I. A double-blind, placebo-controlled investigation of the effects of two doses of a valerian preparation on the sleep, cognitive and psychomotor function of sleep-disturbed older adults. Phytother Res. 2004 Oct; 18(10):831–6.

33. Coxeter PD, Schluter PJ et al. Valerian does not appear to reduce symptoms for patients with chronic insomnia in general practice using a series of randomised n-of-1 trials. Complement Ther Med. 2003 Dec; 11(4):215–22.

34. Glass JR, Sproule BA et al. Acute pharmacological effects of temazepam, diphenhydramine, and valerian in healthy elderly subjects. J Clin Psychopharmacol. 2003 Jun; 23(3):260–8.

35. Volz HP. [Phytochemicals as means to induce sleep] Z Arztl Fortbild Qualitatssich. 2001 Jan; 95(1):33–4. [Article in German]

36. Murphy K, Kubin ZJ et al. Valeriana officinalis root extracts have potent anxiolytic effects in laboratory rats. Phytomedicine. 2010 Jul; 17(8–9):674–8. Epub 2009 Dec 29.

37. Hubner R, van Haselen R et al. Effectiveness of the homeopathic preparation Neurexan compared with that of commonly used valerian-based preparations for the treatment of nervousness/restlessness - an observational study. Scientific World Journal. 2009 Aug 11; 9:733–45.

38. Benke D, Barberis A et al. GABA A receptors as in vivo substrate for the anxiolytic action of valerenic acid, a major constituent of valerian root extracts. Neuropharmacology. 2009 Jan; 56(1):174–81. Epub 2008 Jun 17.

39. Tang JY, Zeng YS et al. [Effects of Valerian on the level of 5-hydroxytryptamine, cell proliferation and neurons in cerebral hippocampus of rats with depression induced by chronic mild stress] Zhong Xi Yi Jie He Xue Bao. 2008 Mar; 6(3):283–8. [Article in Chinese]

40. Awad R, Levac D et al. Effects of traditionally used anxiolytic botanicals on enzymes of the gamma-aminobutyric acid (GABA) system. Can J Physiol Pharmacol. 2007 Sep; 85(9):933–42.

41. Khom S, Baburin I et al. Valerenic acid potentiates and inhibits GABA(A) receptors: molecular mechanism and subunit specificity. Neuropharmacology. 2007 Jul; 53(1):178–87. Epub 2007 May 13.

42. De Feo V, Faro C. Pharmacological effects of extracts from Valeriana adscendens Trel. II. Effects on GABA uptake and amino acids. Phytother Res. 2003 Jun; 17(6):661–4.

43. Hariya T, Kobayashi Y et al. [Effects of sedative odorant inhalation on patients with atopic dermatitis] Arerugi. 2002 Nov; 51(11):1113–22. [Article in Japanese]

44. Andreatini R, Sartori VA et al. Effect of valepotriates (valerian extract) in generalized anxiety disorder: a randomized placebo-controlled pilot study. Phytother Res. 2002 Nov; 16(7):650–4.

45. Cropley M, Cave Z et al. Effect of kava and valerian on human physiological and psychological responses to mental stress assessed under laboratory conditions. Phytother Res. 2002 Feb; 16(1):23–7.

46. Hosoi J, Tanida M et al. Mitigation of stress-induced suppression of contact hypersensitivity by odorant inhalation. Br J Dermatol. 2001 Nov; 145(5):716–9.

47. Hendriks H, Bos R et al. Central nervous depressant activity of valerenic acid in the mouse. Planta Med. 1985 Feb; 51(1):28–31.

48. Arushanian B, Mastiagina OA et al. [Peculiarities in the effect of tofisopam and valerian extract on short-term memory and anxiety states in healthy humans] Eksp Klin Farmakol. 2004 Nov-Dec; 67(6):23–5. [Article in Russian]

49. Dimpfel W, Suter A. Sleep improving effects of a single dose administration of a valerian/hops fluid extract—a double blind, randomized, placebo-controlled sleep-EEG study in a parallel design using electrohypnograms. Eur J Med Res. 2008 May 26; 13(5):200–4.

50. Brattström A. Scientific evidence for a fixed extract combination (Ze 91019) from valerian and hops traditionally used as a sleep-inducing aid. Wien Med Wochenschr. 2007; 157(13–14):367–70.

51. Koetter U, Schrader E et al. A randomized, double blind, placebo-controlled, prospective clinical study to demonstrate clinical efficacy of a fixed valerian hops extract combination (Ze 91019) in patients suffering from non-organic sleep disorder. Phytother Res. 2007 Sep; 21(9):847–51.

52. Morin CM, Koetter U et al. Valerian-hops combination and diphenhydramine for treating insomnia: a randomized placebo-controlled clinical trial. Sleep. 2005 Nov 1; 28(11):1465–71.

53. Schellenberg R, Sauer S et al. The fixed combination of valerian and hops (Ze91019) acts via a central adenosine mechanism. Planta Med. 2004 Jul; 70(7):594–7.

54. Müller D, Pfeil T et al. Treating depression comorbid with anxiety—results of an open, practice-oriented study with St John's wort WS

5572 and valerian extract in high doses. Phytomedicine. 2003; 10 Suppl 4:25–30.

55. Müller CE, Schumacher B et al. Interactions of valerian extracts and a fixed valerian-hop extract combination with adenosine receptors. Life Sci. 2002 Sep 6; 71(16):1939–49.

56. Füssel A, Wolf A et al. Effect of a fixed valerian-Hop extract combination (Ze 91019) on sleep polygraphy in patients with non-organic insomnia: a pilot study. Eur J Med Res. 2000 Sep 18; 5(9):385–90.

57. Müller SF, Klement S. A combination of valerian and lemon balm is effective in the treatment of restlessness and dyssomnia in children. Phytomedicine. 2006 Jun; 13(6):383–7. Epub 2006 Feb 17.

58. Gramowski A, Jügelt K et al. Functional screening of traditional antidepressants with primary cortical neuronal networks grown on multielectrode neurochips. Eur J Neurosci. 2006 Jul; 24(2):455–65.

59. Rezvani ME, Roohbakhsh A et al. Anticonvulsant effect of aqueous extract of Valeriana officinalis in amygdala-kindled rats: possible involvement of adenosine. J Ethnopharmacol. 2010 Feb 3; 127(2):313–8. Epub 2009 Nov 10.

60. Cuellar NG, Ratcliffe SJ. Does valerian improve sleepiness and symptom severity in people with restless legs syndrome? Altern Ther Health Med. 2009 Mar-Apr; 15(2):22–8.

61. Wang J, Zhao J et al. Chemical analysis and biological activity of the essential oils of two valerianaceous species from China: Nardostachys chinensis and Valeriana officinalis. Molecules. 2010 Sep 14; 15(9):6411–22.

62. Letchamo W, Ward W et al. Essential oil of Valeriana officinalis L. cultivars and their antimicrobial activity as influenced by harvesting time under commercial organic cultivation. J Agric Food Chem. 2004 Jun 16; 52(12):3915–9.

63. Sudati JH, Fachinetto R et al. In vitro antioxidant activity of Valeriana officinalis against different neurotoxic agents. Neurochem Res. 2009 Aug; 34(8):1372–9. Epub 2009 Feb 4.

64. Ebringerová A, Kardosová A et al. Mitogenic and comitogenic activities of polysaccharides from some European herbaceous plants. Fitoterapia. 2003 Feb; 74(1–2):52–61.

65. Hromádková Z, Ebringerová A et al. Ultrasound-assisted extraction of water-soluble polysaccharides from the roots of valerian (Valeriana officinalis L.). Ultrason Sonochem. 2002 Jan; 9(1):37–44.

66. Lin S, Shen YH et al. Revision of the Structures of 1,5-Dihydroxy-3,8-epoxyvalechlorine, Volvaltrate B, and Valeriotetrate C from Valeriana jatamansi and V. officinalis. J Nat Prod. 2010 Sep 20. [Epub Previous.]

67. Occhiuto F, Pino A et al. Relaxing effects of Valeriana officinalis extracts on isolated human non-pregnant uterine muscle. J Pharm Pharmacol. 2009 Feb; 61(2):251–6.

68. Circosta C, De Pasquale R et al. Biological and analytical characterization of two extracts from Valeriana officinalis. J Ethnopharmacol. 2007 Jun 13; 112(2):361–7. Epub 2007 Mar 20.

69. Fields AM, Richards TA et al. Analysis of responses to valerian root extract in the feline pulmonary vascular bed. J Altern Complement Med. 2003 Dec; 9(6):909–18.

70. Hazelhoff B, Malingré TM et al. Antispasmodic effects of valeriana compounds: an in-vivo and in-vitro study on the guinea-pig ileum. Arch Int Pharmacodyn Ther. 1982 Jun; 257(2):274–87.

71. Yang GY, Wang W. [Clinical studies on the treatment of coronary heart disease with Valeriana officinalis var latifolia] Zhongguo Zhong Xi Yi Jie He Za Zhi. 1994 Sep; 14(9):540–2. [Article in Chinese]

72. Sharifzadeh M, Hadjiakhoondi A et al. Effects of aqueous, methanolic and chloroform extracts of rhizome and aerial parts of Valeriana officinalis L. on naloxone-induced jumping in morphine-dependent mice. Addict Biol. 2006 Jun; 11(2):145–51.

73. Mkrtchyan A, Panosyan V et al. A phase I clinical study of Andrographis paniculata fixed combination Kan Jang versus ginseng and valerian on the semen quality of healthy male subjects. Phytomedicine. 2005 Jun; 12(6–7):403–9.

74. Yao M, Ritchie HE et al. A developmental toxicity-screening test of valerian. J Ethnopharmacol. 2007 Sep 5; 113(2):204–9. Epub 2007 Jun 2.

Water Avens

1. Panizzi L, Catalano S et al. In vitro antimicrobial activity of extracts and isolated constituents of Geum rivale. Phytother Res. 2000 Nov; 14(7):561–3.

2. Tunón H, Olavsdotter C et al. Evaluation of anti-inflammatory activity of some Swedish medicinal plants. Inhibition of prostaglandin biosynthesis and PAF-induced exocytosis. J Ethnopharmacol. 1995 Oct; 48(2):61–76.

Water Speedwell

1. Küpeli E, Harput US et al. Bioassay-guided isolation of iridoid glucosides with antinociceptive and anti-inflammatory activities from Veronica anagallis-aquatica L. J Ethnopharmacol. 2005 Nov 14; 102(2):170–6. Epub 2005 Jul 12.

White Dead-nettle

1. Matkowski A, Piotrowska M. Antioxidant and free radical scavenging activities of some medicinal plants from the Lamiaceae. Fitoterapia. 2006 Jul; 77(5):346–53. Epub 2006 May 19.

2. Bradley, P. 2006. *British Herbal Compendium Volume 2*. British Herbal Medicine Association, Bournemouth.

3. Paduch R, Wójciak-Kosior M et al. Investigation of biological activity of Lamii albi flos extracts. J Ethnopharmacol. 2007 Mar 1; 110(1):69–75. Epub 2006 Sep 17.

4. Zhang H, Rothwangl K et al. Lamiridosins, hepatitis C virus entry inhibitors from Lamium album. J Nat Prod. 2009 Dec; 72(12):2158–62.

Wild Strawberry

1. Mudnic I, Modun D et al. Cardiovascular effects in vitro of aqueous extract of wild strawberry (Fragaria vesca, L.) leaves. Phytomedicine. 2009 May; 16(5):462–9. Epub 2009 Jan 7.

2. Nesterova IuV, Povet'eva TN et al. [Evaluation of anti-inflammatory activity of extracts from Siberian plants] Vestn Ross Akad Med Nauk. 2009; (11):30–4. [Article in Russian]

3. Oktyabrsky O, Vysochina G et al. Assessment of anti-oxidant activity of plant extracts using microbial test systems. J Appl Microbiol. 2009 Apr; 106(4):1175–83. Epub 2009 Jan 30.

4. Kiselova Y, Ivanova D et al. Correlation between the in vitro antioxidant activity and polyphenol content of aqueous extracts from Bulgarian herbs. Phytother Res. 2006 Nov; 20(11):961–5.

Willow

1. WHO. 2005. *WHO monographs on selected medicinal plants. Vol. 4.* World Health Organization, Geneva.

2. Tunón H, Olavsdotter C et al. Evaluation of anti-inflammatory activity of some Swedish medicinal plants. Inhibition of prostaglandin biosynthesis and PAF-induced exocytosis. J Ethnopharmacol. 1995 Oct; 48(2):61–76.

3. Alam MS, Kaur G et al. Evaluation of antioxidant activity of Salix caprea flowers. Phytother Res. 2006 Jun; 20(6):479–83.

4. Sultana S, Saleem M. Salix caprea inhibits skin carcinogenesis in murine skin: inhibition of oxidative stress, ornithine decarboxylase activity and DNA synthesis. J Ethnopharmacol. 2004 Apr; 91(2–3):267–76.

Wood Cranesbill

1. Sigurdsson S, Gudbjarnason S. Inhibition of acetylcholinesterase by extracts and constituents from Angelica archangelica and Geranium sylvaticum. Z Naturforsch C. 2007 Sep-Oct; 62(9–10):689–93.

Yarrow

1. Jónsdóttir G. Áhrif vatnsútdrátta af horblöðku og vallhumli á þroska angafrumna og getu þeirra til að ræsa ósamgena CD4+ T frumur in vitro. University of Iceland. MSc thesis, 2010. Found on 25.11.2010 at http://hdl.handle.net/1946/6959. In Icelandic.

2. Frey FM, Meyers R. Antibacterial activity of traditional medicinal plants used by Haudenosaunee peoples of New York State. BMC Complement Altern Med. 2010 Nov 6; 10(1):64. [Previous Epub.]

3. Kotan R, Cakir A et al. Antibacterial activities of essential oils and extracts of Turkish Achillea, Satureja and Thymus species against plant pathogenic bacteria. J Sci Food Agric. 2010 Jan 15; 90(1):145–60.

4. de Sant'anna JR, Franco CC et al. Genotoxicity of Achillea millefolium essential oil in diploid cells of Aspergillus nidulans. Phytother Res. 2009 Feb; 23(2):231–5.

5. WHO. 2005. *WHO monographs on selected medicinal plants. Vol. 4.* World Health Organization, Geneva.

6. Benedek B, Kopp B. Achillea millefolium L. s.l. revisited: recent findings confirm the traditional use. Wien Med Wochenschr. 2007; 157(13–14):312–4.

7. Pires JM, Mendes FR et al. Antinociceptive peripheral effect of Achillea millefolium L. and Artemisia vulgaris L.: both plants known popularly by brand names of analgesic drugs. Phytother Res. 2009 Feb; 23(2):212–9.

8. Babaei M, Abarghoei ME et al. Antimotility effect of hydroalcoholic extract of yarrow (Achillea millefolium) on the guinea-pig ileum. Pak J Biol Sci. 2007 Oct 15; 10(20):3673–7.

9. Saluk-Juszczak J, Pawlaczyk I et al. The effect of polyphenolic-polysaccharide conjugates from selected medicinal plants of Asteraceae family on the peroxynitrite-induced changes in blood platelet proteins. Int J Biol Macromol. 2010 Dec 1; 47(5):700–5. Epub 2010 Sep 30.

10. Kintzios S, Papageorgiou K et al. Evaluation of the antioxidants activities of four Slovene medicinal plant species by traditional and novel biosensory assays. J Pharm Biomed Anal. 2010 Nov 2; 53(3):773–6. Epub 2010 May 20.

11. Potrich FB, Allemand A et al. Antiulcerogenic activity of hydroalcoholic extract of Achillea millefolium L.: involvement of the antioxidant system. J Ethnopharmacol. 2010 Jul 6; 130(1):85–92. Epub 2010 Apr 24.

12. Raudonis R, Jakstas V et al. Investigation of contribution of individual constituents to antioxidant activity in herbal drugs using postcolumn HPLC method. Medicina (Kaunas). 2009; 45(5):382–94.

13. Csupor-Löffler B, Hajdú Z et al. Antiproliferative effect of flavonoids and sesquiterpenoids from Achillea millefolium s.l. on cultured human tumor cell lines. Phytother Res. 2009 May; 23(5):672–6.

14. Williamson, EM. 2003. *Potter's Herbal Cyclopaedia*. The C. W. Daniel Company, Essex.

15. Santos AO, Santin AC et al. Activity of an essential oil from the leaves and flowers of Achillea millefolium. Ann Trop Med Parasitol. 2010 Sep; 104(6):475–83.

16. Nilforoushzadeh MA, Shirani-Bidabadi L et al. Comparison of Thymus vulgaris (Thyme), Achillea millefolium (Yarrow) and propolis hydroalcoholic extracts versus systemic glucantime in the treatment of cutaneous leishmaniasis in balb/c mice. J Vector Borne Dis. 2008 Dec; 45(4):301–6.

17. Conti B, Canale A et al. Essential oil composition and larvicidal activity of six Mediterranean aromatic plants against the mosquito Aedes albopictus (Diptera: Culicidae). Parasitol Res. 2010 Nov; 107(6):1455–61. Epub 2010 Aug 10.

18. Tariq KA, Chishti MZ et al. Anthelmintic efficacy of Achillea millifolium against gastrointestinal nematodes of sheep: in vitro and in vivo studies. J Helminthol. 2008 Sep; 82(3):227–33. Epub 2008 Apr 18.

19. Khan AU, Gilani AH. Blood pressure lowering, cardiovascular inhibitory and bronchodilatory actions of Achillea millefolium. Phytother Res. 2010 Sep 20. [Previous Epub.]

20. Takzare N, Hosseini MJ et al. The effect of Achillea millefolium extract on spermatogenesis of male Wistar rats. Hum Exp Toxicol. 2010 Jun 1. [Previous Epub.]

Index

A

Abscesses, 9, 12, 20, 48, 144, 166, 174
Achillea millefolium. See Yarrow
Acne, 20, 70, 100, 130, 154, 184
Aðalbláber, 24
Ajuga pyramidalis, 4
Alchemilla alpina, 128
Alchemilla filicaulis, 128
Alchemilla glabra, 128
Alchemilla glomerulans, 128
Alchemilla mollis, 128
Alchemilla vulgaris. See Lady's Mantle
Alchemilla wichurae, 128
Allergies, 46, 54, 90, 94, 190, 210
Allium oleraceum, 4
Alpine Bistort *(Bistorta vivipara)*, 12
Alpine Clubmoss *(Diphasiastrum alpinum)*, 84
Alzheimer's disease, 48, 178
American Wintergreen *(Gaultheria procumbens)*, 132
Amnesia, 190, 240
Amphibious Bistort *(Persicaria amphibia)*, 4
Analgesic, 16, 18, 34, 56, 74, 88, 92, 108, 118, 122, 144, 146, 160, 164, 166, 186, 190, 211, 222, 230, 236, 238
Anemia, 26, 60, 64, 68, 80, 104, 140, 210, 216, 232
Angelica *(Angelica archangelica)*, 14–16, 17, 58, 152
Angelica sinensis. See Dong Quai
Angelica sylvestris, 16, 152
Anthelmintic, 82, 96, 110, 122, 136, 158, 244
Anthoxanthum odoratum. See Sweet Vernal Grass
Anthriscus sylvestris. See Cow Parsley
Anthyllis vulneraria. See Kidney Vetch
Antibacterial, 16, 22, 24, 26, 38, 40, 48, 52, 56, 58, 60, 62, 66, 74, 76, 88, 92, 96, 98, 108, 110, 112, 118, 122, 124, 130, 132, 146, 156, 170, 172, 174, 182, 184, 188, 190, 194, 196, 200, 214, 224, 226, 236, 244
Anti-emetic, 88, 110
Antifungal, 16, 40, 56, 62, 66, 76, 88, 92, 98, 118, 122, 124, 156, 174, 194, 196, 200, 214, 224
Anti-inflammatory, 12, 16, 22, 24, 26, 30, 34, 42, 44, 46, 48, 52, 66, 70, 74, 76, 86, 88, 90, 92, 94, 98, 100, 102, 104, 108, 114, 118, 122, 124, 130, 146, 148, 150, 158, 160, 164, 172, 174, 178, 188, 190, 192, 194, 196, 200, 210, 211, 214, 226, 230, 232, 236, 238, 240, 244
Antioxidants, 26, 62
Antispasmodic, 48, 50, 64, 132, 142, 186, 222
Antitussive, 48, 56, 98, 104, 110, 114, 120, 170, 172
Antiviral, 22, 88, 92, 120, 186, 188, 190, 200, 214, 232, 244
Anxiety, 168, 176, 178, 186, 188, 222, 224
Appetite, 16, 20, 34, 38, 64, 74, 78, 82, 160, 202, 204, 222, 226, 230, 236, 242, 244
Arctic Poppy *(Papaver radicatum)*, 4, 18
Arctium lappa, 192
Arctostaphylos uva-ursi. See Bearberry
Argentina anserina. See Silverweed
Argentina egedii. See Eged's Silverweed
Armeria maritima. See Sea-thrift, Common
Arrhythmia, 126
Arthritis, 16, 20, 22, 28, 30, 32, 34, 42, 58, 68, 74, 76, 77, 82, 92, 96, 102, 106, 108, 116, 118, 126, 134, 136, 142, 144, 148, 154, 156, 162, 164, 182, 188, 190, 204, 210, 214, 230, 234, 236, 240, 244
Asplenium septentrionale, 4
Asplenium trichomanes, 4
Asplenium viride, 4
Asthma, 16, 38, 48, 56, 94, 98, 112, 166, 210, 214
Astragalus membranaceus, 134
Astringent, 12, 24, 28, 44, 60, 66, 86, 88, 92, 104, 108, 122, 146, 150, 164, 174, 176, 182, 194, 200, 212, 226, 230, 232, 236, 240, 244, 246
Atherosclerosis, 16, 26, 90, 100, 178
Athlete's foot, 168
Augnfró, 44
Autoimmune diseases, 34, 244

B

Bacillus subtilis, 58
Back pain, 14, 68, 198, 236, 238
Baldursbrá, 186
Baths, herbal, 10
Bearberry *(Arctostaphylos uva-ursi)*, 20–22
Bed-wetting, 22
Beitilyng, 102

Bellis perennis. See Daisy
Bell's Palsy, 142
Benign prostatic hyperplasia, 16, 52, 108, 210
Beriberi, 230
Betula lenta. See Sweet Birch
Betula nana. See Dwarf Birch
Betula pendula. See Silver Birch
Betula pubescens. See Downy Birch
Bilberry *(Vaccinium myrtillus)*, 24–27
Birch, 18, 70, 74, 76, 108, 169, 180, 240
Birki, 74
Bistorta vivipara. See Alpine Bistort
Biting Stonecrop *(Sedum acre)*, 28–29
Bjöllulilja, 132
Bladder cancer, 178
Bladder stones, 126
Bladderwrack *(Fucus vesiculosus)*, 30–31, 50
Blágresi, 240
Blákolla, 188, 190
Blechnum spicant var. *fallax*, 4
Bleeding, 12, 14, 20, 22, 26, 76, 82, 88, 90, 92,
        94, 98, 106, 108, 122, 124, 126, 128, 130,
        134, 136, 138, 152, 154, 156, 176, 184,
        188, 192, 194, 196, 198, 200, 202, 204,
        210, 212, 218, 226, 232, 234, 236, 238,
        240, 242, 244
Blends, herbal, 10
Bloating, 16, 38, 58, 70, 78, 82, 84, 110, 114,
        118, 146, 210, 216, 242
Blóðarfi, 122
Blóðberg, 56
Blóðkollur, 88
Blood circulation, 16, 42, 198
Blood cleansing, 28, 74, 218, 230, 234, 242
Blood pressure, 26, 28, 38, 40, 100, 116, 124,
        134, 188, 190, 196, 210, 216, 222, 224,
        234, 244
Blood sugar, 24, 26, 30, 46, 70, 108, 118, 152,
        178, 210, 211
Blood-thinning, 16, 27, 30, 34, 115, 148, 169,
        238, 244
Blueberry *(Vaccinium uliginosum)*, 26
Bogbean *(Menyanthes trifoliata)*, 32–34
Boils, 24, 42, 92, 154
Bóluþang, 30
Bones, 20, 68, 92, 94, 108, 128, 134, 138, 146,
        236, 240
Boreal Starwort *(Stellaria borealis)*, 4
Botrychium simplex, 4
Breast, 26, 38, 70, 118, 169, 240

Breast cancer, 26, 118, 166, 169
Breast milk, 38, 42, 70, 210, 211
Brenninetla, 208, 210
Brennisóley, 144
Bronchitis, 16, 38, 48, 56, 66, 94, 98, 100, 104,
        112, 114, 118, 122, 160, 164, 166, 172
Brönugrös, 206
Brucellosis, 98
Bruises, 66, 68, 72, 92, 94, 100, 120, 174, 242
Buerger's Disease, 16
Burnet Rose *(Rosa pimpinellifolia)*, 4
Burnirót, 176
Burns, 20, 42, 68, 88, 114, 120, 126, 144, 168,
        170, 208, 210, 230
Butterwort *(Pinguicula vulgaris)*, 3, 36–37

C

Callitriche brutia, 4
Calluna vulgaris. See Heather
Caltha palustris. See Marsh Marigold
Cancer, 16, 26, 30, 34, 54, 76, 80, 94, 100,
        102, 112, 118, 136, 142, 148, 152, 160,
        166, 168, 169, 174, 178, 188, 190, 192,
        196, 200, 202, 210, 238, 244. *See also
        individual cancers*
Candida, 58
Capillary veins, 26, 100
Capsella bursa-pastoris. See Shepherd's Purse
Caraway *(Carum carvi)*, 38–40, 211
Cardamine pratensis subsp. *angustifolia. See*
        Cuckooflower
Cardiovascular disease, 26
Carex flava, 4
Carex heleonastes, 4
Carminative, 32, 56, 64, 70, 82, 108, 118, 158,
        162, 186, 222
Carum carvi. See Caraway
Cataracts, 26
Cat's Puff *(Mastocarpus stellatus)*, 114
Cervical cancer, 80, 148
Cetraria islandica. See Iceland Moss
Chamerion angustifolium. See Rose Bay Willow
        Herb
Chamomile *(Chamomilla recutita)*, 158, 186
Chickenpox, 148
Chickweed *(Stellaria media)*, 42–43
Children, dosages for, 11
Cholagogue, 16, 32, 70, 82, 96, 118, 154, 244
Cholera, 124

Cholesterol, 152, 166, 168, 204, 210, 211

Chondrus crispus. See Irish Moss

Cirsium arvense, 208

Cochlearia officinalis. See Scurvy Grass

Colds, 14, 16, 20, 28, 32, 56, 58, 60, 80, 86, 92,
94, 102, 106, 114, 116, 118, 122, 144,
146, 148, 158, 160, 170, 176, 178, 180,
210, 226, 236, 242, 244, 246

Cold sores, 212

Cold-weather Eyebright *(Euphrasia frigida),*
44–46

Colic, 32, 34, 38, 58, 82, 188, 210

Colitis, 24, 34, 88, 94, 130, 158, 164, 172, 174,
200, 211, 222

Colon cancer, 26, 40

Colon cramps, 172

Colon spasms, 16, 142

Coltsfoot, 48, 49

Coltsfoot *(Tussilago farfara),* 48–49

Comarum palustre. See Purple Marshlocks

Common Dog Violet *(Viola riviniana),* 4

Common Heath Grass *(Danthonia decumbens),*
4

Common Marsh-Bedstraw *(Galium palustre),* 4

Common Sea-thrift *(Armeria maritima),* 50

Common Twayblade *(Listera ovata),* 4

Compresses, 9

Conjunctivitis, 20, 46, 86, 170, 188

Connective tissue, 108, 122, 124

Constipation, 28, 32, 52, 56, 68, 70, 78, 84, 92,
96, 106, 112, 120, 140, 154, 160, 162,
168, 184, 192, 202

Cooling, 24, 42, 60, 148, 192, 198, 202, 234

Corns, 28, 54, 168, 192, 214, 215, 236

Couch Grass *(Elytrigia repens),* 52–53

Coughs, 16, 36, 38, 48, 56, 66, 72, 94, 102, 104,
112, 114, 120, 122, 160, 166, 172, 178,
214, 216, 246

Cow Parsley *(Anthriscus sylvestris),* 54

Cradle cap, 100

Cramps, 76

Crataegus oxyacantha. See Hawthorn

Creams, 9

Creeping Thistle *(Cirsium arvense),* 208

Creeping Thyme *(Thymus praecox),* 56–58, 200

Crowberry *(Empetrum nigrum),* 60–62

Cryptogramma crispa, 4

Cuckooflower *(Cardamine pratensis* subsp.
angustifolia), 64

Cuminum cyminum, 130

Cystitis, 16, 22, 24, 26, 46, 48, 50, 52, 74, 76, 94,
100, 102, 108, 114, 118, 126, 132, 148,
174, 196

D

Dactylorhiza maculata. See Spotted Orchid

Daisy *(Bellis perennis),* 66

Dandelion *(Taraxacum officinale),* 4, 68–70

Dandruff, 20, 72, 210

Danthonia decumbens, 4

Decoctions, 6–7

Demulcent, 36, 42, 48, 52, 72, 110, 138, 170,
174, 206, 232, 242

Depression, 86, 168, 176, 178, 214, 224

Devil's Bit Scabious *(Succisa pratensis),* 72

Diabetes, 22, 26, 38, 40, 48, 80, 108, 124, 168,
178, 190, 211

Diaphoretic, 16, 74, 96, 100, 108, 126, 140, 146,
160, 192, 226, 244

Diarrhea, 12, 20, 22, 24, 26, 28, 31, 34, 38, 43,
60, 83, 84, 86, 88, 92, 94, 102, 106, 110,
116, 122, 124, 130, 134, 144, 146, 148,
150, 156, 158, 170, 174, 176, 178, 180,
182, 188, 190, 192, 194, 196, 198, 200,
202, 204, 206, 210, 212, 226, 232, 234,
236, 238, 240, 244

Digestion, 16, 24, 34, 38, 42, 64, 68, 78, 82, 112,
114, 186, 204, 216, 244

Digestive system, 31, 40, 66, 82, 130, 152, 153,
170, 174, 212, 244

Diphasiastrum alpinum. See Alpine Clubmoss

Dislocations, 202

Diuretic, 16, 20, 22, 24, 32, 38, 40, 46, 48, 52, 54,
56, 60, 66, 70, 74, 76, 86, 94, 96, 98, 100,
102, 108, 122, 126, 132, 146, 148, 152,
160, 162, 170, 180, 184, 188, 190, 194,
196, 198, 202, 204, 210, 211, 216, 218,
232, 234, 244

Diuretic Tea, 70

Dog bites, 134, 216, 244

Dog Violet, Common *(Viola riviniana),* 4

Dong Quai *(Angelica sinensis),* 12

Dosages, 10–11

Douches, 10

Downy Birch *(Betula pubescens),* 70, 74–76, 77,
169

Drosera peltata, 214

Drosera rotundifolia. See Sundew

Dryas octopetala. See Mountain Avens

Drying tips, 5

Dryopteris filix-mas. See Male Fern
Dulse *(Palmaria palmata),* 78–80
Duodenal ulcers, 83, 112, 114, 146
Dwarf Birch *(Betula nana),* 74
Dysentery, 22, 34, 76, 84, 88, 90, 92, 94, 124, 164, 170, 194, 198, 206, 212, 214, 226, 234, 236, 240, 246

E

Earache, 172
Ear infections, 58, 204
Eczema, 42, 70, 74, 76, 88, 90, 100, 122, 124, 126, 154, 166, 210
Edema, 26, 28, 32, 38, 40, 54, 64, 68, 74, 76, 98, 106, 108, 116, 118, 126, 162, 180, 184, 188, 192, 196, 202, 210, 230
Eged's Silverweed *(Argentina egedii),* 200
EIAV virus, 190
Einir, 116
Elytrigia repens. See Couch Grass
Emmenagogue, 16, 38, 56, 96, 118, 244
Empetrum nigrum. See Crowberry
Emphysema, 48, 108
Endometriosis, 130, 190, 196
Engjamunablóm, 228
Engjarós, 164
Epilepsy, 28, 50, 64, 126, 134, 224
Equisetum arvense. See Horsetail
Equisetum palustre, 108
Equisetum pratense, 106
Escherichia coli, 134
Essential oils, 9
Euphrasia calida, 4, 44
Euphrasia frigida. See Cold-weather Eyebright
Euphrasia officinalis, 44
Euphrasia stricta, 44
Expectorant, 16, 36, 38, 56, 66, 72, 92, 94, 104, 110, 114, 120, 140, 142, 160, 204, 214, 216, 232
Eyebaths, 9–10
Eyebright *(Euphrasia calida),* 4, 44, 46, 246
Eye diseases, 24, 26, 32, 44, 46, 134
Eyesight, 22, 26, 38, 46, 246
Eyewash, 46

F

Fagurfífill, 66
Fatigue, 178, 206

Febrifuge, 32, 34, 72, 108, 146, 192, 194, 202, 234, 236, 244
Fever, 12, 14, 16, 24, 28, 38, 66, 72, 82, 86, 88, 102, 116, 136, 148, 158, 178, 188, 192, 200, 202, 210, 220, 230, 236, 240, 244
Fibromyalgia, 34
Field Garlic *(Allium oleraceum),* 4
Field Gentian *(Gentianella campestris),* 82–83
Filipendula ulmaria. See Meadowsweet
Fir Clubmoss *(Huperzia selago),* 84
Fjallagrös, 110
Fjörugrös, 114
Flatulence, 14, 16, 32, 34, 38, 40, 56, 58, 64, 70, 82, 118, 146, 158, 186, 216, 232
Forked Spleenwort *(Asplenium septentrionale),* 4
Fragaria vesca. See Strawberry, Wild
Fucus vesiculosus. See Bladderwrack
Fungal infections, 94, 124, 154, 156, 174, 232

G

Galactogogue, 210
Galeopsis tetrahit. See Hemp-nettle
Galium palustre, 4
Galium verum. See Lady's Bedstraw
Gallbladder, 34, 70, 82, 86, 168
Gallstones, 70
Garðabrúða, 222
Garðahjálmgras, 104
Gargles, 10
Gastritis, 16, 24, 26, 40, 68, 78, 94, 102, 112, 114, 130, 146, 148, 174, 186, 198, 200, 214, 240, 244
Gaultheria procumbens, 132
Geldingahnappur, 50
Genital diseases, 218
Gentiana lutea, 82
Gentianella amarella, 82
Gentianella campestris. See Field Gentian
Geranium maculatum, 240
Geranium robertianum, 240
Geranium sylvaticum. See Wood Cranesbill
Geranium wilfordii, 240
Geum rivale. See Water Avens
Giardia duodenalis, 26
Gingivitis, 12, 20, 24, 28, 58, 86, 122, 124, 130, 150, 154, 156, 190, 200, 226, 234
Glands, 132, 146, 154, 218
Glandular fever, 188
Glaucoma, 26

Glaucous Dog Rose *(Rosa dumalis)*, 4
Glossy Moonwort *(Botrychium simplex)*, 4
Gout, 34, 38, 52, 66, 70, 74, 102, 118, 124, 144, 168, 188, 192, 203, 216, 234
Grædisúra, 92
Grass of Parnassus *(Parnassia palustris)*, 86–87
Greater Burnet *(Sanguisorba officinalis)*, 3, 88
Greater Plantain *(Plantago major)*, 92–94, 170
Greenland Primrose *(Primula egaliksensis)*, 4
Green Spleenwort *(Asplenium viride)*, 4
Groundsel *(Senecio vulgaris)*, 96–97
Gullkollur, 120
Gulmaðra, 126

H

Hair, 20, 36, 76, 80, 108, 116, 140, 150, 176, 210, 212, 236
Halitosis, 12, 38, 178, 184, 212
Hárdepla, 204
Hard Fern *(Blechnum spicant* var. *fallax)*, 4
Harvesting tips, 3–4
Haugarfi, 42
Hawkweed (*Hieracium* spp.), 98
Hawthorn *(Crataegus oxyacantha)*, 234
Hay fever, 210, 220
Headaches, 14, 16, 20, 29, 34, 56, 64, 68, 83, 84, 106, 126, 144, 148, 170, 176, 188, 194, 214, 222, 236, 244
Heart, 64, 70, 76, 82, 86, 88, 100, 108, 130, 132, 134, 136, 140, 160, 168, 178, 188, 194, 202, 211, 212, 218, 222
Heartburn, 68, 116
Heartsease *(Viola tricolor)*, 100–101
Heather *(Calluna vulgaris)*, 102–3
Heath Grass, Common *(Danthonia decumbens)*, 4
Helicobacter pylori, 16, 24, 26, 40, 112, 148
Helluhnoðri, 28
Hemorrhoids, 12, 26, 88, 94, 122, 124, 130, 174, 182, 188, 196, 200, 210, 226, 230, 232, 236, 244
Hemostatic, 12, 88, 92, 108, 122, 130, 138, 170, 188, 194, 200, 210, 212, 226, 232, 240, 244
Hemp-nettle *(Galeopsis tetrahit)*, 104
Hepatic, 70, 154, 244
Hepatitis, 66, 70, 90, 94, 108, 142, 160, 190, 200, 244
Herb Paris *(Paris quadrifolia)*, 4

Herbs. *See also individual herbs*
dosages of, 10–11
drying, 5
harvesting, 3–4
storing, 5
uses of, 6–10
Hernia, 98, 106
Herpes simplex virus, 22, 114, 120, 186, 190
Hieracium spp. *See* Hawkweed
Hierochloe odorata. See Sweet Grass
High blood pressure, 26, 38
Hippuris vulgaris. See Mare's-tail
HIV, 30, 112, 114, 136, 190
Hjartarfi, 194
Hlaðkolla, 158
Hóffifill, 48
Hófsóley, 140
Holtasóley, 150
Hookworms, 124
Horblaðka, 32
Horsetail *(Equisetum arvense)*, 17, 70, 77, 106–8
Hot flashes, 168, 238
Hrafnaklukka, 64
Hrútaber, 212
Hudson Bay Sedge *(Carex heleonastes)*, 4
Hundasúra, 192
Huperzia selago. See Fir Clubmoss
Húsapuntur, 52
Hymenophyllum wilsonii, 4
Hypertension. *See* High blood pressure
Hypnotic, 34, 222
Hypoglycemic, 24, 40, 210
Hypotensive, 169, 188, 210, 222, 244
Hypothyroidism, 28, 80

I

Icelandic Hawkweed *(Pilosella islandica)*, 98
Iceland Moss *(Cetraria islandica)*, 3, 4, 110–12, 148
Iceland Poppy *(Papaver croceum)*, 18
Ilmreyr, 220
Immune system, 26, 30, 34, 70, 76, 84, 148, 152, 172, 174, 190, 200, 211
Impetigo, 100
Incontinence, 52, 102, 108
Indigestion, 112, 114, 146
Infertility, 128, 130, 212, 244
Inflammation, 42, 66, 72, 82, 86, 114, 136, 148, 158, 172, 174, 178, 192, 210, 240, 244

Influenza, 16, 22, 56, 60, 80, 94, 148, 178, 236, 240, 242, 244

Infused oils, 8–9

Infusions, 6

Insect bites, 94, 134, 172, 210

Insomnia, 18, 28, 56, 64, 102, 176, 178, 220, 222, 224, 232

Irish Moss (*Chondrus crispus*), 114–15

Irritable bowel syndrome, 112

Itching, 20, 26, 42, 46, 72, 88, 100, 122, 124, 130, 140, 154, 156, 158, 190, 210

J

Jarðarber, 234

Jaundice, 14, 38, 52, 68, 70, 82, 116, 124, 154, 160, 162, 164, 166, 242, 246

Joint pain, 32, 42, 74, 76, 102, 118, 211, 220, 222

Juices, 10

Juncus gerardii, 4

Juniper (*Juniperus communis*), 116–18

K

Kidney diseases, 52, 60, 102, 166, 196, 204

Kidney stones, 20, 22, 28, 30, 52, 74, 76, 102, 108, 116, 124, 126, 156, 192, 196, 203, 210

Kidney Vetch (*Anthyllis vulneraria*), 3, 120

Klóelfting, 106

Knotgrass (*Polygonum aviculare*), 122–24, 196

Köldugras, 160

Kornsúra, 13

Krækiber, 60

Krossfífill, 96

Kúmen, 38

L

Lady's Bedstraw (*Galium verum*), 126–27, 169

Lady's Mantle (*Alchemilla vulgaris*), 128–30, 148, 196

Lamium album. See White Dead-nettle

Large-flowered Wintergreen (*Pyrola grandiflora*), 3, 132–34

Large Yellow-sedge (*Carex flava*), 4

Laryngitis, 38, 94, 130

Laugadepla, 230

Laxative, 20, 24, 32, 34, 36, 52, 60, 70, 80, 94, 96, 100, 110, 120, 132, 136, 154, 160, 162, 182, 184, 192, 202, 234

Leg pain, 130

Lepidotheca suaveolens. See Pineappleweed

Lesser Spurrey (*Spergularia salina*), 4

Leukemia, 26

Ligaments, 108

Ligusticum scoticum, 16

Linum catharticum. See Purging Flax

Listera ovata, 4

Liver, 16, 32, 46, 49, 52, 64, 68, 70, 76, 78, 82, 86, 96, 97, 108, 124, 136, 138, 162, 168, 169, 178, 202, 211

Liver damage, 16, 46, 96, 97, 136

Liver disease, 34, 52, 136, 162, 168

Ljósatvitönn, 232

Lófótur, 138

Lokasjóður, 246

Lumbago, 116, 142

Lung diseases, 36, 44, 100, 104, 108, 114, 160, 170, 172, 196, 214, 228

Lungs, 64, 76, 122, 138, 142, 160, 178, 208

Lupine, 152–53

Lupinus alba, 152

Lupinus caudatus, 152

Lupinus nootkatensis. See Nootka Lupine

Lycopodium annotinum. See Stiff Clubmoss

Lycopodium clavatum, 4, 84

Lyfjagras, 36

Lymphatic system, 126, 166

Lymphitis, 214

Lymph nodes, 166, 188

M

Maidenhair Spleenwort (*Asplenium trichomanes*), 4

Malaria, 124, 194

Male Fern (*Dryopteris filix-mas*), 136

Mare's-tail (*Hippuris vulgaris*), 138

Maríustakkur, 128

Maríuvöndur, 82

Marsh-Bedstraw, Common (*Galium palustre*), 4

Marsh Horsetail (*Equisetum palustre*), 108

Marsh Marigold (*Caltha palustris*), 140–42

Mastitis, 42, 58, 188

Mastocarpus stellatus. See Cat's Puff

Meadow Buttercup (*Ranunculus acris*), 144

Meadow Horsetail (*Equisetum pratense*), 106

Meadowsweet (*Filipendula ulmaria*), 77, 124, 146–48

Measles, 148, 244

Melasól, 18
Memory loss, 46, 84
Meningitis, 26, 62
Menopause, 130, 166, 168, 186, 210, 232, 236, 238
Menstrual bleeding, 14, 20, 22, 88, 90, 98, 122, 130, 134, 152, 184, 192, 196, 210, 226, 232, 244
Menstrual cramps, 22, 68, 222
Menstrual pain, 26, 38, 58, 96, 130, 158, 182, 186, 198, 232, 244
Mentha longifolia, 130
Menyanthes trifoliata. See Bogbean
Metabolism, stimulating, 54
Micrococcus luteus, 134
Migraines, 130, 236
Mjaðjurt, 146
Mountain Avens *(Dryas octopetala),* 150
Mountain Sorrel *(Oxyria digyna),* 192
Mouth ulcers, 12, 20, 86, 130, 150, 166, 170, 174, 176, 184, 200, 236
Mouthwashes, 10
Mucus, 38, 48, 56, 94, 142, 160, 204, 208, 214, 216, 232
Muscle pain, 58, 74, 76, 108, 118, 220, 224, 236
Mycobacterium tuberculosis, 118
Myocarditis, 178
Myosotis scorpioides. See Water Forget-me-not
Mýrasóley, 86
Myrrhis odorata. See Sweet Cicely

N

Nails, 80, 108, 180
Nausea, 34, 78, 80, 83, 88, 112, 136, 156, 158, 190, 196, 206, 244
Nephritis, 142, 188
Nerves, 86, 102, 116, 134, 138, 206, 222
Nervine, 222
Nervousness, 126
Nervous system, 50, 204
Nettle, 108, 130, 154, 208, 210, 211, 232, 242
Neuritis, 58
Neurological diseases, 178, 196
Night blindness, 26
Night sweats, 166, 168, 236
Njóli, 154
Nootka Lupine *(Lupinus nootkatensis),* 152–53
Northern Dock *(Rumex longifolius),* 152, 154–56

Nosebleeds, 26, 98, 106, 108, 122, 134, 152, 194, 196, 198, 210, 242
Nourishing, 24, 30, 60, 78, 80, 110, 114, 206, 210

O

Oils
essential, 9
infused, 8–9
Ointments, 9
Olea europaea, 130
Opium Poppy *(Papaver somniferum),* 18
Osteoarthritis, 34, 52, 70, 76, 108, 144, 154, 164, 168, 190, 192, 211, 238
Osteoporosis, 108, 166, 168, 169
Otitis, 26, 62
Ovarian cancer, 166
Oxalis acetosella. See Wood Sorrel
Oxyria digyna. See Mountain Sorrel

P

Pain reliever, 18, 74, 238, 240
Palmaria palmata. See Dulse
Papaver croceum. See Iceland Poppy
Papaver radicatum. See Arctic Poppy
Papaver somniferum. See Opium Poppy
Parasites, 124, 244
Paris quadrifolia, 4
Parkinson's disease, 48, 178
Parmelia omphalodes, 152
Parnassia cabulica, 86
Parnassia nubicola, 86
Parnassia palustris. See Grass of Parnassus
Parsley Fern *(Cryptogramma crispa),* 4
Pedicularis muscicola, 12
Pedunculate Water-starwort *(Callitriche brutia),* 4
Persicaria amphibia, 4
Phlebitis, 244
Pilosella islandica. See Icelandic Hawkweed
Pineappleweed *(Lepidotheca suaveolens),* 158
Pinguicula vulgaris. See Butterwort
Pinus pinaster, 210
Pinworms, 124
Plantago asiatica, 94
Plantago lanceolata. See Ribwort Plantain
Plantago major. See Greater Plantain
Plantago maritima. See Sea Plantain
Plantago ovata, 92

Plantago psyllium, 92
Platanthera hyperborea, 206
Pleurisy, 160
Pneumonia, 26, 62, 76, 160, 178, 240
Poliovirus, 120, 186
Polygonum aviculare. See Knotgrass
Polygonum bistorta, 12
Polypodium calaguala, 160
Polypody (*Polypodium vulgare*), 160–61
Potentilla erecta, 4, 200
Poultices, 9
Powders, 8
Premenstrual tension, 26, 130
Primula egaliksensis, 4
Prostate gland, 17, 52, 102, 106, 108, 169, 174, 210, 232
Protected plants, 4
Prunella vulgaris. See Self-heal
Pseudorchis staminea, 206
Psoriasis, 42, 70, 76, 100, 126, 154, 160, 166
Psoriatic arthritis, 74
Purging Flax (*Linum catharticum*), 162
Purple Marshlocks (*Comarum palustre*), 164
Pyramidal Bugle (*Ajuga pyramidalis*), 4
Pyrola grandiflora. See Large-flowered Wintergreen
Pyrola minor, 132

R

Ranunculus acris. See Meadow Buttercup
Rashes, 12, 20, 36, 42, 72, 76, 92, 100, 106, 108, 112, 120, 126, 154, 156, 160, 164, 178, 188, 192, 204, 206, 210, 212, 218, 235, 240
Raspberry (*Rubus idaeus*), 212
Rauðsmári, 166
Raynaud's Disease, 26
Red Clover (*Trifolium pratense*), 166–69
Relaxing, 224
Restless Leg Syndrome, 224
Restlessness, 86, 102, 178, 222
Retina, 26
Reyrgresi, 218
Rheumatism, 34, 38, 70, 82, 100, 164, 168, 203, 230, 238
Rheumatoid arthritis, 74
Rheum palmatum, 192
Rhinanthus minor. See Yellow Rattle
Rhodiola rosea. See Roseroot

Ribwort Plantain (*Plantago lanceolata*), 170–72
Ringworm, 154, 164, 214
Rosa dumalis, 4
Rosa pimpinellifolia, 4
Rose Bay Willow Herb (*Chamerion angustifolium*), 174–75
Roseroot (*Rhodiola rosea*), 3, 176–79
Rowan (*Sorbus aucuparia*), 180–82
Rubefacient, 28
Rubus idaeus. See Raspberry
Rubus saxatilis. See Stone Bramble
Rumex acetosa. See Sorrel
Rumex acetosella. See Sheep's Sorrel
Rumex crispus. See Yellow Dock
Rumex longifolius. See Northern Dock

S

Salix spp. *See* Willow
Saltmarsh Rush (*Juncus gerardii*), 4
Sanguisorba officinalis. See Greater Burnet
Saxifrage Foliolose (*Saxifraga foliolosa*), 4
Sciatica, 58, 210
Scurvy, 12, 18, 24, 26, 28, 32, 64, 66, 78, 154, 184, 192, 202, 212, 222, 230, 236
Scurvy Grass (*Cochlearia officinalis*), 184
Sea Mayweed (*Tripleurospermum maritimum*), 186
Sea Plantain (*Plantago maritima*), 92
Sea-thrift, Common (*Armeria maritima*), 50
Sedative, 16, 18, 86, 102, 108, 126, 158, 176, 186, 222, 232
Sedum acre. See Biting Stonecrop
Self-heal (*Prunella vulgaris*), 188–90
Selgresi, 170
Senecio ambrosiodes, 96
Senecio aureus, 96
Senecio cineraria, 96
Senecio flaccidus, 96
Senecio jacobaea, 96
Senecio multicapitatus, 96
Senecio vulgaris. See Groundsel
Serenoa repens, 210
Sexually transmitted diseases, 22, 108, 124
Shakes, 10
Sheep's Sorrel (*Rumex acetosella*), 192
Shepherd's Purse (*Capsella bursa-pastoris*), 194–96
Sigurskúfur, 174
Silver Birch (*Betula pendula*), 74, 76

Silverweed *(Argentina anserina)*, 124, 198–200
Sinuses, 46, 172
Sinusitis, 56
Skarfakál, 184
Skin cancer, 166, 170, 172
Skin Cleansing Tea, 169
Skin problems, 22, 34, 52, 64, 66, 70, 76, 100, 108, 126, 134, 154, 166, 168, 174, 202, 210, 244
Skin rashes. *See* Rashes
Skógarkerfill, 54
Skollafingur, 84
Snake bites, 12, 88, 134, 216, 244
Söl, 78
Sóldögg, 214
Sorbus aucuparia. See Rowan
Sores, 22, 36, 76, 88, 92, 102, 116, 120, 140, 152, 158, 164, 176, 188, 194, 204, 206, 210, 212, 226, 240, 244
Sorrel *(Rumex acetosa)*, 202–3
Sortulyng, 20
Spánarkerfill, 216
Spasms, 64, 244
Speedwell *(Veronica officinalis)*, 204–5
Spergularia salina, 4
Spleen, 64, 68, 204
Spotted Orchid *(Dactylorhiza maculata)*, 206–7
Spotting, 106, 226, 232
Stag's-horn Clubmoss *(Lycopodium clavatum)*, 4
Staphylococcus aureus, 58, 76, 134, 178
Stellaria borealis, 4
Stellaria media. See Chickweed
Stiff Clubmoss *(Lycopodium annotinum)*, 84
Stinging Nettle *(Urtica dioica)*, 130, 208–11
Stomach acid, 146
Stomach cancer, 148
Stomach cramps, 32, 34, 38, 102, 118, 150, 164, 186, 194
Stomachic, 64, 216
Stomach pain, 66, 78, 96, 112, 146, 158, 164, 202
Stomach ulcers, 24, 52, 94, 112, 114, 146, 172, 200, 214
Stone Bramble *(Rubus saxatilis)*, 212
Storage tips, 5
Stóriburkni, 136
Strawberry, Wild *(Fragaria vesca)*, 234–35
Streptococcus pneumoniae, 26, 62
Stroke, 90
Stúfa, 72
Succisa pratensis. See Devil's Bit Scabious
Sundew *(Drosera rotundifolia)*, 3, 36, 214–15

Sweet Birch *(Betula lenta)*, 74
Sweet Cicely *(Myrrhis odorata)*, 216
Sweet Grass *(Hierochloe odorata)*, 218
Sweet Vernal Grass *(Anthoxanthum odoratum)*, 220
Syrups, herbal, 8

T

Tágamura, 198
Tapeworm, 124, 136
Taraxacum officinale. See Dandelion
Tea
for arthritis, 77
for cystitis, 22
for diarrhea, 124
diuretic, 70
for flatulence, 40
for gastritis, 148
for hair and nails, 108
making, 6
for menopause, 130
for menstrual bleeding, 196
for menstrual pain, 244
milk-stimulating, 211
for prostate gland, 17
for skin cleansing, 169
Tendons, 56, 240
Throat, sore, 12, 16, 24, 58, 68, 72, 88, 112, 122, 132, 134, 150, 160, 182, 188, 200, 234, 244
Throat infections, 38, 46, 48, 56, 58, 78, 112, 116, 118, 130, 166, 174, 176, 188, 218, 230
Thrombosis, 220
Thyme *(Thymus vulgaris)*, 56, 214
Thymus praecox. See Creeping Thyme
Thyroid, 30, 31, 80, 115, 169, 188
Tillaea aquatica, 4
Tinctures, 7–8
Tinnitus, 188
Toothache, 14, 70, 148, 194
Tormentil *(Potentilla erecta)*, 4, 200
Trifolium pratense. See Red Clover
Tripleurospermum maritimum. See Sea Mayweed
Tuberculosis, 26, 42, 50, 62, 76, 90, 94, 98, 100, 110, 114, 116, 118, 134, 146, 164, 172, 174, 176, 188, 190, 204, 226, 244
Túnfífill, 68

Túnsúra, 202
Tussilago farfara. See Coltsfoot
Twayblade, Common *(Listera ovata)*, 4

U

Ulcerative colitis, 88, 174, 200
Ulmus fulva, 192
Undafífill, 98
Urethritis, 52
Urinary system, 22, 52, 76, 94, 102, 108, 122, 124, 126, 132, 182, 204, 234, 244
Urtica dioica. See Stinging Nettle
Uterine tumors, 130, 196

V

Vaccinium myrtillus. See Bilberry
Vaccinium uliginosum. See Blueberry
Vaginal discharges, 24, 58, 88, 102, 130, 148, 182, 188, 200, 226, 230, 232, 234, 240, 244
Vaginal douches, 10
Vaginal infections, 22
Vaginal itching, 124, 130
Valerian *(Valeriana officinalis)*, 222–24
Vallhumall, 242
Varicose veins, 26, 42, 88, 130, 232, 244
Vascular disease, 26
Vasculitis, 26, 88
Veins, 14, 16, 26, 42, 88, 100, 130, 232, 244
Venereal diseases. *See* Sexually transmitted diseases
Venous system, 24, 130, 244
Vermifuge, 52
Veronica anagallis-aquatica. See Water Speedwell
Veronica chamaedrys, 204
Veronica officinalis. See Speedwell
Veronica serpyllifolia, 204
Víðir, 236
Villilín, 162
Viola riviniana, 4
Viola tricolor. See Heartsease
Vomiting, 22, 28, 29, 34, 43, 52, 80, 83, 84, 96, 104, 120, 136, 140, 156, 158, 180, 190, 196

W

Warts, 28, 54, 68, 70, 140, 142, 144, 192, 214, 215, 236
Water Avens *(Geum rivale)*, 200, 226–27
Water Forget-me-not *(Myosotis scorpioides)*, 228
Water Pygmyweed *(Tillaea aquatica)*, 4
Water Speedwell *(Veronica anagallis-aquatica)*, 204, 230
White Dead-nettle *(Lamium album)*, 232
Whooping cough, 36, 48, 98, 100, 214, 228
Wild Strawberry *(Fragaria vesca)*, 234–35
Willow *(Salix* spp.*)*, 236–38
Wilson's Filmy-fern *(Hymenophyllum wilsonii)*, 4
Wolf's Foot *(Lycopodium clavatum)*, 84
Wood Cranesbill *(Geranium sylvaticum)*, 240
Wood Sorrel *(Oxalis acetosella)*, 4, 192
Worms, 14, 28, 32, 38, 58, 78, 82, 92, 96, 110, 112, 122, 136, 152, 158, 160, 170, 172, 194, 202, 230, 236, 244
Wounds, 12, 20, 22, 24, 28, 30, 36, 42, 48, 50, 54, 58, 66, 68, 70, 76, 86, 92, 94, 98, 106, 108, 112, 114, 116, 120, 122, 126, 128, 130, 132, 134, 136, 138, 140, 146, 148, 152, 154, 156, 158, 166, 170, 172, 174, 176, 182, 186, 188, 192, 194, 196, 198, 200, 204, 212, 216, 218, 226, 230, 232, 234, 236, 240, 242, 244
Wrinkles, 26, 166

Y

Yarrow *(Achillea millefolium)*, 58, 77, 130, 242–44
Yellow Dock *(Rumex crispus)*, 154, 156
Yellow Rattle *(Rhinanthus minor)*, 246

Þ

Þrenningarfjóla, 100

Photo © Berglind Karlsdottir

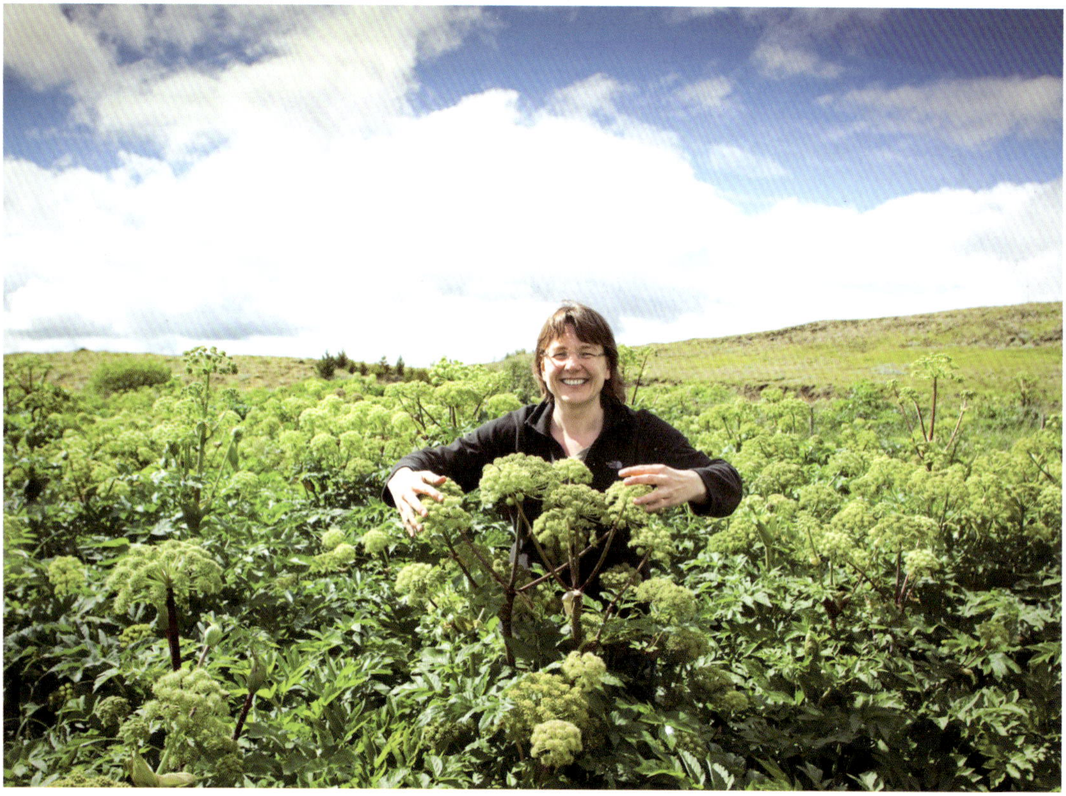

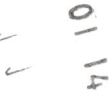

About the Author

Anna Rósa Róbertsdóttir studied medical herbalism at the College of Phytotherapy in England from 1988 to 1992. She also has an ITEC Diploma in massage and a B.Sc. in business from the University of Reykjavík. She is a member of the UK National Institute of Medical Herbalists, which is the oldest herbalist institute in the world, founded in 1894.

Anna Rósa has worked as a consultant in her own herbal practice for over two decades. A frequent lecturer on the use of Icelandic herbs, she has taught in the U.S., Canada, and Europe. Anna Rósa also runs a successful herbal products business producing her own creams, ointments, and tinctures, which are sold in pharmacies and health shops in Iceland. She wild-crafts all the Icelandic herbs used in her production. More information can be found at www annarosa.is.